Health
Promotion
for All

Remembering Susan Forster

For Churchill Livingstone:

Commissioning editor: Ellen Green
Project manager: Valerie Burgess
Project editor: Mairi McCubbin
Project controller: Pat Miller
Copy editor: Sue Beasley
Sales promotion executive: Maria O'Connor
Design direction: Judith Wright
Indexer: Jill Halliday

Health Promotion for All

Edited by

Susan Pike BA MSc RGN RHVT PGCE
Head of School of Health Studies, University of North London, UK

Diana Forster BA MSc RGN RM RHVT RNT
Formerly Head of Health Studies, University of East London, UK

CHURCHILL LIVINGSTONE
EDINBURGH HONG KONG LONDON MADRID MELBOURNE
NEW YORK AND TOKYO 1995

Churchill Livingstone
Medical Division of Pearson Professional Limited

Distributed in the United States of America by
Churchill Livingstone, 650 Avenue of the Americas, New
York, N.Y. 10011, and by associated companies, branches
and representatives throughout the world.

First published 1995

ISBN 0 443 05089 9

British Library Cataloguing in Publication Data
A catalogue record for this book is available from the
British Library.

Library of Congress Cataloging in Publication Data
A catalog record for this book is available from the
Library of Congress.

The
publisher's
policy is to use
**paper manufactured
from sustainable forests**

Produced by Longman Singapore Publishers (Pte) Ltd.
Printed in Singapore

Contents

Contributors   viii

Preface   ix

SECTION 1

An individual and community focus for
health promotion

1. What is health promotion?   3

Introduction   3
The health story   4
Building the blocks of health promotion   9
An individual and personal focus for
    health promotion   9
A community and public health
    approach for health promotion   10
An underpinning of equity and quality   10
An integrating process for health
    promotion   10
An openness to multidisciplinary work as
    part of health promotion   11
Promoting health in a time of turbulence   12
References   12
Further reading   13

2. Why health promotion?   15

Introduction   15
Public health and health promotion   16
The split between public and personal
    health   19
Personal health services and health
    promotion   19

Health promotion and community care   21
Health promotion and gender issues   23
Crisis in the cost of health care   25
References   25
Further reading   26

3. Health promotion now: the
development of policy   27

Introduction   27
International programmes and policy   28
International policy development and
    the World Health Organization   29
Strategies and policy development   30
Health promotion policy in the United
    Kingdom   31
'The Health of the Nation'   33
General practice and community nursing   34
Policy and the user   36
References   38
Further reading   38

4. Health promotion: models and
approaches   39

An integrated approach   39
An integrated approach to planning   41
The preventive model   42
The radical model   45
Psychological theory in health promotion   46
Social marketing   47
Evaluation   48
References   50
Further reading   50

5. Values and ethical issues 51

Introduction 51
Values 52
Agreement: reactive response to sickness 54
Disagreement: proactive health
  promotion 54
Consensus: health promotion to cut
  rising health care costs 55
Health promotion and the nurse's role 56
Professional nursing and interests 56
The whole causal spectrum 59
Professional nursing and personhood 59
UKCC Code (1992) 62
The WHO ethics target 63
Conclusion 64
References 64

SECTION 2

Practising health promotion 67

6. Information and health promotion 69

Introduction 69
Health promotion and resource
  allocation 69
Needs assessment and health promotion 70
Levels of health promotion activity 70
Sources of health information 72
Related information of interest to health
  promotion 77
Accessing information 80
Conclusion 80
References 80

7. Communication for health promotion 81

What is communication? 81
Counselling and communication 83
Language and listening 84
Written communication 87
Nonverbal aspects of communication 88
Conclusion 92
References 92
Further reading 92

8. Groups and teams 95

Introduction 95
Life context and the primary health care
  approach 96

Definition 96
Groupwork skills 96
Group characteristics 97
Leadership 100
Teamwork 102
Self-help groups 105
References 107

9. Education for health 109

Health education as 'freeing' 109
Types of learning 111
Motivation to learn 114
Getting the message across 117
References 122
Further reading 123

**10. A life-cycle approach to health
  promotion** 125

Introduction 125
Infancy and childhood 126
Adolescence 129
Health promotion in adulthood 133
Health promotion in later life 136
References 139
Further reading 140

SECTION 3

Broadening the vision for health
promotion 141

11. Settings for health promotion 143

Introduction 143
Health-promoting schools 144
The health-promoting workplace 148
Health education and the mass media 151
References 154
Further reading 155

**12. Inequalities in health and health
  promotion** 157

Introduction 157
The health of our population 158
Health and lifestyle in contemporary
  Britain 161
Access to health care 161
Social stratification in modern Britain 162
Gender differences in health status 163

Ethnicity and health   164
Social class and inequalities in health   165
Inequalities in health in later life   168
Geographical variations in health   168
Conclusion: the challenge for health
    promotion   169
References   170

13. Health and the environment   171

The environment affects your health   171
Community safety   177
Environmental inequalities   178
Health and the green agenda   178
Transport and health   179
The environmental professions   180
References   183

**14. Towards an integrated model of health
    promotion in nursing practice**   185

Introduction   185

Health promotion in nursing
    philosophy and practice   186
Models of nursing and health
    promotion   188
Multisectoral collaboration and equity
    in health promotion   191
Conclusion   196
References   196

SECTION 4

Further activities   197

**15. Organising information and
    exploring ideas**   199

Introduction   199
Portfolio formulation   200
Applied activities   200
Locality profiling   206
References   208

Index   209

Contributors

Diana Forster MSc BA RGN RM RHVT RNT
Independent writer and consultant in health
psychology and health promotion, London, UK

4. *Health promotion: models and approaches*
7. *Communication for health promotion*
8. *Groups and teams*
9. *Education for health*
10. *A life-cycle approach to health promotion*
11. *Settings for health promotion*

Eileen O'Keefe BSc (Hons)
Senior Lecturer in Philosophy and Health
Policy, University of North London, London,
UK

5. *Values and ethical issues*

David Pike BSc MSc CEng MICE MRTPI
Director of Environment, London Borough of
Camden, London, UK

13. *Health and the environment*

Susan Pike BA MSc RGN RHNT PGCE
Head of School of Health Studies, University of
North London, London, UK

1. *What is health promotion?*
2. *Why health promotion?*
3. *Health promotion now: the development of policy*

Jo Skinner MA PGCEA RGN RM CPT
Principal Lecturer in Health Studies, University
of North London, London, UK

14. *Towards an integrated model of health promotion
    in nursing practice*
15. *Organising information and exploring ideas*

Christina R. Victor BA MPhil PhD HonMFPHM
Senior Lecturer, Department of Public Health
Sciences, St. Georges Hospital Medical School,
Cranmer Terrace, London, UK

6. *Information and health promotion*
12. *Inequalities in health and health promotion*

Preface

Health promotion is central to the work of the 'new nurse' and to all health workers, and this book views health promotion as an expanding area within nursing and health care generally.

Health Promotion for All reflects the shift in focus towards care in community settings and the recent emphasis on public health. An integrated approach is developed throughout, reflecting the central position that health promotion occupies in the activity of nursing, and, indeed, all health work. Personal and public health issues, equity and multi-sectoral working are central to these activities.

The book's major concern is with health promotion in the United Kingdom, but the integrated approach adopted is based on World Health Organization (WHO) health promotion initiatives, acknowledging the global nature of many of today's health problems. The WHO Targets for the European Region highlighted at the tops of chapters 2–13 represent the focus for this approach.

Health is not only part of the current medical and health care system, but something far wider. It extends from people's views of themselves and their own health to the environment and the broader contexts of their lives. Health promotion is central to the whole picture of health and caring, not marginal to mainstream care. We seek to develop a framework and a series of debates, which can inform health promoting activities and encourage the development of reflective practitioners.

About this book

The book is organised into four sections.

Section 1 looks at the fundamental questions of what health promotion is and why it is necessary. Individuals are presented in the context of their own community setting, at the centre of health promoting work. Relevant WHO and national policy initiatives and changes are introduced; a variety of approaches to health promotion are examined and the section is completed by an innovative debate about values and ethical issues.

Section 2 emphasises the practice of health promotion, including health education and the requirement for sound information and clear communication.

Section 3 seeks to broaden health promoting horizons. The necessity to tackle widening inequalities in health experiences is debated; the impact of environment and its key place on the health promotion agenda is examined in detail; and the importance of health within a variety of organisational settings is considered. Finally, a strategy to facilitate the development of health promotion as a central activity of nursing is presented. These debates are transferable to other health occupations.

The book also provides a comprehensive approach to study skills and each chapter makes extensive use of activities and exercises.

Section 4 provides practical advice on setting up a portfolio, as well as a full set of additional activities that students may use in compiling their material.

How to use this book

Chapter 15 is intended to be of use to both students and tutors and we suggest the reader first refers to this chapter.

Although *Health Promotion for All* is particularly directed towards Project 2000 students, other health practitioners keen to develop their understanding of health promotion and changes in health care, will find it useful and relevant.

'By the year 2000, people should have the basic opportunity to develop and use their health potential to live socially and economically fulfilling lives'

(World Health Organization 1993)[1]

---

[1]World Health Organization 1993 Health for all targets: the health policy for Europe, updated edition. WHO Regional Office for Europe, Copenhagen

ACKNOWLEDGEMENTS

We would like to thank Mary Reynolds for her practical assistance and Jenny Newbury for her helpful comments. We also wish to thank all our colleagues and students both past and present for their help in the formulation of our ideas. Thanks are due to Gordon Forster for his unstinting support and to both our families for their forbearance and encouragement.

An individual and community focus for health promotion

SECTION CONTENTS

1. What is health promotion?   3

2. Why health promotion?   15

3. Health promotion now: the development of policy   27

4. Health promotion: models and approaches   39

5. Values and ethical issues   51

This section begins by examining the fundamental basics of health promotion and why it is needed, with a chapter on how policy is developed. Different models and approaches are considered, and the values and ethical issues are placed in an international and a national context.

CHAPTER CONTENTS

Introduction   3

The health story   4
   Health and curing   4
   Quality of life and differing views of health   5
   Prevention is better than cure   5
   Health and individual choices   6
   Health and education   7
   Broader health issues   8

Building the blocks of health promotion   9

An individual and personal focus for health promotion   9

A community and public health approach for health promotion   10

An underpinning of equity and quality   10

An integrating process for health promotion   10

An openness to multidisciplinary work as part of health promotion   11

Promoting health in a time of turbulence   12

References   12

Further reading   13

1

What is health promotion?

Susan Pike

INTRODUCTION

Health promotion at its simplest involves improving people's health and keeping them healthy. It is central to the work of nurses and other health workers and is the major health challenge for the year 2000.

There have been many attempts to define health (see Boxes 1.1 and 1.2) and, increasingly, much debate about the meaning of health promotion. The way in which health is defined will determine the sort of health promotion approach that is adopted, and consequently the two are defined together within this chapter. Many of the issues are very complex and some of the key areas

---

Box 1.1   Ways of defining health (Aggleton 1990)

- Health as the absence of disease
- Health as an ideal state
- Health as physical and mental fitness
- Health as a commodity
- Health as a personal strength or ability
- Health as the basis for personal potential

Box 1.2   Defining health as human potential

Seedhouse (1986) suggests that the most useful way of conceptualising health is to see it as providing the 'foundation for human achievement'. It is a means to an end rather than a fixed state that a person can or should aspire to. Thus, with the appropriate resources for health, people are more easily enabled to achieve their potential.

are expressed through the idea of a 'story of health' presented below. In the story, aspects of health are seen to build on one another. They are not discrete but are related both to each other and to ways in which health is maintained, improved and promoted.

THE HEALTH STORY

Health is a state of complete physical, mental and social well-being and not merely the absence of disease or infirmity

(WHO 1946)

This World Health Organization (WHO) definition of health is now quite old and well known. There are a number of problems associated with it. First, it suggests a state that very few people could aspire to and secondly it assumes there is one particular state that equals being healthy. It is therefore limited in its scope. But the idea of health contained within the statement is still a very important one. What it does is attempt to move thinking away from concepts of health which are solely to do with the physical and with what has sometimes been termed a biomedical model of health. It brings in mental and social aspects, it brings in ideas about well-being, and it suggests that there is more to being healthy than just not being sick. It therefore extends ideas about health and introduces the whole person rather than the physical problem from which the person may be suffering.

This is quite easy to write about and accept literally, but, even all these years later, it is a view that is sometimes difficult to move into the centre of our thinking. Hart (1985) makes the point that it is quite difficult to think about health without thinking about medicine, as many of our formal thoughts about health are firmly based with doctoring and with hospitals. Writers such as Illich (1976) and Navarro (1976) have argued very eloquently that our society has become over-medicalised and that physical and technological aspects of health care are dominant. Many people suggest that the National Health Service has always been a national medical service, concerned mainly with symptoms and organic signs of disease; when we think about health we think

Box 1.3   The health story
● Cure
● Care/quality of life
● People's own views about health
● Prevention
● Education

about people being 'cured'. The health story (Box 1.3) begins therefore by addressing health and curing. The health story is based loosely around case studies of Joshim, Josie, Danny, Mrs McDonald and Paul.

Health and curing

Joshim has a migraine; he wants it to go away. Josie has a broken arm; she wants it mended as soon as possible. Danny has recently been diagnosed as having a serious heart condition; he is waiting for bypass surgery in order to return to work and a normal life. Cure is thus very important. Some things may mend on their own, but others need medical intervention, maybe drugs, a plaster cast or complex surgery. The problem is that for many people, often nurses, doctors and other health care workers included, this has been seen as the necessary and sometimes only focus for health and health care. But many problems of today are not amenable to cure (see Ch. 2). For large numbers of people with chronic illnesses that do not have a neat beginning and end the concept of 'care' and the idea of living as independently as possible in spite of their problems may be a far more appropriate way of looking at health.

Activity 1.1

Working individually or in small groups, discuss:

a. what health means to you personally
b. what health promotion means to you.

Write down four points from your discussion of (a) and four from (b).

Summary

- Medicine and curing as approaches to health are important but limited.
- Many people have contact with hospitals and other acute health care settings, and with a variety of health professionals. These places and people have an important role to play in health-promoting work.

Quality of life and differing views of health

Mrs McDonald is 84 and has arthritis; 8-year-old Paul has learning disabilities and is confined to a wheelchair. Both may recognise that cure is not a very strong possibility. Also they may not only need care and help to enjoy relatively independent lives; they may also wish to think of themselves as healthy. Health to them will seem very much more than merely the absence of disease or disability and, although there are limitations on their lives, they, in common with most other people, will wish to lead full lives. Medical interventions may be useful to them at times, but they are limited and are only one small part of what is needed to enable Mrs McDonald and Paul to improve the quality of their lives. The way in which people view their own health, whether they are elderly, have a disability, are athletes, are plump or thin and so on, may be as important to understanding health, and consequently their health promotion needs, as are the views of health professionals about them. Research into people's views about their own health (Blaxter & Paterson 1982, Blaxter 1990, Calnan 1987, Pill 1991) suggests that this is certainly the case. Quality of life issues and well-being, as in the WHO definition, are thus very important to views of health and of health promotion.

Summary

- Caring and quality of life issues are important aspects of health care.
- It is vital to take into account people's own views of health and their perceptions of need.

- Health is not just one particular state, it will mean different things to different people.

Prevention is better than cure

Another stage in the story of health requires that we stop to look at prevention. Just as the story moved on from cure to care and to differing views of health and quality of life, so preventing illness is also a key element. Some writers have argued that our current approach to health care appears constantly reactive rather than proactive (Macdonald 1993). Or put another way it results in a 'system of medicine which responds, which waits to pick up the pieces' (Kennedy 1981). But illness and disease may be more usefully seen as one end of a much longer continuum, where interventions which may well not be medical in nature would often be better introduced at an earlier stage. The examples of Joshim, Josie and Danny were examined at the point at which they required curing via medical intervention of one sort or another, but it is also possible to look further back in their individual histories.

Joshim is a student. Whenever assignments come up or he has an argument with his girlfriend, his headaches start. They are not helped by alcohol and cigarettes either, which he turns to when under pressure. His doctor thinks he has a predisposition to migraines, as his mother and his brother also have them. Josie's broken arm and a degree of bruising were sustained while riding her bike. She swerved to miss a large pothole in the road, lost her balance and fell heavily on to the kerb. Danny was a bus driver until his illness. He gets little exercise and often eats a rather unhealthy diet; he used to smoke heavily but gave up some time ago. He is under a great deal of stress as he lives in a small flat with his wife, three children and his mother-in-law; finances are very tight. Could these crises for Joshim, Josie and Danny have been prevented or at the least minimised? It is useful to see them as part of a continuum of individual histories (see Fig. 1.1).

We can see from these case studies that there are a variety of factors leading up to each individual crisis, and it would be possible to construct many more. Some of the factors will be

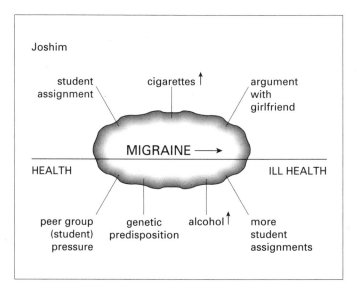

Figure 1.1 Health/illness continuum.

biological and genetic, others may be brought about by particular lifestyles, and yet others by factors outside of the control of the individuals concerned. Looking at their lives at the far right-hand side of the continuum (Fig. 1.1), focuses only at the point of crisis and the need for intervention by the health care system. Illness prevention is clearly about absence of disease. It is thus an important part of the WHO (1946) definition of health and a vital aspect of health promotion. However, it stops short of promoting well-being and becoming a positive force for health.

Summary

- Many conditions may be preventable, and the impact of others may be lessened if they are looked at early enough.
- Prevention is an important part of promoting health, but does not specifically address well-being and quality of life, which are also extremely important.

Health and individual choices

Joshim, Josie and Danny, Mrs McDonald and Paul are all individuals; they can all to some extent or another make choices and take responsibility for their own health. Will Joshim smoke? Will Josie ride a bike or be assertive enough to go to the local council to make a complaint about potholes? Will Mrs McDonald be really depressed about her arthritis or determined to get about and enjoy life as much as she can? They will all have more control and choice over some factors than they will have over others.

Some of the factors are known as 'lifestyle' factors. Quite simply, these are about the way or the style in which people choose to live their lives: what they eat or drink; whether they smoke; how they look after different parts of their bodies; and what risks they choose to take with their health as reflected in their behaviour. But the examples of Joshim, Josie and Danny can be used to demonstrate that responsibility for health and making healthy choices is quite complex.

First, quite a number of the factors affecting their health are outside their individual control: a badly maintained road; pressures of the educational system; inadequate local housing stock. Joshim, Josie and Danny, as part of local or national groups, may be able to influence change in such factors, just as Mrs McDonald and Paul, or their carers, may be able to campaign for better facilities for people with disabilities, but as individuals their control is very limited.

There are many social and environmental factors affecting health over which an individual can have little or no control. While some environmental factors may affect everyone, for example air and water pollution, some social factors, such as low income, poor housing, inability to afford a car, will affect some groups of people far more than others and will mean that making healthy choices is far easier for some people than it is for others (see Ch. 12). It also indicates that responsibility for health cannot rest solely with the individual. It will be the responsibility of other agencies at local, regional, national and international level to enable Joshim, Josie and Danny, Mrs McDonald and Paul to make healthy choices more easily.

Secondly, lifestyle factors are themselves often complex. Why does Joshim still smoke even though he knows it is bad for his health? Why does Danny eat fatty food even though he understands it is linked with coronary heart disease? Davison (1994) notes that behaviour does not exist in a cultural vacuum. Peer group pressures, stress and a huge number of other issues may be important in the choices people make. Davison cites an example of the importance of cream as a celebratory food in a South Wales mining valley. Most people there know of its possible link with coronary heart disease but its symbolic importance in birthday cakes, as treats and as part of the language, 'creaming off the best bits' for example, makes its relationship with something unhealthy quite complex. Graham (1986) notes that for many women smoking is an escape from fraught domestic lives. Lea (1975) suggests that everyone has 'support systems' which may or may not be unhealthy, but which have to be recognised. Nurses and other health promoters may themselves find making healthy choices just as difficult as do many of their clients. It is important to recognise and acknowledge this. Healthy choices are tied up with people's value systems (see Ch. 5 for full discussion). The link between individual

lifestyle health factors and the rest of the social and environmental context of people's lives is firmly forged.

Summary

- Making choices about being healthy or not is more complex than it seems.
- Many factors are outside an individual's control.
- Healthy choices are easier to make for some people than for others.
- Individual choices that people do make are affected by their cultural background and the social context in which they live.
- Nurses and other health promoters need to acknowledge their own difficulties in making healthy choices.

Health and education

Health education is brought in at this stage of the health story as again, like prevention, it is often allied to the discussion of choices in the last part of the story. Effective education about health is important. Children and adults need to know how their bodies work, and how best to look after them. Joshim might well have been helped by education which enabled him to understand why he turned to cigarettes and alcohol under stress, and education might have helped Danny to understand how a healthy diet might have improved his quality of life. But, as the section above showed, just telling them it was bad and expecting them to stop would probably not have very much effect. Research suggests that most people do know at least the basics about what keeps them healthy. Their reasons for continuing an unhealthy lifestyle are complex and associated with both psychological and external factors (see Ch. 5). Peter Draper and colleagues, as far back as 1980, distinguished three kinds of health education:

- Type 1 health education: education about the body and how to look after it
- Type 2 health education: provision of information about access to, and the most appropriate use of, health services

---

Activity 1.2

What choices do you make that comfort you but are not necessarily healthy? Try to think through why you make these choices. Discuss with your fellow students.

- Type 3 health education: education about national, regional and local policies and structures and processes in the wider environment which are detrimental to health (Draper et al 1980).

There has been much work on health education since this early work, but the essentially simple issues of differing levels of information and education, are still very important (see Ch. 4). Health education is directed at individuals; it can revolve around both preventing ill health and facilitating well-being and more positive approaches to health. It needs to be part of a broader public policy framework, which can tackle the factors outside the control of individual people.

Summary

One of the major approaches within health promotion therefore is to:

- give people appropriate information to make choices
- enable people to examine choices which they make
- help people develop skills to analyse and recognise alternative choices which are open to them.

Health education is one very important, but not the only, part of health promotion.

Broader health issues

The final piece in our story of health requires summing up and broadening out the picture. All the aspects below are important to our understanding of health and all have to be taken into account in the approach to health promotion. First, from the earlier parts of the story it will be clear that hospitals and health services in the community, in other words the whole health care

---

Activity 1.3

Why are (a) the prevention of ill health and (b) health education only parts of a whole picture of health promotion?

---

sector, are vital to health care. Joshim, Josie and Danny, Mrs McDonald and Paul all need good quality professional health services. The health services are important places for health promotion work.

Secondly, much of the care, even that required by Danny as he recovers, will not be in hospital. Care will be needed from what are known as the community, primary health and social care services, that is all the care services that are outside a hospital setting (see Chs 2 and 3). Also very importantly, Joshim and the others are part of social networks in the community, made up of families and friends. It is these who will probably provide the major part of caring, maintaining and improving the health of all the people we have referred to in the story (Graham 1984, Finch & Groves 1985). The community as a location for care and health promotion is thus very important.

Thirdly, as we have seen, many factors outside the health services determine these people's health. Some of these are about their individual psychology and lifestyle. Others centre around social and economic concerns involving whole communities and populations rather than just individuals, for example road repair and transport affecting Josie's accident, housing policies and work environment affecting Danny's health, restrictions on smoking in public places affecting Joshim.

Many basic health requirements to do with food, shelter, clean water, finance, etc. will have far more effect on people's health than even the most appropriate health care system. Medicine cannot provide us with many answers to the world's health problems today, whether we are talking about the need for clean water to combat disease in parts of Africa, the needs of someone in Glasgow with a severe physical disability requiring care and assistance to live independently, or the health needs of a young, single woman in Birmingham expecting her first child. These social and economic factors are sometimes known as health prerequisites or, in other words, the requirements on which good health can be built. If healthy choices are to be made easier, then health promotion will need robust public health policies to address these matters. The many

```
┌─────────────────────────────────────────────┐
│                                             │
│   Activity 1.4                              │
├─────────────────────────────────────────────┤
│                                             │
│   Pick two or three points from the story of health which │
│   you find most difficult to understand or to accept. │
│   Discuss these difficulties with your fellow students. │
│   Are there any other points which you think are important? │
│                                             │
└─────────────────────────────────────────────┘
```

factors affecting health mean that a wide variety of work and types of workers are involved and not just those in the health care sector.

Summary

- Good quality professional services are necessary for curing, caring and promoting people's health.
- Most caring and health-promoting work is carried out in the community.
- Families and social networks are major players in caring for people and maintaining and improving their health.
- Many things that affect people's health are outside the health services (health prerequisites).
- Things that affect people's health are a combination of lifestyle and community or environmental factors.
- Healthy public policies are required to make healthy choices easier.
- A wide variety of different professionals may be involved in health work.

BUILDING THE BLOCKS OF HEALTH PROMOTION

The story has tried to show that when health is thought of as something much wider than a medical and curing approach, then maintaining and improving people's health becomes something that pervades all aspects of health care. The way we define health promotion in other words is closely bound up with the way we define health.

The word 'promotion' itself, does not really convey the full intention or meaning of the word as it is used in health promotion. From the story, it is clear that it links with curing, caring, quality of life, making choices, prevention, education, policy and individuals and communities. The

area or domain (Dines & Cribb 1993) for health promotion is thus potentially very wide. Health can become 'all things to all people' (Dines & Cribb 1993), or become merely 'a virtue' (Tones & Tilford 1994) or moral stance, or it may be taken over by any interest group with a particular message to peddle (Green & Raeburn 1988).

In order to avoid these dilemmas and to demonstrate how very powerful the concept of health and health promotion can become, the approach adopted here follows the initiatives spelled out in the World Health Organization's Ottawa Charter (WHO 1986) and the WHO targets for 'Health for All' (WHO 1993). The Charter is about enabling individuals and groups to increase control over and improve their health, and this serves as a rationale for this book. The WHO targets introduce most chapters of the book (see Ch. 3 for a fuller discussion). The approach adopted here identifies key themes, some of which are part of the WHO philosophy. Others, we believe, are required to address the need for nurses and health professionals to develop a realistic and operable approach to health promotion throughout their work. The themes build from the health story and are as follows:

- an individual and personal focus for health promotion
- a community and public health approach for health promotion
- an underpinning of equity and quality
- an integrated process for health promotion
- an openness to multidisciplinary approaches to health-promoting work
- health-promoting work in a time of turbulence.

These themes are introduced below; they permeate through the chapters of the book and are addressed in differing ways and in more depth in all of them.

AN INDIVIDUAL AND PERSONAL FOCUS FOR HEALTH PROMOTION

The first theme places the individual or user of services at the centre of health promotion. Health and health care services, it is argued, have to be user focused and in addition have the whole person, rather than any sick part of him, at their core. The individual is seen as a 'doing' person, rather than as a person who is 'done to'. Consequently, people as individuals, or as members of groups and communities, will want to have control over many aspects of their health. The nurse or other health professional is there to facilitate this. At times it may be very difficult; this is the challenge facing health professionals.

One way of understanding the process is for the nurse to recognise that she herself is both an individual and a user as well as a professional. Being a professional gives an expertise and sound knowledge base; acknowledging herself as an individual, a user and an ordinary citizen enables the nurse to better understand health from the viewpoint of the user with whom she is working.

A COMMUNITY AND PUBLIC HEALTH APPROACH FOR HEALTH PROMOTION

A second central theme of the approach links to a more public and community focused dimension. There is much debate about the usefulness of the term 'community'. It may mean geographical locality and/or a set of social networks based for example on age, religion, ethnicity or class. As the health story demonstrated, working with locality and social networks is important for health-promoting work.

Traditionally in health care, the hospital has been one category and everything outside the hospital has been termed 'the community'. We would argue that this is no longer appropriate. The hospital here is viewed as firmly within the community setting and health promotion is seen as a key part of all health activities wherever they take place. Although 'community' is not an easy concept and can become merely a 'catch-all' word, it can be useful in defining a locality, a set of social networks and the 'ordinary life' concerns of most people. It can also be useful as a reference point for understanding the concept of 'prerequisites for health' and the need for a broader public health and population approach to health promotion. It is clear that dimensions of the contexts of people's lives and of the wider

environment have a major impact on the health of people and of nations.

This theme is given equal prominence to that of the personal; the two have to be seen as interdependent. As the health story showed, the social, cultural and economic context is a part of people themselves. An approach which seeks to maintain and improve people's health and develop their potential (Seedhouse 1986) must acknowledge and work with this if it is to be effective.

AN UNDERPINNING OF EQUITY AND QUALITY

Inequalities and difficulties with making healthy choices have been seen to underpin many aspects of health. The approach taken here, in keeping with the WHO initiatives, has a theme of equality closely tied to all health-promoting activities. If individual and personal approaches to health promotion are not tied to equity issues we may end up with health promotion strategies which do not consider the difficult contexts of people's lives, and which will consequently be ineffective for large numbers of people.

It becomes increasingly clear that many of the major health problems experienced in the United Kingdom today, and in other parts of the world, are closely tied up with disadvantage and with poverty of varying degrees. Services of whatever sort should be appropriate, effective and of as high a quality as possible for all groups of people. This concept of quality is one which can enable services to address all groups of people; it is implied but not directly addressed in WHO initiatives to date. Nurses are in a unique position to see at first hand the necessity for equitable health-promoting services. A recent RCN document on nursing and public health states: 'nurses witness daily the effects of poverty and the wider environment on the health of individuals and families' and 'nurses have much to contribute to the public health movement' (RCN 1994).

AN INTEGRATING PROCESS FOR HEALTH PROMOTION

In introducing the building blocks approach to

health promotion, reference was made to the pitfalls of appearing to have no boundaries at all in health promotion because its content is potentially so wide. But the major message which the health story tried to convey was that health matters needed to be *seen* in a different way. In other words, it is the process of doing health promoting work rather than the content which must come to the forefront of the health professional's work.

Health promotion can be conceptualised as a way of *seeing* health differently and a way of *doing* health work differently. What do we mean by this?

Health-promoting work is not a series of tasks which are less important than clinical concerns and thus are tacked on at the end of 'real' clinical doctoring and nursing activities. 'Remember to tell them not to smoke at the end of dressing the leg ulcer'! Rather, maintaining and promoting health becomes an integral and central part of all medical, nursing and clinical activities. The way in which the nurse, for example, approaches health promotion may be better viewed as being about engaging in regular nursing tasks in different sorts of ways, perhaps as facilitator, teacher, supporter or advocate, helping to make health choices a little easier. Conceptualising health promotion as an integrating process for seeing and doing health work is a key part of the approach taken in this book; it links closely with the other themes (see Ch. 13 particularly).

AN OPENNESS TO MULTIDISCIPLINARY WORK AS PART OF HEALTH PROMOTION

The health story showed that for all the people concerned, health was tied up with issues both inside and outside the health services and with a range of agencies concerned with promotion and public health (see Box 1.4). Health promotion work needs to be carried out in a variety of settings and will require involvement from a wide network of workers.

Community-based health service staff

These include community nurses, health visitors, midwives, nurses in general practice, health

Box 1.4   Agencies for a public health strategy (Jacobson et al 1991)
• Government • Health promotion agencies • The communications media • Training institutions • Local authorities • Health authorities • Primary health care • Employers, industry and trade unions

education/promotion specialists, doctors, dentists and dietitians. These workers will often be at the forefront of health promotion, working in a variety of types of health teams.

Hospital-based health service staff

'Those who work in rehabilitation and care tend to see health as their (an individual's) ability to function fully in their environment, whereas those who work in the acute hospital sector tend to view health from a more biological perspective, viewing health as an absence of disease.' (Gwent Profile of Illness and Health 1990).

It is often more difficult within strongly medically focused settings for hospital-based nurses and doctors to see their role as health promoters (Macleod Clark et al 1992). Seeing and doing health work in different health-promoting ways and working together in multidisciplinary teams, often with colleagues from the community services, presents a very real challenge for hospital-based nurses and staff.

Health service and other groups of workers

Just as health workers in the NHS will be collaborating together more positively and frequently, so nurses and other health workers will need to develop ways of working with social workers, community and youth workers, voluntary organisations, and sometimes with housing officers and local authority planners. The multidisciplinary dimension suggests that there will be many players in health promotion. In some contexts the nurse will be the key player, in others he or she will be one part of a larger team. In yet other health-promoting activities, the nurse may play very little part. All practitioners and planners of health care will have to address barriers to joint working, such as closed professional cultures, which are often present even between different groups of nurses. Dalley (1993) refers to 'professional tribalism' which often locks people within their own disciplines.

Users and carers

Users and carers will be right at the forefront of new ways of working. There will be many teams concerned with planning, operating and evaluating services, in which users and carers have a vital part to play. Being a member of a multidisciplinary team offers a way of sharing and exchanging knowledge with other workers both inside and outside the health service and with people who use services. Health is not only the province of professional experts. People themselves or their family and friends who help them maintain their health and independence are often expert on matters relating to their own health.

If nurses and health workers are to play a central part in health promotion, then their roles need to be made clear. Health workers will need to examine their own views of health and health promotion, discuss concepts of responsibility for health, and develop a confident and reflective approach to work which recognises when to act and when to seek help and support from colleagues both within and outside their own areas of work.

PROMOTING HEALTH IN A TIME OF TURBULENCE

All of these aspects of health-promoting work have to be viewed within the context of rapid change. Health care, like many other aspects of social life at present, is complex and often confusing. There is no doubt that health-promoting work at the current time is both exciting and daunting. The debate about health promotion is by no means fixed; there is much to be added to our knowledge and understanding. Many of the issues developed here are tentative. They will be discussed, revised and added to over the years to come. Education for nurses and all health professionals will need to enable them to develop a thoughtful and critical approach, which views the many problems faced as challenges rather than barriers. A recent review of both pre- and post-registration educational programmes for nurses, midwives and health visitors (Lask et al 1994) proposed three principal recommendations:

- there is a need for nurses, midwives and health visitors, to develop their own conceptualisation of health promotion
- health promotion needs to be addressed throughout educational programmes
- nursing facilitators should be introduced to help students apply health promotion theory to practice.

This chapter and the others in the book are intended as a contribution to the development of a strategy for health promotion for nurses and other health professionals, which is realistic and recognises the need for change and for consolidation.

Activity 1.5

Repeat the exercise of Activity 1.1 when you have finished reading this chapter. Have any of your points changed? If so, why do you think this is, and if not, why not?

REFERENCES

Aggleton P 1990 Health. Society Now Series, Routledge, London
Blaxter M 1990 Health and lifestyles. Tavistock/Routledge, London

Blaxter M, Paterson L 1982 Mothers and daughters: a three generational study of health attitudes and behaviour. Heinemann, London
Bunton R, Macdonald G (eds) 1992 Health promotion:

disciplines and diversity. Routledge, London

Calnan M 1987 Health and illness: the lay perspective. Tavistock, London

Dalley G 1993 Professional ideology or organisational tribalism? In: Walmsly J et al (eds) Health welfare and practice. Open University & Sage, London

Davison C 1994 Conflicts of interest: lifestyle, anthropology, ill health. Nursing Times 90(13): 40–42

Dines A, Cribb A (eds) 1993 Health promotion: concepts and practice. Blackwell Scientific Publications, Oxford

Draper P et al 1980 Three kinds of health education. British Medical Journal 16 (August): 493–495

Finch J, Groves D 1985 Community care and the family: a case for equal opportunities? In: Ungerson C (ed) Women and social policy. Macmillan, London

Graham H 1984 Women, health and the family. Harvester Press, Sussex

Graham H 1986 Women, smoking and family health. Paper presented at the British Sociological Association Medical Sociology Group Conference, September, York

Green L W, Raeburn J M 1988 Health promotion. What is it? What will it become? Health Promotion 3(2): 151–159

Gwent Profile of Illness and Health 1990 Consultation on the annual report of the Director of Public Health Medicine. Gwent Health Authority, Gwent

Hart N 1985 The sociology of health and medicine. Causeway Press, Lancashire

Illich I 1976 Medical nemesis. Bantam Books, New York

Jacobson B, Smith A, Whitehead M 1991 The nation's health: a strategy for the 1990's, 2nd edn. King's Fund, London

Kennedy I 1981 The unmasking of medicine. Allen & Unwin, London

Lambert H, McPherson K 1993 Disease prevention and health promotion. In: Davey B, Popay J (eds) Dilemmas in health care. OUP Health and Disease Series, Book 7, Open University Press, Milton Keynes

Lask S, Smith P, Masterson A 1994 A curricular review of pre- and post-registration education programmes for nurses, midwives and health visitors in relation to the integration of a philosophy of health: developing a model for evaluation. Institute of Advanced Nursing Education RCN, English National Board, London

Lea M 1975 Health and social education. Heinemann, London

Macdonald J 1993 Primary health care: medicine in its place. Earthscan, London

Macleod Clark J, Wilson-Barnet J, Latter S, Maben J 1992 Health education in nursing: a study of practice in the acute areas. Executive summary of a 2 year research project, Department of Nursing Studies, King's College, London

Navarro V 1976 Medicine under capitalism. Croom Helm, London

Pill R 1991 Issues in lifestyles and health. In: Badura B, Kickbusch I (eds) Health promotion research: towards a new social epidemiology. WHO, Regional Office for Europe, Copenhagen

Pill R, Stott N 1986 Concepts of illness causation and responsibility. In: Curer C, Stacey M (eds) Concepts of health, illness and disease: a comparative perspective. Berg, Leamington Spa

Royal College of Nursing 1994 Public health: nursing rises to the challenge. RCN Public Health Special Interest Group Publication, RCN, London

Seedhouse D 1986 Health: the foundations for achievement. John Wiley, Chichester

Tones K, Tilford S 1994 Health education: effectiveness, efficiency and equity, 2nd edn. Chapman & Hall, London

World Health Organization 1946 Constitution. WHO, Geneva

World Health Organization 1978 Report on the International Conference on Primary Health Care, Alma Ata, 6–12 September. WHO, Geneva

World Health Organization 1986 Ottawa Charter for health promotion. An International Conference on Health Promotion, November 17–21. WHO Regional Office for Europe, Copenhagen

World Health Organization 1993 Health for all targets: the health policy for Europe, updated edn. WHO, Regional Office for Europe, Copenhagen

FURTHER READING

Aggleton P 1990 Health. Society Now Series, Routledge, London

Seedhouse D 1986 Health: the foundations for achievement. John Wiley, Chichester

Tones K, Tilford S 1994 Health education: effectiveness, efficiency and equity, 2nd edn. Chapman & Hall, London

CHAPTER CONTENTS

Introduction   15

Public health and health promotion   16
The epidemiological transition   16
Explaining the changing patterns   16
Florence Nightingale and the health visitors   17
Environmental issues today   18

The split between public and personal health   19

Personal health services and health
promotion   19
Developing individual responsibility for health   19
The Peckham experiment: an innovation in
promoting personal health   20
Health promotion and the National Health
Service   20

Health promotion and community care   21
Demographic change   21
Chronic illness, degenerative conditions and
disability   21
Inequalities in health and health promotion   22

Health promotion and gender issues   23
Women as health promoters in the informal health
sector   23
Women as health promoters in the formal health
sector   24

Crisis in the cost of health care   25

References   25

Further reading   26

2

Why health promotion?

Susan Pike

---

*By the year 2000, all people should have the
opportunity to develop and use their own health
potential in order to lead socially, economically
and mentally fulfilling lives.*

(Target 2: Health and quality of life, WHO 1993)

INTRODUCTION

The influence of the medical sector was shown
in Chapter 1 to have limited use in defining
health and determining directions for health
promotion. Health promotion, it was suggested,
encompasses health education and the prevention of ill health; it emphasises the importance
of individuals and personal health services as
well stressing the enormous importance of social
and contextual issues.

Current legislation in the health area has
strong emphasis on health promotion and this is
mirrored in documentation concerning the education of nurses, midwives and health visitors.
The United Kingdom Central Council and the
National Boards of England, Scotland, Wales and
Northern Ireland all stress the need for nurses
now and into the next century to include health
promotion as a central part of their education and
training (UKCC 1986, ENB 1985). This chapter
examines major reasons for that stress on health
promotion; it examines the context for health
promotion using both historical and present-day
examples. Many of the issues raised have great
significance for the day-to-day activities of nurses
and other health service workers, other issues

concern nurses working only in particular sectors, while yet others may not directly concern the day-to-day work of nurses but have implications for any national or local strategy for health which nurses will be part of.

PUBLIC HEALTH AND HEALTH PROMOTION

The epidemiological transition

The Manchester and Salford Sanitary Association (MSSA) was formed in 1852, with the aim of promoting knowledge of health and temperance and aiding the Board of Health in giving effect to regulations for sanitary improvement.

(Davies 1988)

The quotation above makes it clear that health promotion is not a new concept, even though the term 'health promotion' would not have been used in the nineteenth century. There was a very great necessity at that time to improve the health of the working classes in London and in all the growing industrial towns of Britain by providing a better environment, better housing and increased understanding of health issues. Infectious diseases were the major cause of death through the last century. A visit to an old cemetery will show clearly the huge numbers of babies and young children who did not live to adulthood. Sometimes all of the children within one family, and this could be five, six or more, might have died very young. Contraception was not in any way in the advanced state that is familiar today and infant mortality was very high (see Box 2.1). Infants and children who had not developed any immunity were the most vulnerable to diseases such as typhoid, cholera and tuberculosis. Many babies were born but many did not survive to adulthood and fewer still to old age; consequently

---

Box 2.1   Infant mortality rate

The infant mortality rate is the number of children under 1 year old dying during a year, related to the number of live births in the same year. (For further discussion see Walker 1992.)

Box 2.2   Populations and demography

Demography is the study of information about human populations and is extremely important to the understanding of approaches to health promotion both past and present. Basic information about populations includes:

- size of the population
- age and sex structure.

The information may concern a population of a country, a region or a group.

---

there were far fewer older people in the populations than today (see Box 2.2). Through the latter part of the last century and on into the twentieth century the fall in the infectious disease rate was enormous and rapid. The infant mortality rate tumbled and as a consequence many more people survived into middle and old age.

Explaining the changing patterns

These changes were brought about by social, environmental and medical advances, but it is generally accepted that the key factors were environmental rather than medical. Thomas McKeown (1979) and other epidemiologists (see Box 2.3) have argued that nutritional and agricultural improvements, leading to a much better food supply for the population, were vital in building immunity to infectious diseases. Other key factors identified by McKeown were similar to those noted by Edwin Chadwick, a social reformer of the last century. Chadwick gave first priority to:

- water supply
- house drainage
- street drainage
- main sewerage (Webster 1990).

Box 2.3   Epidemiology

Epidemiology is concerned with the distribution of disease within populations. An epidemiological approach seeks to give an overview of the major health problems in a community or population and to identify causes and help prevent disease. (For further discussion see Walker 1992.)

Chadwick produced his 'Report on the Sanitary Condition of the Labouring Population' in 1842, in which he set out a picture of intolerable conditions of urban decay and poverty, and the Public Health Acts of 1848 and 1875 paved the way for improvements in Chadwick's priority areas, which he and other social reformers had fought long and hard to secure. Inadequate housing was also a key factor in the spread of disease. The industrial revolution had created urban squalor where contagious diseases flourished. Ashton & Seymour (1988) instance the case of central Liverpool where in the 1830s the first medical officer of health in the country, Dr Duncan, discovered that: 'one-third of the population [of Liverpool] were living in the cellars of back-to-back houses with earth floors, no ventilation or sanitation and as many as 16 people to a room.'

McKeown argues that although medical innovations such as vaccination, immunisation and drug therapy were certainly important, particularly to the individuals and families being protected and treated, they were not in the main the key to change. For example, the numbers of people in the population dying from tuberculosis were falling rapidly before the discovery of the tubercle bacillus and well in advance of the development of chemotherapy and the BCG vaccine (Walker 1992). Thus factors other than medical and curative interventions have been vital to improvements in the health of the people. This does not undermine the enormous contribution which modern medicine has made to health; it rather points to its limitations in meeting all health needs and perhaps provides a real understanding of how an effective health promotion agenda of yesterday and today must really begin to take on board a wide range of issues affecting health.

Florence Nightingale and the health visitors

Florence Nightingale

An historical example of a nursing approach to health promotion and environmental issues is provided through an examination of the work of Florence Nightingale. Ms Nightingale was very interested in the built environment of the hospital care setting, although it is interesting to note (Versluysen 1980) that she has regularly been portrayed in soft and gentle feminine terms as the 'lady with the lamp' bringing comfort to the young men who were casualties of the Crimean war during the 1850s. In fact, she was an extremely astute administrator and organiser of health care and one of her major tasks was to reform the hospital environment. Food, sanitation, ventilation, and the state of the hospital generally were particular concerns for her. The delivery of appropriate nursing care depended in large part on the environment in which it was delivered. The nursing task did not start and end at the patient's bedside; health promotion in the form of environmental concerns was very much the role of the nurse.

The health visitors

Although all nurses are now seen as becoming health educators and promoters, the group of nurses who have traditionally been seen as having the greatest potential for health promotion are health visitors. Health visitors were not originally required to be nurses and whether or not this should be the case has been a debate carrying on through this century (Wilkie 1979).

Health visitors are closely associated with both the public health and the personal health tradition of health promotion. The Manchester and Salford Sanitary Association was responsible for sending out the first lady 'sanitary visitors' (later called health visitors) in 1862. By 1894, Manchester Corporation (the local authority) were paying the salaries of a number of them and health visiting was well on its way (Davies 1988). These visitors had responsibilities for monitoring the sanitary conditions in domestic homes and also were

---

Activity 2.1

How might a nurse or other health worker today use the example of Florence Nightingale to introduce environmental change into patient/client care?

very much involved with infant welfare, reflecting the concern for the high infant mortality rate at this time. They were expected to both educate women in appropriate infant care and have skills to understand and advise on drainage, cleanliness and sanitary conditions generally within the home. Davies reports that in Glasgow and later in a number of other cities (Leeds, Sheffield, Bradford and St Helens) women health visitors were employed as trained sanitary inspectors, overseeing factories as well as domestic environments and child welfare; the job was seen as a real mix of the public and domestic health spheres.

However, there was no consensus on this role of the health visitor and Davies documents the conflicting arguments. Many people saw health visiting as an extension of the caring domestic role of women into the public arena, and considered that the more 'scientific' work required from a factory inspector was better carried out by a man. By 1911 the roles were split and health visitor concerns were firmly placed in the domestic/private arena. Health visiting, and as a corollary of this health promotion, was to an extent a casualty of battles to prevent the full participation of women in the world of public work.

Nevertheless, many health visitors today would argue that their health promotion work does still have a strong environmental dimension. Working with mothers and children and many other groups within the community necessitates a broad view of health needs and a requirement very often to cooperate closely with other sectors and workers from both the statutory and voluntary services, as well as working closely with women and families themselves. The major emphasis on health promotion and environmental issues is outlined in the four principles of their work:

- the search for health needs
- the stimulation of the awareness of health needs
- the influence on policies affecting health
- the facilitation of health-enhancing activities (Council for the Education and Training of Health Visitors 1977).

Environmental issues today

Many health promotion commentators would argue that environmental issues linked with public health issues are the most important to be tackled today and that health promotion and public health have very similar aims and goals (Bracht 1990, Griffiths & Adams 1991, Ashton & Seymour 1988). Draper (1991) identifies six features of healthy public policy; these are:

- the need for policy to work across different sectors
- the need to involve private, business and voluntary sectors as well as health and local authorities
- the need to recognise the international dimensions of health
- an aim to be educational and persuasive rather than dictatorial or puritanical
- the need to involve small community projects as well as policy on a wider scale
- the need to recognise the political dimensions of public health.

These features or characteristics match very neatly with the World Health Organization (WHO) approach to health promotion, outlined in Chapters 1 and 3. The WHO 'Healthy Cities' movement, forms the basis for much of the activity around health promotion and environmental issues today (see Ch. 13).

While many of the old public health battles concerning legislation around clean water, sanitation and clean air have been won, new problems have arisen. Health today is affected by factors as diverse as poor housing, street environments and traffic pollution through to acid rain, toxic waste and the depleting ozone layer. There is increasing concern about environmental issues being expressed by individuals, pressure groups and governments, though many in what has come

---

Activity 2.2

Pick any one of Peter Draper's six features of healthy public policy and try to work out what it might mean. Write down four points which you think relate to the particular feature and discuss these with a colleague.

to be known as the 'green' movement would argue that these issues are not yet being treated seriously enough.

Nurses and other health workers may be directly or indirectly involved with environment-related concerns. While global and national policy debates will probably be outside professional experiences, local and immediate factors will not. A nurse working in a community setting may very well soon find her- or himself working in a joint team where issues of mobility for older people, people with physical or learning disabilities, or those with HIV and AIDS are not confined to clinical and psychosocial dimensions but also include ways of accessing work, shopping, transport and services. As part of the joint team the nurse will be expected to participate. Similarly, nearly 150 years on from Florence Nightingale, environmental issues in relation to the built environment, to places where services are delivered and patients and clients looked after, are still of much concern to the health worker. Policies such as no smoking in public places, seat belt legislation and new environmental controls on industry (such as those now coming into effect in a number of European countries) are of interest and concern to everyone in their roles as citizens and stewards of the future environment.

THE SPLIT BETWEEN PUBLIC AND PERSONAL HEALTH

From the preceding sections it is easy to see that engineers, builders and town planners were at least as important, if not more so, in the early approaches to what could now be called health promotion as were doctors and nurses. Doctors, nurses and other health workers are very much more associated with personal health services

and individual care, although health visitors and nurses have quite frequently crossed the divide between the public and the private. However, by the beginning of the twentieth century the public and the personal health services were becoming separate. The 'real' health sector was starting to be seen as personal or individual care delivered by doctors and nurses mainly in hospitals. Medical Officers of Health who had first overseen many of the public health initiatives now became much more involved with individual care, particularly the health of mothers and children, and less with environmental issues. From a health promotion perspective these two important facets of improving the nation's health were moved apart. This was certainly the case from a governmental viewpoint, and the two also became separate in the eyes of the general public and of workers in the health and medical services. Monitoring, recording, surveillance and generally keeping track of individual health was becoming a major preoccupation by the turn of this century.

PERSONAL HEALTH SERVICES AND HEALTH PROMOTION

Developing individual responsibility for health

Tracing the links between personal health and health promotion is more difficult than in the case of public health, where the effects of health-improvement measures were large scale and very visible. In the mid-1800s there was an emphasis on organised sports and on the importance of exercise and physical health. But this was essentially a class-based phenomenon, with only middle- and upper-class people really participating (Open University 1985). Domestic health and cleanliness became a focus for concern and municipal baths and wash houses also grew in number from the mid-1800s, with Liverpool again being a city that led the way, assisted by the developing and marketing of soap by William Lever at Port Sunlight in the 1850s. Exhortations towards cleanliness, hygiene, abstention and the curbing of 'bad habits' became increasingly the direction of health education as it emerged into

---

Activity 2.3

It has been identified by older people living on a housing estate that personal mobility and access to local services and shops is a major problem. Identify what sort of workers might be involved in a care team to tackle this issue and what sort of plan might evolve.

the twentieth century, and there was often little attempt to hide the religious and moral overtones. The concept of individual responsibility for health was emerging quite strongly and in 1927 the Central Council for Health Education (later to become the Health Education Council) was established. The Health Education Journal, started in 1943, originally carried many articles directed towards mothers as being at fault for not imparting appropriate health information to their children (Thorpe 1993). Much health education material was filled with doom and gloom and seemed directed towards changing bad habits started in childhood, which unless 'cured' would result in juvenile delinquency as well as poor health. A notion of blame and fecklessness was often firmly bedded in the discourse.

Individual responsibility, as has been argued in Chapter 1, can be directed in either a positive or a negative way. It can develop into either an empowering or a 'victim-blaming' approach. By 1927, however, there was little official acknowledgement of the need to locate bad habits and lack of cleanliness within the conditions under which people were living. There was also little articulation of the idea that for some people healthy choices were very much easier to make than they were for others. Some of these ideas still have resonances today in the more extreme versions of the 'lifestyle' approaches to health and health promotion, which often fail to take into account the complex social issues that inform people's lives.

The Peckham experiment: an innovation in promoting personal health

There were some attempts within the personal health field to really improve the health of ordinary people and to develop what today would be called a health promotion approach. The Dawson Report published in 1920 drew on emerging notions of 'holistic' medicine and envisaged the setting up of 'health centres' where both preventive and curative services would be provided. But these ideas were not taken up on any large scale. An example of one celebrated attempt to put these ideas into practice was the Pioneer Health Centre

set up in Peckham in South London in 1935. It was started by a number of committed people who were interested in extending opportunities for positive health, initially particularly in the areas of birth control and child welfare for the poorer people of Peckham. Stallybrass (1989) describes the five main 'conditions' of the project. First, the building itself was not built to resemble a hospital setting as many health centres are today. Rather it was intended to be comfortable and very much more of a community centre. It contained a swimming pool and a gymnasium, a cafeteria, a playground and comfortable meeting areas as well as a medical centre and consulting rooms. Secondly, 'health overhauls' which today would be considered as part of primary prevention (see Ch. 4) were available to all members. Thirdly, membership was open to all the local community within what was considered 'pram walking distance' from the centre. All members paid a small family subscription, which was the fourth important condition and was tied to notions of responsibility and ownership and to the fifth condition which was what Stallybrass refers to as 'a sort of anarchy'. This meant that both adults and children were allowed to follow whatever activities they wished to do within the centre and, to an extent, determine themselves the way in which the centre should operate.

Arguably the project was a fairly paternalistic approach to the poor working classes and not a true reflection of the 'user' approach described in Chapter 1. It nevertheless demonstrates a very real attempt to provide a positive and health-promoting approach to the health of individuals and communities and to see individuals as whole people. It again clearly reflects the WHO approach to local initiatives in primary health care and health promotion. The Peckham Pioneer Health Centre was never financially supported by Welfare State finances, though its supporters tried hard to bring this about. It finally closed at the start of the 1950s.

Health promotion and the National Health Service

In the 1940s, the Beveridge report provided the

underpinnings for the emerging post-war Welfare State and in particular the National Health Service set up in 1948. The NHS (see Ch. 1) has never really had a broad health agenda or had health promotion as a central aim. With its concentration on hospitals and on medicine it has often been referred to as a national medical service. It is only very recently, as the examination of policy in the next chapter shows, that the pendulum has begun to swing towards health promotion.

Nurses and other health care workers are very clearly regularly involved, as a major and increasing part of their work, with health promotion for individuals and communities. One of the main issues for health workers working in the personal health services is to see the personal as encompassing the whole person and to see personal and public areas of health as clearly interlinked. So, for example, health promotion and education programmes around coronary heart disease could become very much more concerned with general physiological, psychological, social health and quality of life issues and less with dietary and exercise regimes. Similarly, the prevention of accidents in childhood would encompass both the built environment of home and school and the traffic environment, rather than concentrating on a health education programme directed solely towards children and their parents.

HEALTH PROMOTION AND COMMUNITY CARE

The past few years have seen a distinct shift in orientation towards a community basis for the delivery of care. This is the case in the health sector and in social work and social care. Large institutions such as those where people with mental health problems were housed, institutions for the learning disabled, large homes for older people and many of the grand hospital institutions which were a legacy from the last century have been disappearing. The community or much smaller units are thought to be more appropriate places for the care of people. Institutions take away people's independence and often they are far too expensive to run. Community care is in part a recognition that many conditions today

are amenable to a caring rather than a curing response. Health promotion and the enhancement of health for many people are closely tied to the types of care that they need and the quality of life that they want to experience. The work of nurses and other health care workers will have to become increasingly responsive to these needs, and this will be the case whether the setting for their work is in the community itself or in an institution or hospital within the community. What has brought about the focus on community and on health promotion?

Demographic change

The fall in incidence of infectious diseases was, as we have seen, in large part responsible for the rapid rise in the numbers of older people in the population. This has clear implications for community issues and for health promotion.

A major concern is with the numbers of 'very elderly' people who will require an increasing amount of support as they become more dependent. It is interesting to note that this is something occurring across the western industrialised world and increasingly in what have come to be called third world countries. Health promotion strategies have to take on board both the large numbers of older people generally and the increasing dependency of 'very elderly' people. It can be argued that as a society we have not begun to tap into the positive aspects of growing older or the potential arising from the increasing numbers of active older people. Health care professionals tend to concentrate on the ailments of older people, which can often be alleviated at least in part, rather than on improving their quality of life. The increasing numbers of dependent older people and the levels of care they will need pose serious problems for societies and communities today, and positive approaches to health to accompany much needed comfort and care will be a requirement for both older people and their carers.

Chronic illness, degenerative conditions and disability

The great reduction in infectious diseases also

brought along with it an increase in the numbers of people suffering from chronic illnesses, degenerative conditions and disability. This has been due to a number of factors. For example, as people live longer so various parts of their bodies are more likely to show signs of wear and tear. Disability figures, which are considered to be very much underestimated, show that approximately 75% of those people who are known to be suffering from disability are over the age of 65 years. Similarly, genetic predispositions to certain conditions such as diabetes, hypertension, coronary heart disease and arthritis are more likely to surface and increase in the population as the majority of people survive into adulthood and older age. Physical and learning disabilities are believed to be on the increase, as are mental health problems concerned with depression, stress, and alcohol and drug abuse. Accidents on the road and in the home, and occupational hazards are a very real threat in our industrialised world. As suggested in Chapter 1, many of these conditions may be preventable or, at the very least, the burdens of disability and discomfort may be alleviated and people's quality of life improved.

The majority of people suffering from chronic illnesses and disability are for most of the time looked after in the community and not in institutions or hospitals, although the focus of interest and resources on the hospital sector until very recently has tended to mask this fact. This is a major reason for the shifts in policy towards a greater community focus for health and social care and for the changes in nurse education brought about initially by Project 2000 (UKCC 1986). The authors of Project 2000 recognised that health needs into the next century would require a nurse who had skills and knowledge to work with children and adults with chronic and disabling conditions, as well as those needing acute care; who could work with people in their own domestic and work environments as well as in hospital settings; and who recognised that the prevention of ill health and the promotion of health for all patients and clients was a key aspect of the role of the new nurse. Increasingly, other health professions have also adopted this approach.

Activity 2.4

Give reasons why the community has become important as a basis for both health and social care. How are community care and health promotion linked together?

Inequalities in health and health promotion

Reducing inequalities in health experiences and opportunities is a central principle of health promotion. It is also a cornerstone of the WHO health promotion strategies of 'Health for All' and 'Healthy Cities' (see Chs 3 and 13). As was described earlier, Chadwick in London and Dr Duncan in Liverpool, along with many other reformers, linked poverty and ill health as far back as the middle of the last century, as did Beveridge in the 1940s. Inequalities are still very much with us today and this recognition is the cornerstone of many local health promotion programmes.

Inequalities exist in relation to:

- social class
- race
- gender
- ageing
- disability
- region and locality
- access to services
- health outcomes.

In 1980, the report of the Working Group on Inequalities in Health (known as the Black Report after its Chairman, Sir Douglas Black) was published. This was followed by a second report, 'The Health Divide', published in 1987 (Whitehead 1987). The reports confirmed that ill health was not randomly distributed through the population but was experienced differentially by various groups. Furthermore, there was: 'generally little sign of health inequalities diminishing and in some cases they may be increasing.' (DHSS 1980). Other studies have shown similar startling findings (Wilkinson 1986, Marmot & McDowall 1986, Townsend et al 1988).

A particularly important issue for health promotion was the finding made by Black and subsequent studies that inequalities in terms of access to health services seemed to be greatest in the preventive and promotive services. Such areas as dental services, family planning and maternity services, and screening services such as breast screening and cervical screening were used least by those who were most disadvantaged (see Ch. 12 for an in-depth discussion). The research and evidence also indicated clearly that it is the actual conditions of people's lives that affect their health and not just the health services that they are offered. For example, a pregnant woman may have access to excellent antenatal care, or she may have poor or mediocre services in her area. This will obviously be very important for her psychological well-being and for the welfare of the baby, particularly if there should be any complications. But the health of the woman before she becomes pregnant, for example her general nutrition, smoking habits, alcohol consumption, living conditions and general psychological state, will have more effect on the outcome of her pregnancy than will the quality of the antenatal care. What this example highlights is that good services are very necessary, but also that it is factors apart from the provision of services which in large part determine health status and health outcomes.

Black recommended three major objectives:

- an anti-poverty strategy for children and their families
- the mobilisation of prevention and education activities to encourage good health
- a greater emphasis on the health needs and quality of life of people with disabilities who now make up such a considerable section of the population.

There is now an increasing recognition, by governments across the western industrialised world, of whatever political persuasion, that if health problems of today are to be tackled realistically, action must start before people become sick, and that health promotion has a key part to play in any current and future health programmes. What is not always part of this consensus is the approach taken to health promotion. Thus, Black argued for the emphasis to be placed on improving the conditions of people's lives and reducing

inequalities, while much UK government policy to date has focused rather more on individual lifestyles. These policies will be examined in more depth in Chapter 3.

HEALTH PROMOTION AND GENDER ISSUES

Gender issues and health promotion relate both to specific needs for health promotion which men and women may have and to the setting for health promotion in which women's roles play a key part. On the first point it is notable for example that men tend to die earlier than women and that women tend to experience more sickness through their lives than do men. Rose (1991) argues that while men and women's needs for a health-promoting environment are the same in many ways, gender structures our lives in terms of differential patterns of mortality and morbidity, and that women do have very specific needs. Women use health services far more often than do men both for themselves and in their role as parents. On the second point, in relation to women's roles, it is clear that women are the key players in both the maintenance and promotion of health in our society, both as parents, wives and carers in the informal health sector and as nurses, midwives, health assistants, etc. in the formal, paid health sector. O'Keefe et al (1992) argue that women are far more likely to be both service users and providers than are men. The setting for health promotion is influenced significantly by these roles and it is this aspect of health promotion and gender that is examined here, while Chapter 12 looks more closely at the differential health experiences of women and men.

Women as health promoters in the informal health sector

Earlier in this chapter, the links between health promotion and community care were examined. Women are a further important link in this chain. Many feminists and other writers in the area of community studies have suggested that the concept of community care is itself not straightforward and that it cannot be separated from generally held views of women as the 'natural' carers and nurturers. Caring and, as an extension of this, the promotion and maintenance of health are largely the province of women. Community it is argued equals families, equals women (Finch & Groves 1985). When talking about community care, Finch & Groves argue that we are not just talking about care in the community, but care by the community, given largely by women looking after frail elderly people and people with physical and learning disabilities and mental health problems, in their capacities as wives, mothers, friends and neighbours. Similarly, Graham (1985) argues that women not only largely make up this vast army of unpaid carers, but are also responsible for health maintenance, health education and health promotion within families. Women buy and prepare food, and they deal in the main with the physical care of their families, with dental health, with visits to the school doctor and general practitioner, with family ailments and with the health-maintaining and health-promoting needs of more sick and disabled members of the family.

There are many issues within this analysis which it is important for nurses and health workers, who inevitably work very closely with women as carers, wives, partners, daughters and mothers, to address. It is important that nurses do not assume that women will be willing or able to take on the role of chief health maintainer and promoter within their families. Many women now go out to work from choice or necessity which may place added pressures on them. It is increasingly the case that some women who may be sole carers and providers of tertiary health promotion to frail family members may themselves be older and infirm. In addition, for women in low income families the responsibility for family health can be both very onerous and some-

times detrimental to the woman's own health (Graham 1984). Charles & Kerr (1986), in a study drawing on the experiences of 200 women in Yorkshire, noted that women were almost solely responsible for food buying and preparation within their families. They were also very aware of what was nutritious and what was not, but their efforts to provide a 'good' diet were thwarted by the strongly held tastes of husbands and by the costs of many nutritious foods. Many women were also very anxious but confused about media coverage of dangers arising from the consumption of food additives. Generally, these women felt responsible and often guilty at being unable to deliver the best possible diet for their families.

It is a very real challenge for health workers to recognise ways in which gender stereotypes may pressurise women and to develop mechanisms of support within health promotion programmes for individuals and families, which address and minimise the problems. From the above discussion it is clear that the informal and unpaid health sector is an important locus for health promotion in the community. It is sometimes easy for health professionals to assume that they are the health promoters and to fail to see the important contribution of women and families.

Women as health promoters in the formal health sector

Women are also the major health promoters in the formal, paid health sector. The majority of nurses are women and, as has been discussed, health promotion is increasingly becoming a major part of their role. Similarly, in many of the paramedical professions women predominate, and within community health services, where health promotion is a key aspect of all health work, a far higher percentage of doctors and dentists are women (O'Keefe et al 1992).

As general practitioners become increasingly involved with health promotion (see Ch. 3), practice nurses will have an increasing role to play, as will occupational health nurses who were clearly identified by the WHO as having an important role in health-promoting activities.

Activity 2.5

Watch the advertisements on television on any two evenings. Observe and document ways in which women may be more pressurised to be aware of health than are men. Compare and discuss with colleagues.

Health promotion is not always clearly identifiable by nurses, midwives and professions allied to medicine in their work. For example, it is only fairly recently that district nurses have examined their role with patients and discovered that although a great deal of their work is clinically based much of it is not. District nurses spend a great deal of their time with patients, carers and parents discussing issues such as diet, physical environment, mobility, transport, social and leisure activities, negotiating health and social care services and filling in benefit claim forms, all of which has far more to do with health maintenance and health promotion than with clinical issues.

This army of new nurse health promoters joins the health visitor whose past and ongoing role has already been examined.

CRISIS IN THE COST OF HEALTH CARE

No discussion of the setting for health promotion would be complete without recognising the crisis in financing health care which has occurred across the whole of the western industrialised world. Costs of health care along with people's rising expectations have been soaring over many years. Hospital costs and costs of high technology in acute care have increasingly caused concern. These concerns coupled with resource constraints brought about by national and international recession have resulted in a major emphasis on costs and on efficiency and effectiveness.

Prevention and health promotion have been viewed until quite recently as the remit of health care outside the hospital. The community health services were the place where health promotion was practised. These services have traditionally received only a very small slice of the resources within the NHS (Ottewill & Wall 1990). Thus, to date, only a relatively small amount of resources have been put into prevention and health promotion.

The crisis in costs, coupled with the issues of demographic change, shifting patterns of health and disease, plus a recognition that much ill health can be prevented, is leading to a far greater emphasis on community and on health promotion. Hospital care and technological innovation and intervention are still much needed but the recognition of changing health needs is beginning to shift the focus of interest. There is a danger, however, that health promotion can be seen as a cheap option; this will undoubtedly not be the case if it is to be taken seriously. But preventive and promotive activities will be required to stand up to rigorous examinations of efficiency and effectiveness.

Prevention and health promotion are no longer seen just as the province of the community health services. Health promotion in hospital nursing care becomes increasingly important as indeed it does within all institutional settings. All health workers will be required to see promotion as a key part of their work.

REFERENCES

Ashton J, Seymour H 1988 The new public health. Open University Press, Milton Keynes
Blaxter M 1990 Health and lifestyles. Tavistock/Routledge, London
Bracht N (ed) 1990 Health promotion at the community level. Sage Publications, Newbury Park CA
Chadwick E 1842 The sanitary condition of the labouring population of Great Britain. Republished 1965, Flinn M W (ed), Edinburgh University Press, Edinburgh
Charles N, Kerr M 1986 Issues of responsibility and control in the feeding of families. In: Rodmell S, Watt, A (eds) The politics of health education: raising the issues. Routledge and Kegan Paul, London
Council for the Education and Training of Health Visitors 1977 An investigation into the principles of health visiting.

CETHV, London
Davies C 1988 The health visitor as mother's friend: a woman's place in public health, 1900–14. In: The Society for the Social History of Medicine, January 1988
Department of Health and Social Security (DHSS) 1980 Inequalities in health (Black Report). HMSO, London
Dingwall R 1976 Collectivism, regionalism and feminism: health visiting and British social policy, 1850–1975. Journal of Social Policy 63
Draper P 1991 Health through public policy. Green Print, Merlin Press, London
English National Board for Nursing, Midwifery and Health Visiting (ENB) 1985 Consultation paper: professional education/training courses. ENB, London
Finch J, Groves D 1985 Community care and the family: a

case for equal opportunities? In: Ungerson G (ed) Woman and social policy. Macmillan, London

Gott M, O'Brien M 1990 The role of the nurse in health promotion. Health Promotion International 5(2): 137–143

Graham H 1984 Women, health and the family. Health Education Council, London

Graham H 1985 Providers, negotiators and mediators: women as the hidden carers. In: Lewin E, Olesun V (eds) Women, health and healing.

Griffiths J, Adams L 1991 The new health promotion. In: Draper P (ed) Health through public policy. Green Print, Merlin Press, London

Land H 1992 The confused boundaries of community care. In: Gabe J, Calnan M, Bury M (eds) The sociology of the health service. Routledge, London

McKeown T 1979 The role of medicine: dream, mirage or nemesis? 2nd edn. Basil Blackwell, Oxford

Marmot M, McDowall M 1986 Mortality decline and widening social inequalities. Lancet ii: 274–276

O'Keefe E, Ottewill R, Wall A 1992 Community health: issues in management. Business Education Publishers, Sunderland

Open University 1985 Caring for health: history and diversity. U205, Course Team, Book VII, Open University Press, Milton Keynes

Orr J 1991 Community nursing. In: Draper P (ed) Health through public policy. Merlin Press, London

Ottewill R, Wall A 1990 The growth and development of the community health services. Business Education Publishers, Sunderland

Rose H 1991 Gender politics in the new public health. In: Draper P (ed) Health through public policy. Merlin Press, London

Stallybrass A 1989 Being me, and also us: lessons from the Peckham experiment. Scottish Academic Press, Edinburgh

Thorpe L 1993 Spinning webs of words: a glance through some back issues of the HEJ. Health Education Journal 52(3): 120–124

Townsend P, Davidson N 1982 Inequalities in health: the Black Report. Penguin Books, London

Townsend P, Phillimore P, Beattie A 1988 Health and deprivation: inequality and the north. Croom Helm, London

United Kingdom Central Council for Nursing, Midwifery and Health Visiting 1986 Project 2000: a new preparation for practice. UKCC, London

Versluysen M C 1980 Old wives tales? Women healers in English history. In: Davies C (ed) Rewriting nursing history. Croom Helm, London

Walker M 1992 Patterns of ill health. In: Kenworthy N, Snowley G, Gilling C (eds) Common foundation studies in nursing. Churchill Livingstone, Edinburgh

Webb C 1986 Feminist practice in women's health care. John Wiley, Chichester

Webster C 1990 The Victorian public health legacy: a challenge to the future. The Institution of Environmental Health Offices, The Public Health Alliance, Birmingham

Whitehead M 1987 The health divide: inequalities in health in the 1980s. Health Education Council, London

Wilkie E 1979 The history of the Council for the Education and Training of Health Visitors. Allen & Unwin, London

Wilkinson R M (ed) 1986 Class and health: research and longitudinal data. Tavistock, London

World Health Organization 1993 Health for all targets: the health policy for Europe, updated edn. WHO, Regional Office for Europe, Copenhagen

FURTHER READING

Ashton J, Seymour H 1988 The new public health. Open University Press, Milton Keynes

Blaxter M 1990 Health and lifestyles. Tavistock/Routledge, London

Whitehead M 1987 The health divide: inequalities in health in the 1980s. Health Education Council, London

CHAPTER CONTENTS

Introduction   27

International programmes and policy   28

International policy development and the World
   Health Organization   29
   The Lalonde Report and the Alma Ata
      Declaration   29
   'Health for All': the 38 targets   29
   The Ottawa Charter   30

Strategies and policy development   30

Health promotion policy in the United
   Kingdom   31
   Changes in the National Health Service   31
   Containing costs   32
   Working towards a UK strategy for health
      promotion   32

'The Health of The Nation'   33

General practice and community nursing   34
   General practice   34
   Community nursing   35

Policy and the user   36
   Consumerist approach   36
   Empowerment approach   37

References   38

Further reading   38

3

Health promotion now: the development of policy

Susan Pike

---

*By the year 2000, all Member States should
have developed, and be implementing, policies in
line with concepts and principles of the European
health for all policy, balancing lifestyle,
environment and health service concerns.*

(Target 33: Health for all policy development, WHO
1993)

INTRODUCTION

This chapter sets out some of the important areas
of development in health promotion policy.
While actual practice and 'doing' health promotion are vital and basic, the need to have an overview, a direction and a focus for practice rather
than muddling through is increasingly important. What is the size and the nature of the health
promotion issue being tackled? Who is or ought
to be involved in it? What might be the implications of one course of action rather than another?
What are the key priorities and what resources
are available? These are just some of the questions
which constitute what we mean by policy, and
policy can be formulated at many levels, for
example at international, national, local, hospital
ward, health centre or community group level.
Milio (1991) suggests that public policy can become 'a prime approach to creating the conditions and relations that can nurture health'.

The process of policy-making is fundamental
and so is the content. As Chapters 1 and 2 have
implied, policies will need to take on board the
enormous demographic and epidemiological
changes taking place across the world. They will

need to examine what is an appropriate balance of resource allocation amongst cure, care, prevention and promotion, and address contentious considerations such as whether individual or environmental, medical or broader approaches to health and health promotion should be paramount. These are matters which nurses and other health workers cannot ignore. Policy is not just the province of politicians and top managers. Hard and difficult decisions have to be made and, as both professionals and citizens, health workers increasingly need to be both aware of and a part of policy- and decision-making processes.

This chapter examines:

- international risk factor intervention programmes
- World Health Organization approaches to health promotion which have provided a direction for promoting health at international, national and more local levels
- what is meant by strategies and policy development
- policy in the United Kingdom that addresses the shift towards a clearer focus on promoting health
- 'Health of the Nation' strategy and the targets which are providing the framework for much current health promotion activity
- general practice and community nursing as the focus for health promotion
- the increasing emphasis on users and on public participation in the health sector.

INTERNATIONAL PROGRAMMES AND POLICY

Many international health promotion approaches have been directed towards coronary heart disease (CHD) which is now the main cause of premature death (deaths under 65 years of age) across all industrialised countries (see Ch. 6). These have tended to be substantial intervention studies such as the Stanford and Minnesota programmes in the United States, and the North Karelia (NK) project in Finland. The goals of these programmes are primarily those of preventive medicine, and they are based on reducing risk factors such as smoking and obesity by a combination of approaches including health education and often use of the mass media. The NK project arose from great concern in the local population about the high rate of premature death from CHD. In the 1970s, this area of Eastern Finland headed the World Health Organization's league table of deaths for CHD and a 10-year programme to reduce these deaths was initiated, supported by the WHO.

The NK project places more emphasis on socioeconomic and environmental issues than do many of the US projects (Tones & Tilford 1994) and the programme was far-reaching, involving all health care workers, many local organisations, schools and the mass media. Nutrition was a key issue and the high intake of dairy produce and other fatty foods was considered to be an important causal factor. CHD did begin to reduce significantly in NK and it was clear that as a result of the mobilisation of so many community resources there was an increased awareness across the population of how lifestyle and behaviours affected health. At the same time, however, deaths from CHD were declining anyway in Finland generally and, as Tones & Tilford (1994) note, the answer to the most important question of how much the programme itself actually reduced deaths from CHD remains unclear—the impact of specific health promotion activities is difficult to determine. Issues such as whether risk factors themselves should be the major focus or whether more general factors affecting both lifestyle (see Maori example later in the chapter) and environment should provide the concentration for health-promoting policies are often strongly debated. There have not been such comprehensive studies in the UK, although 'Heartbeat Wales' (Welsh CHD programme) has provided a substantive set of initiatives, as has the Northern Ireland 'Change of Heart' project (Tones & Tilford 1994). UK programmes have also focused on areas of clinical prevention such as screening for breast cancer and cervical cancer in women. These prevention policies are an important aspect of health promotion; they clearly focus on disease issues and on specifically medically based screening services.

The World Health Organization has sought

to widen policy on health promotion and to shift from concentrating on specific programmes towards developing regional and national strategies. These are discussed through this chapter.

INTERNATIONAL POLICY DEVELOPMENT AND THE WORLD HEALTH ORGANIZATION

The importance of the World Health Organization (WHO) in developing health-promoting policies has been discussed in Chapter 1. It has had, and continues to have, enormous influence at both national and international levels. Even where the steering and guidance of the WHO is not used wholeheartedly by governments, its influence is inescapable. The WHO has developed from having a major focus on the individual towards a far greater emphasis on public health and environmental issues. Its current position, as Target 33 at the beginning of this chapter indicates, is firmly in line with developing and maintaining a balance between lifestyle and environment and health service issues.

The Lalonde Report and the Alma Ata Declaration

A report on the health of Canadians, known as the Lalonde Report, was produced in 1974. It argued for a new perspective on the health of the Canadian population based on preventing disease and on promoting health. Ashton & Seymour (1988) argue that it was a turning point in international policy development, and rediscovered a new public, rather than only a personal, approach to health. This was followed in 1978 by the Alma Ata Declaration of the WHO, which recognised primary health care as a key to achieving a healthy population. Thus it was not the curing of disease and the hospital environment that needed to be tackled first, but the health of people and groups living in community settings. This was vital for many third world countries and regions where clean water and basic health requirements need to be at the top of any health agenda. But it was also very relevant to the more industrialised countries and regions where chronic and

Activity 3.1

Why was primary health care at the top of the agenda for regions of the Third World and the industrialised world?

degenerative diseases were increasingly prevalent (see Ch. 2). The WHO was beginning to place great emphasis on the idea of prerequisites for health, on housing and work, on environment, and on social and economic factors as necessary conditions for good health, rather than concentrating on purely medical or individual concerns.

'Health for All': the 38 targets

In the early and mid-1980s, a series of WHO documents were produced on health promotion which began to push policy forward and attempt to influence governments. In 1985, the WHO European Region produced 38 targets to achieve 'Health for All', to which the majority of European governments including the United Kingdom were signatories. They were revised in 1993 (see Ch. 1). The targets are divided into a number of sections. As the phrase 'health for all' suggests, equity provides an underpinning for all of them. They are not about health for 'some' (David 1994), the some who have usually been the more affluent members of society, but rather the targets seek to embrace more specific and often marginalised groups, such as older people, ethnic minority groups, people with disabilities and mental ill health, and particularly groups disadvantaged by poverty. Thus, the 'all' also does not view society as homogeneous, but recognises that different groups in society may have quite different needs.

The targets are divided into sections, which cover:

- the need for a policy framework
- lifestyle
- appropriate forms of care
- environmental issues.

Thus, health promotion at the level of international policy development was put firmly at the forefront of the WHO's new health agenda into the twenty-first century, and there was an increasing emphasis on the need for political commitment at all levels of government.

The Ottawa Charter

One of the criticisms of WHO approaches to promoting health has been that at times they have seemed over-idealistic and unrealistic. The Ottawa 'Charter for Action' was issued as a clear attempt to make health promotion operational and to give it a much firmer and more realistic base, taking the ideas of prerequisites firmly on board. The Ottawa Charter has become extremely influential and the 'Healthy Cities' movement (see Ch. 13) is an important offshoot of the Charter.

The Charter linked a need for healthy public policy with a need for robust personal and individual involvement in health promotion. It was firmly based on principles of equity and social justice and on achieving 'Health for All' by the year 2000. The Charter encompassed five major elements which were to provide guidance for the development of strategies for action. These were:

- building healthy public policy
- creating supportive environments
- enhancing community health action
- developing personal health skills
- re-orienting health services to new health-promoting functions.

The strategies for action were intended to make health choices easier, whether the 'chooser' was an individual or an organisation or group of some kind. Ziglio (1993) states that the WHO approach sought to support 'ordinary people, local communities and member states (i.e. national governments)'.

The strategy emphasises both personal/individual, and community/public dimensions of health promotion and the need to see these as operating together. It stresses that the contexts of people's lives and the need for a real public approach to health are vital to health promotion. It emphasises the need for individuals to be able to have real choice and real control over their own lives, and to be helped to develop skills which enable them to use such choice and control. The need for different groups of professionals

and users of services to work together is clearly articulated and, in addition, the whole approach is underpinned by the imperative to tackle inequalities. The strategy does not assume that health issues have no boundaries, or that health becomes the major focus for all public policy, but rather that all sectors and all public policies 'should take into account the health interests of the public' (Milio 1991).

STRATEGIES AND POLICY DEVELOPMENT

A strategy can be visualised as a plan or map that gives an overarching rationale and direction. All sorts of approaches may be possible within the overarching strategy, so long as they are compatible with the overall aims of the plan. Carefully thought out policies are then needed to make the strategy happen, or to make it operational.

The WHO provides a strategy or large-scale plan for health promotion and, as Milio (1991) argues and the introduction to this chapter suggests, the sort of policies required to develop the strategy and put it into operation will need to be at a number of different levels. These levels will include central government, regional areas, local government and health agencies, and organisations and groups. There will be a necessity for researching relevant information by collecting data both about individual lifestyles and about groups and populations (see Ch. 6), and there will be a need to give out information to all concerned. Box 3.1 suggests some stages of the development of health promotion policy. The stages are intended to be viewed as continuous and ongoing rather than as something which is completed and an end in itself. The process also does not necessarily follow a linear pattern; it may well be that bits of one stage are going on alongside another.

Box 3.1 Stages of policy development (Milio 1991)

- Initiation
- Adoption
- Implementation
- Evaluation
- Reformulation

Policy development and the implementation of strategies can be very complex processes. They may well be fraught with difficulties: there may be many competing sets of interests; some aspects of the process will be far easier than others; inevitably some aspects will be more successful than others. Whatever the case, there will be a need for much thought and reflection, both in setting up and in evaluating the process and the outcomes. What initially seems an obvious route to follow may sometimes be improved by approaching the problem from a different and more imaginative angle. The approach cited by Ziglio (1991) is a very powerful example of this (see Box 3.2). The policy development and strategy that are described have drawn on the WHO approach.

Policies developed specifically within the UK and a UK strategy for health promotion are discussed next.

Box 3.2   An approach to policy (Dyall 1986/1987; cited in Ziglio 1991)

Although the Maori population and particularly Maori women, have amongst the highest rates of lung cancer and heart disease in the world, these are not our health priorities at present. Instead, we are concerned about rebuilding and strengthening our culture. The biggest health problem facing Maori people is cultural alienation. To be healthy young people need to feel proud of who they are . . . . Maori people are now rebuilding those institutions which provide the foundation for good health. From our perspective, these are: language, strengthening family and tribal links, rebuilding Maori meeting places, regaining ownership of land and water resources and transmission of cultural values and beliefs.

HEALTH PROMOTION POLICY IN THE UNITED KINGDOM

Changes in the National Health Service

The National Health Service, which still provides the majority of health care services, was set up in 1946 to provide everyone with services that were supported by taxation. Since that time it has undergone many changes. These changes have been remarkably rapid since the mid-1980s, particularly in the process of delivery. The services now operate in a climate that is far more influenced by the principles of business management. One significant feature of this is the introduction of an internal market with a clear division between providers of health care and purchasers or commissioners, who plan and authorise services on behalf of patients and clients. The thinking behind this latter development is that, if commissioners do not have to be responsible for actually delivering services, they will be better able to assess the health needs of their local populations in a more independent way and require appropriate services to be developed and delivered. Contracting processes were also introduced as a key part of these new developments. General practitioners (family doctors) now all have contracts which require them to provide specific prevention and health promotion services, for example regular health checks for older people on their lists and cytology services for women. They in turn may be part of fundholding practices or joint purchasing groups which contract with local hospitals (often now hospital trusts) to provide acute and rehabilitative services for the patients of their practice or group of practices. Health promotion departments of community health services are also involved in this internal market. Where do these changes stem from and how do they tie up with promoting health and with international approaches such as those of the WHO?

Containing costs

One of the major pressures in the UK to change health services has been a perceived necessity on the part of government to contain costs (see also Chs 1 and 5), and this is reflected in the move towards the business-oriented climate of the NHS. The need for economies to be made in the face of spiralling health care costs has resulted in a far greater emphasis on the need for efficient and effective services. This emphasis has provided a strong rationale for policy change in all industrialised countries and is clearly acknowledged within international forums such as the WHO. Prevention of ill health and health promotion are tied up with economic policies. It makes sense to try to curtail huge spending on high-technology hospital treatment by stopping people getting sick in the first place and acknowledging the enormous burden of preventable diseases. While it is by no means proven that to provide good and effective preventive and health-promoting services is necessarily a cheap option, there are strong economic and social reasons (as noted in Chs 1 and 2) for shifting the balance of resources from hospital to primary care (see Box 3.3) and from treatment to prevention and health promotion. These views are firmly accepted by the WHO strategy and they are now fairly widely accepted within UK policy, but interpretations of the type of developments and plans required to move towards a preventive and health-promoting orientation for health care can be very different.

Working towards a UK strategy for health promotion

A growing emphasis on health promotion in the UK has been evident in government documentation since the mid-1970s and the pace of change has increased rapidly since the late 1980s. An important early government document entitled 'Prevention and Health: Everybody's Business' was published in 1976. It suggested that the public health battles of the nineteenth century

> **Box 3.3 Primary and secondary services**
>
> ● Primary care services are health services provided in a range of non-hospital settings; they are called primary because they are at the first point of use for people. Settings include patients' own homes, doctors' surgeries, health centres and clinics. The services include:
>
> — Family practitioner services: general practitioners, dentists, pharmacists, opticians
>
> — Community health services: district nurses, health visitors, community midwives, school nurses, community psychiatric nurses, professions allied to medicine, e.g. chiropodists, speech therapists.
>
> Primary health care may also be envisaged in a wider context to include areas outside traditional health care such as: social care, education, leisure, transport.
>
> ● Secondary health services are so called because people move on to them from primary care. They are those services provided in hospital and institutional settings.

had been won and the environment and public health issues were therefore less important, and, as Jacobson et al (1991) note, it laid a heavy emphasis on the responsibility of individuals for their own health. This view is one which is obviously challenged by the WHO approach. Within the Ottawa Charter and the 'Health for All' targets there is a strong emphasis on the individual, but there is also a clear link between the individual and the context in which he or she lives. This is a different approach to responsibility for health than that expressed in 'Prevention and Health'.

The WHO approach is concerned with enabling individuals to have more control over their health through support from public policies and actions that make it easier for them to make choices about health. For example, it is difficult for individuals to have control over their own health or take responsibility for it where healthy foods are too expensive, where housing is very poor, where work conditions are unhealthy or people are unemployed, where there are high levels of traffic pollution, or where a group of people with physical disabilities live in houses with steps but no ramps. The link between people and the lives they live is almost indivisible, and health promotion at all levels has to take account of this. This also highlights the important fact that people have to be seen as being part of groups and communities as well as just individuals. A distinguishing feature of a public health approach, is that it adopts a collective view of health (see Box 3.4) and this is interdependent with work with individuals. So primary health care, public health and health promotion with individuals have to be seen as parts of a continuum. Furthermore, although the hospital and institutional setting is often characterised as separate from this (see Box 3.3; secondary services), it is clear that people have many similar needs and wants whether they are in hospital or not, and there is both a necessity and a challenge to embrace the hospital setting within a more seamless approach (see Ch. 5 on values and ethical issues).

Although UK government policy has undergone much change since 1976, it may be argued that many remnants of the central focus on individual health promotion remain, and that the push and pull between individual and social and environmental factors in health promotion policy are still to be resolved.

Jacobson et al (1991) suggest that, while there has been much improvement in the health of the UK population over the last century, there is little room for complacency, and that progress inthe UK may compare less favourably with other countries in north-western Europe. Recent documentation from London (O'Keefe & Newbury 1993) and Sheffield (Sheffield HAs

1994) highlighting how residents of areas of high unemployment and poverty are far more likely to die prematurely than those in the more affluent areas, supports this view. In the first edition of their book in 1988, Smith & Jacobson began the development of a comprehensive strategy for health for the UK, drawing very much on the necessity to align an individual and public or community approaches to health promotion. This was part of a movement which had been growing in the UK for some time. The need to develop a more comprehensive health policy directed towards primary health care and health promotion was well recognised by many people working in and with the health care field.

Many government reports and policy documents have been influential in the move towards a stronger focus on primary health care. A few which have had key roles in mapping out the recent changes have been:

- 'Promoting Better Health' (DHSS 1987)
- 'Working for Patients' (DoH 1989a)
- 'Caring for People' (DoH 1989b).

The NHS and Community Care Act of 1990 provided the legislation to implement the plans put forward in these reports, and it is within this framework of rapid and significant change that the focus on primary health care and the health promotion developments have taken place and have become closely tied to the developments in social and community care discussed in Chapter 2.

A very important part of the changes has been government recognition of the need for a far broader approach to health and the emergence of the government's health strategy for England. A series of government papers spelt out the strategy for promoting health, reducing mortality and morbidity, and preventing premature death, and 'The Health of The Nation' was finalised and published in 1992 (DoH 1992).

'THE HEALTH OF THE NATION'

'The Health of The Nation' goes some way to accepting the views expressed in the WHO Ottawa Charter. It recognises that a strategy of

---

Box 3.4 Public health responsibilities (Billingham 1994)

- Monitoring and describing the population's health
- Identifying those groups most in need of health support, guidance and treatment
- Identifying the social, economic and environmental factors that impact on people's health
- Taking health action to promote and protect the population's health
- Assessing the impact of health care on health

See Chapter 6 for more in-depth discussion.

health for the nation must have preventing illness and promoting better health at its centre and, as O'Keefe & Newbury (1993) note, it goes some way towards accepting a social definition of health alongside the need for a medically oriented approach. The strategy has five key target or priority areas related to what it considers to be the major national health problems. These areas are:

● cancer
● heart disease and stroke
● mental illness
● HIV/AIDS and sexual health
● accidents.

The strategy is both about addressing length of life, particularly by tackling those diseases which cause early or premature death (adding years to life), and about enhancing the quality of people's lives by limiting the amount of illness and suffering (adding life to years). Important aspects of the strategy are the stress on the need for different government departments to work together to implement the targets and the proposal to initiate joint working at local level between health authorities, local authorities, and voluntary sector agencies. The setting up of 'healthy alliances' was envisaged between these sectors and within different settings—schools, workplaces, hospitals and prisons for example. The mass media are also envisaged as having a key role (see Ch. 11).

The strategy is extremely important as it forms a major contribution to the new focus on health promotion. Although 'Health of the Nation' is an English initiative, the development of strategies for health has also been underway in Wales, via the NHS Welsh Health Planning Forum and the Health Promotion Planning Authority for Wales, and in Scotland and in Northern Ireland. Baggott (1994) argues that these other UK initiatives have attempted to follow more closely the WHO approach to health promotion.

There have also been criticisms of the approach taken in the 'Health of the Nation' strategy (for a summary of this see Baggott 1994). One criticism in particular is that the UK strategies themselves are too narrow and, in conjunction with this, that although there is some movement away from lifestyle factors alone, the targets are still too

---

> **Box 3.5 'Health of the Nation': an example of a healthy alliance between North Staffordshire Health Authority and Stoke-on-Trent City Council (National Association of Health Authorities and Trusts and City University 1994)**
>
> A multi-agency alliance set up on local housing estates comprising:
>
> ● health promotion service
> ● local authority housing
> ● leisure department
> ● social services
> ● youth and community education
> ● voluntary sector
>
> Schemes: home from school network, community neighbourhood forum, quit smoking group, play scheme, women's health group.

---

medically focused and still take too little account of health prerequisites, of the context of people's lives and inequalities and of the group and community dimensions stressed by the WHO. But if the strategy is seen as a beginning of the planning or mapping that goes towards forming an overall framework, then 'Health of the Nation' clearly has the potential to broaden its base, both by extending the scope of the current targets and by opening up other areas and possibilities for development. It is clear that many local and community initiatives are already taking place which build on the first formulations (see Box 3.5).

GENERAL PRACTICE AND COMMUNITY NURSING

General practice

The 'Health of the Nation' strategy articulates very closely with a UK government approach to health promotion focused on the role of the general practitioner (GP), and to date much of the impetus for the delivery of health promotion has been located with GPs. 'Promoting Better Health' (1986), was the government White Paper which confirmed this approach (see Box 3.6). Its health-promoting direction, as expressed in the foreword was to: 'shift the emphasis in primary care from the treatment of illness to the promotion of health and the prevention of disease'.

Box 3.6 'Promoting Better Health' (Baggott 1994)

Health promotion/illness prevention
- Targets (with financial incentives) for GPs to encourage immunisation, vaccination, and screening
- Fees for GPs performing health checks on new patients
- Amendments to GPs' terms of service to clarify their role in relation to health promotion and prevention of ill health

Consumer choice
- The procedure for changing doctors to be altered
- The procedure for making complaints against family practitioners to be simplified
- More information on practices to be made available

The White Paper was firmly directed towards general practitioner services and provided GPs with a set of health promotion targets linked to financial incentives and to their new contractual position within an increasingly market-oriented health service. Two of its key objectives were to:

- promote health and prevent illness
- make services more responsive to the consumer.

A variety of developments have since expanded and consolidated this direction.

It is both necessary and desirable for general practitioners, who are at the forefront of much primary health care delivery, to become closely involved with health promotion. But it can result in health promotion having only a medical base. Furthermore, GPs have traditionally had an extremely individual patient bias which does not address health prerequisites and, although based in the community, the group practice approach has rarely embraced localities or community group approaches. This raises the question of whether general practitioners are best placed to lead health promotion teams.

Community nursing

It is nevertheless clear that health professionals are uniquely placed to take forward the shift in emphasis from curative to preventive and health-promoting services. It has been argued that com-munity nurses could have a more central role to play than they have currently been afforded in government policy and could provide a vital link in the chain linking individual and broader approaches to health promotion. Chapter 2 demonstrated this via the role of health visitors, who have a firm geographical base and whose work via localities, communities and groups recognises the link between poverty and ill health. The work of other groups of nurses such as district and psychiatric nurses, as the Cumberledge Report (DoH 1986) demonstrated, increasingly offers the potential for effective and efficient community work. Ford & Repper (1994) report on an innovative care management and contact programme by community psychiatric nurses to sustain and support people with severe mental illness in the community, where previous GP referral processes had repeatedly failed.

Billingham (1994) argues that the public health role of the nurse is ripe for development. She suggests that via the nursing role a broader view of health promotion, encompassing social and non-medical prerequisites to health that are often seen as peripheral, could flourish. This would provide the basis for a wider approach, building on the 'Health of the Nation' strategy, which could be strongly locality and population based while developing and maintaining multidisciplinary work with individuals. The Royal College of Nursing has also been influential in debating nursing's public health role (RCN 1993) (see Box 3.7). Naish (1994) again views nursing as being central to the link between public health and individual health care at the policy and practice level. She suggests that a public health approach with far more emphasis on social aspects of health is a key part of the ideology and skill base of community nursing. Health promotion work, to be really effective, requires policies which enable problems to be addressed in the settings in which they arise, in the home, workplace, school, street or shopping centre, as well as in medical and health centres (see Chs 11 and 13). Billingham and Naish both stress the need for health-promoting policies within the health services and outside in a variety of settings (see particularly Ch. 13 on environmental policies and concerns), and for

---

Box 3.7 Key activities for public health work in nursing (Royal College of Nursing 1993)

- Assess the health needs of local populations through compilation of health profiles
- Support people to participate in the life of their community to influence factors which affect their health
- Build healthy alliances and a supportive infrastructure to provide information, resources and practical help for community initiatives
- Increase health resources in communities by establishing local networks
- Engage with the local statutory and voluntary groups to work towards health-related policies and actions
- Increase uptake of health services by ensuring they are accessible, offered appropriately and effectively targeted

---

Activity 3.4

Describe one project or activity where (a) a hospital-based nurse and (b) a community-based nurse might be involved in health-promoting work involving a public and individual health approach and team work. Who would be in the team?

---

professionals working in all settings to develop and maintain ways of operating collaboratively.

Hospital and community nurses and other health workers need to be working together with social workers and voluntary groups to provide specific services for older people from ethnic minority groups; general practitioners and practice nurses need to be working with local authority planners to address pollution levels and asthma control; and psychiatric nurses and social workers need to be networking with a range of user, carer, voluntary and professional groups to maintain housing, hostel, medical and a variety of other support services for groups of people with mental health problems. Such approaches to working will also need education and training that facilitates joint initiatives. The future for the 'Health of the Nation' strategy will require not one approach but many to address the pressing and immensely complex health problems facing us today and in the future.

Activity 3.5

Having read this chapter, why, if at all, does the nurse or other health worker need to be involved in policy debates?

POLICY AND THE USER

As was argued earlier in this chapter, there has recently been very much more emphasis in health policies on giving the user of services (the patient, client or customer) a very much more important role and far more control over his or her own health. Previously, it is often argued, the professional (the nurse or doctor for example) has decided what the person being dealt with needs or even wants. New services therefore need to find out much more from users about what they need and want. It is clear firstly that all needs and wants will not be able to be met; there is a finite sum of resources which cannot stretch to meet all requirements. Secondly, and associated with this, there is a need to sort the needs and wants and to determine priorities. But it is possible for the views of users, and particularly those who have not traditionally been heard, to feed into this complex process in a more powerful way (for a much fuller articulation of this see Ch. 5 and discussions of personhood).

Two approaches within current policies towards the user can be isolated: a consumerist approach and a more user-centred or empowerment approach (Walker 1993).

Consumerist approach

A consumer-oriented approach has become a hallmark of much recent UK government policy and is linked with the more commercial approach to health care and promotion discussed previously. The 1991 Patients' Charter initiative (DoH 1991) was part of the government's broader Citizens' Charter initiative which sought to set standards and to provide benchmarks for quality care of individuals. It represents an important step forward in the move to make services more responsive to consumers, but it has very little to say in the important area of health promotion. This is partially because in the main the Charter is dealing only with consumer satisfaction in relation to services received; the consumer has little control over the planning or development of the services themselves, which may or may not be appropriate. This has been a major criticism of the current approach.

An independent watchdog over the rights of individuals in health care has been the Community Health Councils (CHCs). Members are appointed from local people and they are independent of both providers and purchasers. They investigate complaints and act as advocates for local people where necessary. Again they do not have rights to participate in the planning or contracting process. Many local CHCs have been very active in health-promoting activities and have initiated projects and research.

Empowerment approach

The empowerment or user-centred approach, attempts to develop an approach to the user which moves beyond consumerism (also discussed in Ch. 9). It is the sort of approach and policy direction taken by the WHO and the Ottawa Charter. The Charter emphasises the need for processes of health promotion which enable people to 'increase control over their health' (WHO 1986). Hence, individuals (or their carers or advocates) will have more influence or power in expressing their needs and wants; they will be 'guaranteed a "voice" in the organisation and management of services' (Walker 1993).

Parsons & Day (1992), discuss the impact of a multi-ethnic advocacy project which aims to improve the health of women from inner city areas. Whittaker (1993) describes how a group of young people with learning difficulties were helped to play an effective role in meetings at their work centre and challenge assumptions that their contributions could only be minimal. The changes in communication required were difficult for the young people who had learned to be passive. They were also difficult for the workers in the centre who, although kind and caring, had learned to take directive and controlling roles.

There are many examples of how such user-focused approaches have influenced local policy (also see Ch. 8).

'Community development' was a term which developed from a practice of enabling third world communities to become more self-sufficient. It was adopted in the United States in the 1960s and has since had growing importance in Britain. The approach has been concerned with the need to address inequalities in health, and most community development projects have taken place in poor inner city areas, where community development workers have been employed to enable local groups to identify and evaluate their own needs and to access decision-making processes (Watt 1986).

The approach of community development is sometimes referred to as being 'bottom-up'. In other words it seeks to start with people themselves and have them involved in the planning of health-promoting programmes right from their beginnings, and it seeks to encourage self-sufficiency. This approach is a very specific use of the term 'community development', but the empowerment approach may be embedded in a range of other approaches to health promotion. Some may be effective, others less so.

Policies which seek to increase user involvement may thus be relatively limited, as with the consumerist approach, or may attempt to bring the user in right at the centre. While the former may need to be developed further, it is important to note that user participation is often difficult to implement in practice. Who are the users? How do you ensure that not only the loudest voices get heard? How do health workers deal with user participation if they disagree with the way in which users want to move forward? Policies and strategies to involve users require much thought, and debate in this area will be ongoing for many years to come.

Activity 3.6

What is the difference between a consumerist and an empowerment approach to users?

REFERENCES

Ashton J, Seymour H 1988 The new public health. Open University Press, Milton Keynes

Baggott R 1994 Health and health care in Britain. MacMillan, London

Billingham K 1994 Beyond the individual. Health Visitor 67(9): 295

David A 1994 Health targets: devising strategies to achieve them. Nursing Times 90(30) (July 27): 40–41

Department of Health and Social Security 1976 Prevention and health: everybody's business. HMSO, London

Department of Health 1988 Community care: agenda for action. HMSO, London

Department of Health 1989a Working for patients' Cm 555. HMSO, London

Department of Health 1989b Caring for people. Cm 849. HMSO, London

Department of Health 1991 The Patients' Charter. Department of Health, London

Department of Health 1992 The health of the nation: a strategy for health in England. Cm 1986. HMSO, London

Department of Health and Social Security 1986 Neighbourhood nursing a focus for care. Report on the Community Nursing Review (Chairman: Julia Cumberledge). HMSO, London

Department of Health and Social Security 1986 Primary health care: an agenda for discussion. Cmnd 9771. HMSO, London

Department of Health and Social Security 1987 Promoting better health. Cmnd 249. HMSO, London

Department of Health and Social Security 1988 Public health in England: report of the Acheson committee of inquiry into the future development of the public health function. Cm 289. HMSO, London

Dyall L 1986/1987 The Tangata Whenua: Maori people and their health. Radical Community Medicine Winter: 9–13

Ford R, Repper J 1994 Taking responsibility for care. Nursing Times 90(31) (August 3): 54–57

Health Lines 1994 Health Education Authority May/Issue 2: 13

Jackson C 1994 Strelley: teamworking for health. Health Visitor 67(1): 28–29

Jacobson B, Smith A, Whitehead M 1991 The nation's health: a strategy for the 1990s, 2nd edn. King's Fund, London

Lalonde M 1974 A new perspective on the health of Canadians. Government of Canada, Ottawa

Milio N 1991 Making healthy public policy. In: Badura B, Kickbusch I (eds) Health promotion research: towards a new epidemiology. WHO Regional Office for Europe, Copenhagen

Naish J 1994 The growth of public health nursing. Nursing Standard 10(8): 32–34

National Association of Health Authorities and Trusts 1994 A clear future for the NHS: NHS chief executive's speech to NAHAT conference. NAHAT Briefing No. 72

National Association of Health Authorities and Trusts and City University 1994 Quality through healthy alliances. NAHAT and City University, London

O'Keefe E, Newbury J 1993 Divided London: towards a European public health approach. University of North London Press, London

Parsons L, Day S 1992 Improving obstetric outcomes in ethnic minorities: an evaluation of health advocacy in Hackney. Journal of Public Health Medicine 14(2): 183–189

Royal College of Nursing 1993 Public health: nursing rises to the challenge. RCN report: public health special interest group. RCN, London

Sheffield HAs 1994 A health profile of Sheffields electoral wards. Report from Sheffield Health and Family Health Services Authorities, Sheffield

Smith A, Jacobson B 1988 The nations health: a strategy for the 1990s. King's Fund, London

Tones K, Tilford S 1994 Health education: effectiveness, efficiency and equity, 2nd edn. Chapman & Hall, London

Walker A 1993 Community care policy: from consensus to conflict. In: Bornat J et al (eds) Community care: a reader. Macmillan & Open University Press, London

Watt A 1986 Community health education a time for caution. In: Rodmell S, Watt A (eds) The politics of health. Routledge and Kegan Paul, London

Whittaker A 1993 Involving people with learning difficulties in meetings. In: Bornat J et al (eds) Community care: a reader. Macmillan & Open University Press, London

World Health Organization 1981 Global strategy for health for all by the year 2000. WHO, Geneva

World Health Organization 1993 Health for all targets: the health policy for Europe, updated edn. WHO, Regional Office for Europe, Copenhagen

Ziglio E 1991 Indicators of health promotion policy: directions for research. In: Badura B, Kickbusch I (eds) Health promotion research. WHO, Europe

Ziglio E 1993 Visions of the future. Health Education Journal 52/3: 182

FURTHER READING

Ashton J, Seymour H 1988 The new public health. Open University Press, Milton Keynes

Baggott R 1994 Health and health care in Britain. MacMillan, London

David A 1994 Health targets: devising strategies to achieve them. Nursing Times 90(30) (July 27): 40–41

Department of Health 1992 The health of the nation: a strategy for health in England. Cm 1986. HMSO, London

Jacobson B, Smith A, Whitehead M 1991 The nations health: a strategy for the 1990s, 2nd edn. King's Fund, London

CHAPTER CONTENTS

An integrated approach 39
Levels of health promotion 40
Enhancing positive health 40

An integrated approach to planning 41
Back to a medical model? 41

The preventive model 42
Primary prevention 42
Secondary prevention 43
Tertiary prevention 44

The radical model 45
Empowerment 46

Psychological theory in health promotion 46
Health belief model 46
The theory of reasoned action 47

Social marketing 47

Evaluation 48
Evaluating a community health promotion
programme 49

References 50

Further reading 50

4

Health promotion: models and approaches

Diana Forster

By the year 2000, in all Member States, a wide range of organizations and groups throughout the public, private and voluntary sectors should be actively contributing to the achievement of health for all.

(Target 37: Partners for health, WHO 1993)

AN INTEGRATED APPROACH

The integrated approach proposed in this book regards health promotion as an ongoing process; it is not a series of unrelated activities. The position adopted here is that health promotion is any planned measure which promotes health or prevents disease, disability and premature death. It therefore encompasses health education and much more. Health promotion is an integral part of the goal of achieving health for all, referred to in the target above. It is an essential element of the health and well-being goals of nursing discussed in Chapter 14, where clinical problems are seen as part of a broader focus, and health promotion is viewed as a constant aspect of nursing assessment and care planning—with patients, clients, carers and others. Applied to a wide sphere of health and social care policies considered in Chapter 3 and inequalities in health (Ch. 12), health promotion may be regarded as inseparably linked to health needs. It is also, ideally, an integral part of health care throughout the life span (Ch. 10) and of the environmental aspects of health (Ch. 13), thus relating to the whole range of experience of individual people and groups in their social setting. This focus conforms to the principles of equity, participation and empowerment contained in the Ottawa Charter (WHO 1986) which is discussed in Chapter 3.

Levels of health promotion

In the integrated approach to health promotion considered above four levels may be identified:

- environmental
- social
- organisational
- individual.

Kelly et al (1993) suggest that these four levels may be used as a check list when health promotion interventions are planned, so that all aspects impinging on the individual are taken into account. Ideally health promotion should not be confined to one level but the integrated approach should be adopted, in which the relationships between the four levels and the outcomes at all levels should be considered and analysed. Beattie (1991) points out that there are a range of health promotion options to be considered, some of which focus upon the individual and involve the professional, and others of which are targeted at populations or communities.

Enhancing positive health

The World Health Organization definition of health promotion, 'the process of enabling people to increase control over and to improve their health' (WHO 1984), suggests the integration of educational, social and political themes. This fits in with the model for defining, planning, and 'doing' health promotion developed by Tannahill (1985). Health promotion according to this model consists of three interrelated areas of activity:

- health protection
- health education
- prevention.

Downie et al (1990) propose the following definition based on the model: 'Health promotion comprises efforts to enhance positive health and prevent ill-health, through the overlapping spheres of health education, prevention and health protection.'

The specialisms in community nursing and midwifery illustrate these three different, but overlapping, approaches and are an example of the need for collaboration and teamwork in providing an integrated health promotion service (Cowley 1994).

The health protection sphere

The health protection sphere is concerned with legal and fiscal measures, operating at an environmental and social level to achieve policies which target positive health. The aim in this sphere is to empower people to make healthy choices. Health visitors contribute to this aim through developing health profiles highlighting a community's needs, and encouraging people to influence policies affecting their health potential. The environment can, for example, be a handicap for disabled people. Sometimes schools, homes and workplaces need to be adapted so that people with disabilities can function on an equal basis with others, emphasising their normality rather than their differences (Cowley 1994). Occupational health nurses can encourage the implementation of a workplace smoking policy and other health-protecting initiatives at the organisational level. Community health service staff can be said to have a duty to ensure that policy makers at both environmental and social levels are made aware of ways in which damage to health can be avoided, for instance by providing low-cost housing to prevent homelessness. Community participation in the planning, management and monitoring of health-promoting strategies is an important principle, so health workers have to find ways of working with, rather than for, communities—perhaps by facilitating groups and helping to set up projects, as discussed in Chapter 8.

The health education sphere

Health education is viewed as one component of the overarching entity of health promotion. In Tannahill's (1985) model the health education sphere overlaps closely with that of health protection considered above. Health visitors, for example, focus on empowering people through enhancing social skills and life skills as well as offering education at an individual level. School nurses are at the forefront in health education, and are influential in determining attitudes to health in future generations. Nurses working with people who have learning disabilities educate clients individually, but can also influence the wider cultural environment by helping them to be integrated into society (Cowley 1994). Health education efforts are also made to encourage the take-up of preventive services, thus forming links with the third sphere, prevention.

The preventive sphere

The preventive sphere includes health surveillance and prevention, carried out for instance by:

- community nurses
- general practice nurses
- midwives
- school nurses
- occupational health nurses
- nurses for people with learning disabilities
- other members of the primary health care team.

Screening, developmental surveillance and immunisation are examples which fall into this sphere. District nurses and community psychiatric nurses carry out treatment, rehabilitation and palliative care in the realm of tertiary prevention, to be discussed later. Community psychiatric nurses may also be involved in community outreach work, for instance with people who misuse drugs or alcohol. Needle exchange schemes may be helping to prevent the spread of HIV, and also provide an opportunity for education. District nurses and health visitors may offer drop-in sessions for homeless people and provide health education and preventive care with any treatment needed (Cowley 1994).

AN INTEGRATED APPROACH TO PLANNING

Downie et al (1990) propose an integrated approach to planning health promotion initiatives, whereby comprehensive programmes of health education in key settings and with key groups in the community are dovetailed with specific preventive services and health protection measures, tailored to the needs of the communities concerned (this is also discussed in Ch. 8). Key settings, defined locally, include:

- primary health care
- hospitals
- schools
- other educational institutions
- places of work
- deprived communities.

Key groups, which are also defined locally, may include:

- old people
- unemployed people
- parents
- ethnic minority groups.

Back to a medical model?

The model proposed by Tannahill (1985) and taken further by Downie et al (1990) has been criticised for being located in, and drawing from, a medical model of health which limits its usefulness (see Box 4.1).

Instead, Adams (1994) puts forward the following aim adopted by Sheffield Health Authorities for their health promotion activities:

Health promotion aims to contribute to the improvement of health of the people and significantly reduce health inequality. This includes reducing premature death and a wide range of preventable physical and mental illnesses and disabilities, the promotion of positive physical and mental well-being and quality of life.

However, the themes arising from such an aim

Box 4.1 A medical approach to health promotion

A medical approach to health promotion focuses on medical intervention to prevent or ameliorate ill health, aiming to free people from medically defined diseases and disability such as cancer and heart disease, and expecting patients to comply with preventive medical procedures for benefits defined for them by medical practitioners.

are not being equally applied in health promotion at the present time, as will be discussed in Chapter 12. Adams (1994) criticises 'The Health of the Nation' (DoH 1992) for its emphasis on behaviour change as a key strategy to improve health; for example, 'Health education initiatives should continue to ensure that individuals are able to exercise informed choice when selecting lifestyles which they adopt'. He questions whether people really can exercise free choice, especially those who are living in disadvantaged circumstances. Indeed, health education and health promotion interventions may increase inequalities in health by enabling people who are better off and better educated to make use of the messages and improve their health, while there is no impact on those most in need. The key underlying causes of ill health include poverty and deprivation, and Adams (1994) argues that therefore inequality and income distribution should be at the top of the public health and health promotion agenda. He proposes a social model of health promotion (see Box 4.2).

Tones (1993) also criticises 'The Health of the Nation' (DoH 1992) strategy, claiming that the medical model has reached its high point with this publication. However, elsewhere (Tones & Tilford 1994) the authors stress that the document accepts the importance of public policy and the need for intersectoral collaboration and interagency working. O'Keefe et al (1992) point out that although there is a serious failure to acknowledge that poverty is one of the major causes of ill health and of inequalities in health status, there are many positive features in the document. For example, two of the key policy objectives and guiding principles underpinning the detailed proposals are:

- 'to focus as much on the promotion of good health and the prevention of disease as on the treatment, care and rehabilitation of those who fall ill or need continued support'
- 'to recognise that as health is determined by a wide range of influences—from genetic inheritance, through personal behaviour, family and social circumstances to the physical and social environment—so opportunities and responsibilities for action to improve health are widely spread from individuals to government as a whole' (DoH 1992).

O'Keefe et al (1992) assert that both of these quotations reflect a view of health care which is similar to that of WHO (1993) but which differs from the biomedical and curative approach which has been so influential in the past.

THE PREVENTIVE MODEL

Preventive health may be described as improving public health not only by adding years to life—increasing life expectancy and reducing premature deaths—but also through adding life to years—improving the quality of life by minimising the effects of illness and disability, promoting healthy lifestyles and improving social and physical environments. It operates at three levels:

- primary
- secondary
- tertiary.

Primary prevention

Primary prevention means averting the onset of a disease or condition, for instance by immunisation to prevent children from developing many diseases, including measles, mumps, rubella, tetanus and tuberculosis. Primary health education also involves genetic counselling, perhaps for a couple whose future baby might be at risk of developing a genetic disorder such as sickle cell anaemia or Down's syndrome. In the realm of mental health, support may be suggested from appropriate local self-help groups or voluntary groups, advice centres or social services for people considered vulnerable to becoming depressed, including those who are:

Box 4.2   A social model of health promotion

A social model of health takes the view that social and economic factors exert the greatest influence in terms of health. The aim is to identify ways to change the social processes that make almost all the major causes of disease and death more common in poor people. This may be achieved by working with local people to meet health needs, aiming to reduce inequalities and improve the public health.

- bereaved
- physically disabled
- elderly
- socially isolated
- suffering from chronic, painful or life-threatening conditions (Armstrong 1993).

Examples of educative efforts directed towards primary prevention also include:

- weight control to prevent the onset of diabetes
- nutrition education, to help maintain normal systolic and diastolic blood pressure
- 'stop-smoking' programmes to help prevent cancer of the lung and cardiovascular disease
- education concerning the danger of overexposure to sunlight as a risk factor for malignant melanoma.

Policies for primary prevention include measures such as the provision of shade through planting trees near swimming pools to help prevent exposure to the sun, and campaigns for safer roads and speed reduction in the prevention of accidents.

Secondary prevention

In secondary prevention the emphasis is upon halting or reversing the development of a disease or disorder through early diagnosis and effective treatment. It involves the identification of conditions in susceptible people before they themselves are aware of the problem. Screening programmes such as regular assessments of child development and screening for testicular cancer and breast cancer are examples of secondary prevention. Health promotion interventions at the secondary stage, when a metabolic disorder is present, can have dramatic effects—for example, the diet imposed from babyhood for those with phenylketonuria results in the possibility of normal development with no further manifestations of the disease. Hypothyroidism has now virtually disappeared due to the use of thyroid supplements. In the past these conditions resulted in learning disability, but universal screening programmes have almost eliminated this possibility. Criteria for a screening programme to be justified are shown in Box 4.3.

Traditional screening and surveillance roles in

Box 4.3   Criteria for screening

- The disease must have a significant effect on the length or the quality of life.
- The disease must have a sufficiently high prevalence rate to justify the cost of the screening programme.
- The disease must have been shown to have better therapeutic results if detected in the early stages, and worse results if detection and treatment are delayed.
- The disease must have a significant symptom-free period which allows an opportunity for detection and treatment that will reduce mortality and morbidity rates.
- Screening tests must be sensitive and specific in early detection, avoiding false positive and false negative results.
- Screening procedures must be acceptable to those being tested.
- The disease must have an effective and acceptable method of treatment.

---

nursing can be developed to consider a neighbourhood focus as well as an individual one, thus integrating the environmental, social and individual levels of health promotion considered earlier. Gott & O'Brien (1990) point out that assessing child growth and development and child rearing practices remains important, but there needs to be a move away from an almost exclusively individual focus towards recognising the importance of context on outcomes. For example, the incidence of regional inequalities in perinatal mortality rates (see Ch. 12) calls for changes in the provision of services. Positive discrimination in favour of disadvantaged groups of people would involve increasing the level of input of health services and surveillance to those identified groups.

Research in secondary prevention

Secondary prevention of melanoma provides an example of the need for continuing research programmes to develop the most effective curative strategies—in this instance for malignant melanoma; at present treatment regimens can be disappointing. People can be taught to recognise early melanoma and to attend for treatment at a stage when the prospects for cure are good—as with several other types of malignancy. Public education campaigns are needed to explain the signs of the disease in question and promote positive attitudes towards seeking immediate treatment. A public education campaign carried out in Scotland was associated with a statistically significant fall in the average tumour thickness of melanomas in the whole of Scotland. This shows that public education can alert people to features of possible early melanoma (MacKie 1992).

Secondary promotion in an aspect of mental health

A simple mental-state examination using three questions can provide the necessary clues to the requirement for further investigation in the secondary prevention of depression:

- How are you feeling in your spirits?
- Have you been worrying a lot?
- How have you been sleeping?

There may be particular problems in recognising depression in some ethnic minority groups, as its manifestations vary from culture to culture. Some groups are more prone than others to describe psychological distress in terms of bodily symptoms. It is necessary for health care workers to be sensitive to transcultural differences in their locality, and to be aware of advocates, groups and agencies with whom they may work in helping to empower clients and families to influence their own health care (Armstrong 1993).

Tertiary prevention

The function of tertiary prevention is to prevent complications where disease already exists, promoting rehabilitation and preventing relapse so that the best possible level of health might be achieved. The development of primary nursing roles in both hospital and community would facilitate this. Health education and counselling in the tertiary stage can help patients and their carers, relatives and friends to adjust to terminal illness, with the goal of keeping the patient as comfortable as possible. Palliative care, which has developed out of the hospice movement, aims to maintain the patient's ability to function and maximise the quality of life, and includes:

- providing continuing care and support
- symptom control
- rehabilitation
- respite services for relatives and carers
- encouragement to talk over fears and feelings
- providing honest answers to questions and requests for information, e.g. regarding treatment choices.

People with a disabling condition can be empowered to adopt a lifestyle which minimises limitations, through adaptations to their homes or the introduction of mechanical and electronic devices.

The NHS in Wales (Welsh Office 1992) emphasises the importance of health promotion for people with learning disabilities, and summarises current trends (see Box 4.4).

Health care workers can help to make a reality of community care by enabling people with learning disabilities to achieve some self-determination and self-reliance, reducing the consequences of their disabilities and enhancing their health status (Sines 1993). Ways of doing this include:

Box 4.4 Trends affecting health promotion needs for people with learning disabilities (Welsh Office 1992)

- The presence of learning disability in older age groups is likely to increase for at least the next 30 years owing to increased survival; there is little difference in respect of mortality for this group than for the general population.
- Improved life expectancy will bring attendant medical problems. Older people with learning disabilities are more vulnerable to age-related physical and sensory impairment.
- There has been a marked reduction in institutionalised care throughout the UK (over a 50% reduction in Wales alone during the past 10 years); this has resulted in a major increase in people with learning disabilities expecting to have their health care needs met by community health services.
- Some 80–90% of infants born with HIV infections will become developmentally disabled; within 5 years, HIV is expected to become the largest infectious cause of learning disability.

- social training programmes
- skills development strategies
- educational provision
- interpersonal skills awareness training
- survival skills
- rehabilitation.

As discussed in Chapter 3, it is clear that Government policy concerning health promotion and disease prevention emphasises a move toward the primary health care team—meaning a GP-led model based upon screening for individual risk factors and advising on health and lifestyle, either opportunistically or within the more structured setting of a health promotion clinic:

> Through their regular contacts with families and patients, family doctors and other members of the primary health care team such as health visitors, community nurses and practice nurses are well placed to promote good health and to prevent ill health by giving advice on lifestyle, by providing screening for certain conditions for example high blood pressure and by improving take-up of vaccination and immunisation.
>
> (DHSS 1987)

Beattie (1991) describes such an approach as 'top-down' or prescriptive. He claims that this constitutes a 'health persuasion model' in which professionals attempt to shape and modify individual behaviour through health education and persuasion.

He advocates an alternative strategy which puts clients and professionals in a more negotiated, participative relationship. In this model, clients are invited to engage in active reflection (see Ch. 9) and review their lifestyles and the scope for change in a personal 'counselling for health' model. This links in with the holistic approach to health in which all aspects of the person and influences upon her are considered, while she remains in control of the professional/client interaction and the agenda to be followed. Beattie (1991) also discusses a 'community development for health' approach, in which the agenda is determined by collective negotiation, and which fits in with the Ottawa Charter (WHO 1986) model of equity, participation and empowerment.

THE RADICAL MODEL

As we have already seen, the preventive model has been criticised for containing elements of the medical model, focusing upon disease and its prevention rather than on positive health promotion.

The radical approach, described by Tones & Tilford (1994), attempts to tackle the determinants of health and disease at the social level rather than at an individual level. An example of how the root causes of disease, disability and death lie not in the unhealthy lifestyles of individuals and families, but in the social and environmental situations in which people find themselves, is provided by Pearson (1986). In some areas many families, particularly those from ethnic minorities, live in high rise flats or inner city housing where there is little space for children to play. Concern is often expressed about the high number of road traffic accidents among Asian children in large cities, and this sometimes prompts the circulation of leaflets about road safety. However, many children have nowhere to play apart from narrow, traffic-filled streets. Health and safety could be promoted far more effectively through the provision of adequate housing and traffic-free play areas. This illustrates the radical approach, which rejects the medicalisation of health and its 'victim-blaming' overtones. The focus is not upon individuals and their behaviour but upon the social, economic and political factors which promote unhealthy practices and produce such items as unhealthy foods and hazardous products.

Another example of the classic victim-blaming approach is the attempt to persuade people to eat wisely, while ignoring the environmental circumstances which either promoted the consumption of unhealthy food or prevented people from adopting a healthy diet. Effective radical nutrition education would be judged by such measures as:

- a decrease in poverty
- a successful battle with food manufacturers seeking to promote junk food and empty calories in western countries, and formula baby milk and diarrhoea medicines in developing countries

- providing a full range of healthy foods (preferably subsidised) at retail outlets and in the context of institutional catering
- proper food labelling (Tones & Tilford 1994).

Empowerment

The integrated approach to health promotion incorporates the values upon which theories under discussion are based (see also Ch. 5). An essential component of health promotion is of course empowerment, which seeks to enable individuals and communities to participate fully in determining the health and lifestyles to which they aspire. The underlying goal of health promotion is considered to be the achievement of equity—a fair distribution of power and resources. Tones & Tilford (1994) point out that an empowered community facilitates the development of self-empowerment in its members and depends upon a reciprocal relationship between people and their environment. The environment can exert a powerful controlling influence on people, but people can also influence their environments—for instance by lobbying or negotiating for needed health and social policies. The major purpose of an empowerment model is linked to the educational aspects of raising awareness of key issues and equipping people with skills, which are more fully discussed in Chapter 9. Empowered decision-making is also underpinned by many aspects of psychological theory, two of which are discussed below.

PSYCHOLOGICAL THEORY IN HEALTH PROMOTION

Psychological theory can provide a key underpinning to health promotion theory and programmes at all levels of intervention. Health promotion and psychological theories are constantly developing and changing; Bennett & Hodgson (1992) suggest that it must be to the advantage of both health promoters and psychologists to develop theory and practice in tandem, to better inform future health promotion initiatives and to improve the public health.

Two examples of psychological theories applied to health promotion are the health belief model and the theory of reasoned action.

Health belief model

The health belief model (HBM) (Janz & Becker 1984) is a framework designed to explain and predict health-related behaviours. In attempting to account for a person's readiness to act to change behaviour in relation to aspects of health, the health promoter needs to consider:

- the value of health to the person compared to other aspects of living
- the person's perceived susceptibility to a health problem
- the perceived seriousness of the possible health problem to the individual
- the possible consequences of the health problem—in achieving life-plans for example
- belief in diagnosis and possible therapy.

Thus, people may be more likely to adopt a low-fat diet if they are aware of the consequences of a high-fat diet and think that they are vulnerable to heart disease. The health belief model draws attention to the costs as well as the benefits to someone when anticipating changing behaviour in some way. The immediate costs of changing diet to attain the long-term benefit of avoiding heart disease may not seem worth the effort. It may involve changing cooking methods, eating less-favoured foods and perhaps increased shopping expenses. Cues to action may help to motivate or maintain behavioural changes; for example in relation to diet these may include:

- health warnings
- advertising health aspects of foods
- labelling food as having a high or low fat content (Bennett & Hodgson 1992).

A number of researchers in the area of health promotion and change have noted that people often need to pass through stages of changing attitudes and assimilating information before they make actual changes in their behaviour (Anderson & Wilkie 1992). People wanting to change behaviour to avoid the risk of HIV infection, for example, may need help in acquiring social skills that enable them to adopt safer sexual practices, such as effective condom use. The ability to successfully change habitual practices is also influenced by the social and cultural groups to which people belong and the extent to which HIV and AIDS for instance are regarded as threats to health.

It is well established that people pay much more attention to health promotion messages received from lay or professional educators who share their own social and cultural identity (Anderson & Wilkie 1992). Effective helping requires that habitual practices are viewed from the individual client's own world-view. Actions which carry the risk of HIV infection, with its potential life-threatening, long-term consequences, may be regarded by outsiders as irrational and irresponsible, but to some clients 'unsafe' sex may seem to offer security, love and the satisfaction of desire. The potential threats to health in an already uncertain and unpromising future then appear less important.

An understanding of the influence of health beliefs raises questions about what optimum health promotion strategies might involve. Walker (1993) suggests that encouraging responsible attitudes towards sexuality involves the focus, from an early age, upon the empowerment of young people to resist social pressures, including sexual advances and advertising, and to act upon informed choices. Education in parenting skills and empowerment education in schools may well be the best solution in the long term (see Ch. 9).

The theory of reasoned action

Another model which has been found useful in the health field is the theory of reasoned action (Ajzen & Fishbein 1980). This attempts to explain the links between attitudes and behaviour, stating that behaviour is governed by two broad influences:

- the person's attitude towards a certain behaviour—each attitude consists of a belief (e.g. smoking can cause cancer) and a value attached to that belief
- people's ideas of what important others will think of their behaving in certain ways.

These two influences combine to form an intention to act. The link between attitudes and behaviour is therefore modified by certain influences and people do not always behave in accordance with their expressed attitudes. Bennett & Hodgson (1992) provide the example of an ex-smoker who may have a number of negative attitudes towards smoking. However, he may smoke when out for a drink with friends who smoke, because smoking is an acceptable norm for the group, and drinking alcohol may also interfere with the previous intention of not smoking. Similarly, a person may jump out of an aeroplane attached to a flimsy bit of nylon or silk, despite having a negative attitude towards jumping—including fear at the point of exit from the aeroplane—because she does not want to lose face with friends by going against the norms of the group.

SOCIAL MARKETING

Social marketing may provide the type of strategic and practical tools with which Health for All can be achieved; it is incumbent on each of us to assure that it is applied appropriately and wisely.

(Lefebvre 1992).

Social marketing is concerned with introducing and disseminating new ideas and issues, and encouraging the use of specific behaviours among target groups. The actual term 'social marketing' was coined in 1971 to define a process in which marketing techniques and concepts are applied to social issues and causes instead of products and services (Lefebvre 1992). There may be much tobe learned from the world of commerce and advertising. For instance, commercial companies research a community for ways in which to influence its consumer needs and then use this knowledge to sell their product. Nurses and other health promoters, particularly those working in the community, also need to know the social, class, ethnic and other relevant profiles for the areas in which they work. They then need to identify health needs and hazards to health and make the relationship of these hazards to health known to the public, service colleagues and policy makers (Gott & O'Brien 1990).

The social marketing approach includes the use of the mass media to diffuse the message as widely as possible. At the heart of a marketing approach are the consumers one wishes to reach and influence. Two approaches are possible:

- the passive approach which seeks to understand wants and needs in the context of 'doing something for them'
- the active approach which seeks to build relationships and offer opportunities to interact with programme staff (Lefebvre 1992).

The passive approach tends to meet short-term goals of raising levels of knowledge and awareness and sometimes changing behaviour, but these are not sustained. The active approach allows for interaction between lay representatives of the public or audience and programme developers. They can also act as sentinels, drawing attention to programmes that may not be appropriate for community members because of social, cultural and political norms not apparent to programme planners.

Limitations

In the use of the mass media, health information may easily be confused with health education—educating for health is not the same as disseminating information widely (see Ch. 9).

Tones & Tilford (1994) review the limitations of the role of the mass media in health promotion:

1. They will not convey complex messages and create understanding of complicated issues such as the interrelationships of risk factors in coronary heart disease.

2. They cannot easily teach complex motor or social interaction skills, such as breast self-examination or assertiveness in coping with interpersonal pressures.

3. They will not produce attitude change in people who hold resistant views, or provide the necessary support for those motivated to change behaviour but whose physical and social circumstances make this difficult.

However, mass media can deliver straightforward, simple messages and possibly trigger positive behaviour changes in motivated people. Programmes must of course be constructed in accordance with good communication practice if they are to be effective (see Ch. 7).

EVALUATION

As a process, evaluation is concerned with assessing an activity against values and goals so that results can be used in the making of future policy and decisions (Tones & Tilford 1994).

There are many challenges facing nurses, midwives and health visitors in meeting 'Health of the Nation' targets. These include learning how to harness the experience of others by identifying good practice elsewhere and by using the skills available to assist in setting up and evaluating practice (DoH 1993). Box 4.5 lists examples of key people who can be helpful in evaluating current practice.

The establishment of a district-wide rehabilitation service for the mentally ill, an example of tertiary prevention, which included the development and implementation of a care programme approach was evaluated using the following procedures:

- an audit of minimum standards of care (adopted from minimum standards of community care) for use during clinical supervision and at client reviews to monitor the achievement of their goals
- satisfaction surveys conducted annually through a random sample of clients by post, home visits and telephone contact

---

Box 4.5 Key people in evaluating practice

- Quality assurance nurse/coordinators
- Clinical audit coordinators
- Research nurses
- Directors of information
- Academic departments of health and nursing
- Statisticians
- Health economists
- Directors of public health
- Environmental health officers
- Management services staff
- Directors of finance and other finance staff

- annual audit of a random sample of records undertaken externally
- feedback to staff on performance using data collected on individual client assessment forms—to show how clients had developed in terms of health and social functioning (Floodie 1993).

Evaluating a community health promotion programme

The most fundamental decision to be made about any evaluation is the choice of question to be addressed. Pirie (1990) presents a list of questions which could usefully be asked about a community health promotion programme, following the planning, implementation and outcomes approach to be discussed in Chapter 9:

- Planning
  - Should this programme be developed at all?
  - Are the educational materials appropriate?
- Implementation
  - Is the programme being implemented as planned?
  - Is the programme reaching its target audience?
  - Who is the programme failing to reach, and why?
  - Are the programme's participants satisfied with their experience?
  - Are the participants complying with actions requested of them?
- Outcomes
  - Is the programme having the effect it is designed to have?

This list of questions about programme operations is lengthy, and no single programme would necessarily be evaluated on all of them. The process of determining which of these questions needs to be answered to improve a particular programme will depend on the specific programme and issues and concerns raised by participants, facilitators, leaders and organisers. Evaluation requires a clear understanding of the goals of the programme, and methods of data collection and design of the evaluation (e.g. questionnaire, interview, observation) should reflect these goals.

Where possible, participatory styles of evaluation should be used, to help in particular with qualitative data, as programme participants' views are relevant to improving and developing programmes.

Evaluation, as we have seen, is used to develop standards of good practice and to help to assure quality in health promotion. Evans et al (1994) suggest the following questions which evaluation strategies would help to address at the wider, health authority level:

- How do health promotion specialists convince potential purchasers that the quality of their work is of a standard acceptable to purchasers and end-users?
- How do purchasers of health promotion services select the most suitable providers for health promotion interventions?
- Are there quantifiable standards for all aspects of health promotion work?

At the community level, the following changes planned for in health promotion programmes, may be assessed by questionnaires, interviews, discussion, and observation with individuals or groups:

- changes in health awareness—e.g. recording how many people enquired about preventive services
- changes in knowledge or attitudes—e.g. discussing how people apply knowledge to real-life situations
- behaviour change—e.g. noting numbers of people bringing infants for immunisation
- policy changes—e.g. policy statements and implementation relating to healthy food choices in workplaces and schools
- changes to the physical environment—e.g. measuring changes in levels of air pollution
- changes in health status—e.g. analysis of trends in routine health statistics such as infant mortality rates (Ewles & Simnett 1992).

In evaluating health promotion initiatives and their planning, process, implementation and outcomes, the future priorities for promoting health for all may be determined and, it is hoped, acted upon.

REFERENCES

Adams L 1994 Health promotion in crisis. Health Education Journal 53(3): 354-360

Ajzen I, Fishbein M 1980 Understanding attitudes and predicting behaviour. Prentice-Hall, New Jersey

Anderson C, Wilkie P (eds) 1992 Reflective helping in HIV and AIDS. Open University Press, Milton Keynes

Armstrong E 1993 Promoting mental health. In: Dines A, Cribb A (eds) Health promotion: concepts and practice. Blackwell Scientific Publications, Oxford

Beattie A 1991 Knowledge and control in health promotion: a test case for social policy and social theory. In: Gabe J, Calnan M, Bury M (eds) The sociology of the health service. Routledge, London

Bennett P, Hodgson R 1992 Psychology and health promotion. In: Bunton R, Macdonald G (eds) Health promotion: disciplines and diversity. Routledge, London

Cowley S 1994 Collaboration in health care: the education link. Health Visitor 67(1): 13–15

Department of Health 1992 The health of the nation: a strategy for health in England. Cm 1986. HMSO, London

Department of Health 1993 Targeting practice: the contribution of nurses, midwives and health visitors. Department of Health, London

Department of Health and Social Security 1987 Promoting better health: the government's programme for improving primary health care. HMSO, London

Downie R S, Fyfe C, Tannahill A 1990 Health promotion: models and values. Oxford University Press, Oxford

Evans D, Head M J, Speller V 1994 Assuring quality in health promotion: how to develop standards of good practice. Health Education Authority, London

Ewles L, Simnett I 1992 Promoting health: a practical guide, 2nd edn. Scutari, London

Floodie S 1993 Establishing a rehabilitation service. In: Department of Health (ed) Targeting practice: the contribution of nurses, midwives and health visitors. Department of Health, London

Gott M, O'Brien M 1990 The role of the nurse in health promotion. Health Promotion International 5(2): 137–143

Janz N K, Becker M H 1984 The health belief model: a decade later. Health Education Quarterly 11(1): 1–47

Kelly M P, Charlton B G, Hanlon P 1993 The four levels of health promotion: an integrated approach. Public Health 107(5): 319–326

Lefebvre C 1992 Social marketing and health promotion. In: Bunton R, Macdonald G (eds) Health promotion: disciplines and diversity. Routledge, London

MacKie R M 1992 Malignant melanoma—the story unfolds. In: Heller T, Bailey L, Pattison S (eds) Preventing cancers. Open University, Milton Keynes

O'Keefe E, Ottewill R, Wall A 1992 Community health: issues in management. Business Education, Sunderland

Pearson M 1986 Racist notions of ethnicity and culture in health education In: Rodmell S, Watt A (eds) The politics of health education: raising the issues. Routledge & Kegan Paul, London

Pirie P L 1990 Evaluating health promotion programmes: basic questions and approaches. In: Bracht N (ed) Health promotion at the community level. Sage, Newbury Park CA

Sines D 1993 Promoting health for people with learning disabilities. In: Dines A, Cribb A (eds) Health promotion: concepts and practice. Blackwell Scientific Publications, Oxford

Tannahill A 1985 What is health promotion? Health Education Journal 44(4): 167–168

Tones K 1993 Changing theory and practice: trends in methods, strategies and settings in health education. Health Education Journal 52(3): 125–139

Tones K, Tilford S 1994 Health education: effectiveness, efficiency and equity, 2nd edn. Chapman & Hall, London

Walker J 1993 A social behavioural approach to understanding and promoting condom use. In: Wilson-Barnett J, Macleod Clark J (eds) Research in health promotion and nursing. Macmillan, Basingstoke

Welsh Office 1992 NHS Directorate protocol for investment in health gain—mental handicap (learning disability). Welsh Office Planning Forum. HMSO, Cardiff

World Health Organization 1984 Report of the working group on concepts and principles of health promotion. WHO, Copenhagen

World Health Organization 1986 Ottawa Charter for health promotion. WHO, Geneva

World Health Organization 1993 Health for all targets: the health policy for Europe, updated edn. WHO, Regional Office for Europe, Copenhagen

FURTHER READING

Downie R S, Fyfe C, Tannahill A 1990 Health promotion: models and values. Oxford University Press, Oxford

Wilson-Barnett J, Macleod Clark J 1993 Research in health promotion and nursing. Macmillan, Basingstoke

CHAPTER CONTENTS

Introduction   51
   The menu   51

Values   52
   Traditional communities   52
   Changing Britain   53

Agreement: reactive response to sickness   54

Disagreement: proactive health promotion   54
   Health promotion and business interests   55
   Wide definitions of health and grey areas   55

**Consensus: health promotion to cut rising health
   care costs   55**
   Political consensus on changing lifestyle   56

Health promotion and the nurse's role   56

Professional nursing and interests   56
   Best interest and reactive care   57
   Best interest and health promotion   57
   Population-based health promotion: the greatest
      good for the greatest number   58

The whole causal spectrum   59
   Economy and standards   59

Professional nursing and personhood   59
   Responsible decision-making and imperfect
      knowledge   60
   Health and self-esteem   61
   Personhood and community   61
   Personhood and the nurse   62

UKCC Code (1992)   62

The WHO ethics target   63

Conclusion   64

References   64

5

Values and ethical issues

Eileen O'Keefe

---

*By the year 2000, all Member States should have
mechanisms in place to strengthen ethical
considerations in decisions relating to the health
of individuals, groups and populations.*

(Target 38: Health and ethics, WHO 1993)

INTRODUCTION

Action to provide long-term support for chronic
conditions, to prevent the onset of disease and
disability or to promote health is controversial.
Such controversies are rarely just technical; they
are about values. Nurses need to be able to take
part in making difficult decisions. They have to
do this as individual professionals, as members
of multidisciplinary teams and as citizens.

The menu

In this chapter, materials for making sense of
health promotion and values are explored. Health
promotion is ordinarily thought of as devoted to a
specific range of activities and interventions to
prevent disease and disability. This would give
pride of place to the key areas identified in the
government White Paper entitled 'The Health
of the Nation: a Strategy for Health in England'
(DoH 1992). As argued in Chapter 1, however,
health promotion applies not just to particular
strategic areas, but more generally, to a new way
of being a nurse. One can engage in curative or
palliative or any other kind of nursing in health-
promoting ways. The Audit Commission clearly
has this in mind in depicting nurses as facilitators,

health promoters, supporters and teachers (Audit Commission 1992). They see this as being especially appropriate for nurses in partnership with people living with long-term conditions.

Consequently, value issues arise in relation to health promotion when it is viewed as a specialised form of nursing and applicable to all forms of nursing. In this chapter, values are linked to four issues:

- cultural diversity
- the causal spectrum
- the UKCC Code
- the WHO ethics target.

There will be a particular focus on three concerns in health-related decision-making:

- best interest
- the greatest good for the greatest number
- personhood.

The implications for the nurse's health promotion role will be examined. Focus on interests illuminates the specific health promotion tasks and activities which nurses undertake, while focus on personhood illuminates health promotion as a supportive, facilitative approach in all spheres of nursing. The United Kingdom Central Council (UKCC) Code (1992) is seen as a very limited resource for confronting the value questions that nurses face. The new ethics target in the World Health Organization's (WHO) European regional strategy is considered, since the strategy offers a wider canvas for addressing value issues. Of particular interest here is that the strategy urges a turn towards health promotion to meet some of the deep inadequacies of present health care systems. The ethics target encourages professionals, service users and citizens generally to face up to the value-based nature of health policy and practice. The chapter concludes by looking at the target's framework for tackling these inadequacies. This chapter is not written from a neutral point of view. It is written from the point of view of engagement with the value base adopted by the WHO European strategy which gives pride of place to cutting inequalities in health status, and to treating communities and individuals as active participants in the process of achieving health.

VALUES

Moral values are about what is treated as important when people interact with one another, and especially what worth they place on one another in running their collective affairs. As applied to health, this includes, for instance, whether the health needs of all people should be treated as of equal importance, how important health is compared with other aspects of life, such as prosperity, the relative importance of mental and physical well-being, and how important future health is compared with present health. Values are expressed in terms of how people *should* and *should not* act.

Traditional communities

For most of history, people have lived in communities that initiate children into the values of the group from birth. What should and should not be done are clearly marked out by the role structure and codes which forbid certain kinds of behaviour and require others. Stories, histories, song and dance shape the emotions so that pride, humiliation, indignation and solidarity attach to appropriate role models. Members are praised and blamed accordingly.

Much of the role structure and content of codes is related to health. Tight rules about personal and communal hygiene, the treatment of pregnant and menstruating women, when to have sex and with whom and how, what people are allowed to eat, and the use of intoxicating substances are taken in from birth along with mother's milk and the local language. The family is the centre of a network for access to work, support, social and sexual contact, and economic resources. Workmates, kin and neighbours know one another and have a high level of agreement in their reactions to an individual's behaviour or lifestyle. Significant events, conditions, and activities, including giving birth, being ill or dying, working, learning about sexual activity, preparation and consumption of food, take place amongst people who are not strangers to the individual and to one another. The gossip networks are strong and overlapping. Individuals derive their identity from their position within the community. Values are expressed and experienced as duty (Durkheim 1984, Douglas 1970).

Authority

What should and should not be done has often been expressed in texts treated as sacred, such as the Koran or the Bible. Such texts tell people what is forbidden, for instance that they must not commit murder, eat certain foods or engage in particular sexual practices, or that they should give a specific portion of their wealth for the support of those who are sick or poor and treat strangers in a specific manner. The interpretation of sacred texts in relation to values may be the preserve of experts.

Changing Britain

In contrast to the extremely simplified picture just presented of traditional communities, British society is a world of inescapable cultural diversity. Britain is home to people with roots from across the world. People live in households of many shapes and sizes. Increasing numbers are in small, even single-person households. People seek contact and support from outside families. Friends and acquaintances from work may never meet an individual's family. The people who live next door may not be neighbours. The reactions of friends, family, workmates, next-door neighbours to a person's way of life can vary from horror to enthusiastic endorsement, or from deep concern to indifference. Much contact, even in extremely significant matters, takes place with strangers. The gossip networks may be fragmented. Television, radio, films and other media present images of the variability of behaviour and ways of living in different times, different places and different groups. Those same media convey powerful messages glamorising anonymity, risk-taking, the use of violence, and acting on impulse. Freedom of the individual is celebrated, taking the form of individuals being able to do what they like. Success is often presented as the power to consume. People may feel uncomfortable with the idea of having externally imposed obligations

or duties to others. In this complex and loose social structure many people see themselves and others as only partially members of any given group. They may see themselves as partial members of many groups with distinctive and criss-crossing concerns. They may see themselves exclusively as individuals. They do not see their identity derived from group membership, and they judge groups by the extent to which they meet their needs as they define them. People increasingly expect to make judgements about their lives in general and their health in particular for themselves.

Activity 5.1

List the groups of which you are a member. Which of them did you join voluntarily? Which of them were you born into?

Carry out the same task for a parent.

Questioning

This is of profound significance. Those who claim to speak authoritatively are less often taken as worthy of unquestioning acceptance, whether they are religious or political leaders, scientists or highly trained health workers. Values, along with rules and procedures for discipline and conflict resolution, are less likely to be seen as obvious. They come to be seen by some as human products rather like bridges, prams and guns. As such, they relate intrinsically to human purposes and goals. Values and rules seen in this light are open to reflection, discussion, investigation, revision and principled disagreement.

Science

People may think that science holds the answers to value questions. Scientists have enormous contributions to make in disclosing the impact of parenting, nutrition, pesticides, sexual practices and traffic fumes on measurable health status. At the same time, many scientists are employed in the production of junk food, pesticides and other substances which damage health. Health policy and practice need to be informed by scientific knowledge. But the large majority of medical interventions have never been tested (Dunning & Needham 1993). Furthermore, the knowledge scientists reveal cannot of itself determine how the health services should relate to prostitutes, or how government should relate to the automobile industry.

Confusion and diversity

At the same time, many people experience deep confusion about how they should live, what they should expect of workmates, kin, friends, sexual partner(s) and strangers, and how they should treat them in turn. One teenager may have been brought up supplied with information from home about the use of contraceptives as a matter of routine hygiene, in the knowledge that abortion is an option if contraception fails. Another in the same school may have been taught that sex outside of marriage, contraception and abortion are forbidden. One may see gay and lesbian sexual expression as a matter of what meets the needs of someone's personality while the other takes heterosexuality to be compulsory (Rich 1981). What one household considers to be firm, loving discipline another considers to be child abuse.

All the social forces and currents outlined above affect nurses. They need to be able to work effectively with colleagues and clients who have different values and ways of life from their own, where industry has its own agenda and experts disagree. Nurses carry out their health promotion role against a background where lay people are both users of specific services and stake-holders in the processes of thinking about, understanding, discussing and regulating the circumstances in which they live.

Activity 5.2

What are the three biggest differences in the world you live in compared with when your parent of the same sex was your age?

How similar are the problems facing you as compared with those faced by your parent?

AGREEMENT: REACTIVE RESPONSE TO SICKNESS

It is easier for people to agree on values when health is defined negatively and narrowly confined to treatment of physical conditions. Every society puts a high value on health where health is defined negatively, that is as absence of disease or disability. It values health care because pain, damage to the body, extreme deviance and death are universally feared. Every society has built health care systems to respond when pain or illness has occurred or death appears to be at hand. By the same token, unusual emotional states are treated as important for the health care system if they give rise to behaviour which is clearly dangerous to others.

Acute pain and threat of unexpected death present health conditions which give pride of place to the judgement of the clinician with expert knowledge. Emergency action needs to be taken. The person with the condition is thought of as a 'victim' to whom something has 'happened'. It is widely accepted that the unconscious victim of a traffic accident and the sufferer of a heart attack need professionals to act *for* them in an immediate crisis. Individuals demonstrate the value they give to reactive health care when they are in difficulties. They visit their GPs, demand prescriptions and buy over-the-counter preparations once they are afflicted by painful conditions. This is consistent with the value agreement put on reactive intervention to provide acute care.

DISAGREEMENT: PROACTIVE HEALTH PROMOTION

The emerging patterns of illness and disability change all of this. Major health problems have long lead-in times and derive from a spectrum of causes. Many threats to health go back into the adult's past: eating junk food in childhood or smoking in adolescence. Many causes interact to benefit or damage an individual's health. A proactive approach to prevent chronic disease and disability comes onto the agenda. To intervene in childhood eating to prevent the onset of cardiovascular disease and cancers in later life is a clear example of a proactive approach. Deciding where and how to intervene in the spectrum of causality runs up against disagreement.

Health promotion and business interests

Health promotion has come onto the agenda just at the point when modern societies find it difficult to achieve value consensus for reasons, which were outlined earlier, of the diversity and complexity of the population. The dominant culture leads people to think of themselves as primarily individuals. There is little in their experience that helps them to understand how much their choices as individuals are shaped by large social forces. Consequently, much of the spectrum of causality shaping eating, smoking or sexual activity is obscured from view leaving personal behaviour the bit that all can see. Multinational food and tobacco companies want to ensure that health promotion strategies restrict their profitability as little as possible (Economist 1994). This is of enormous significance; for example, the US Environmental Protection Agency claim that 1 in 1000 cancers might be due to dioxins, with food being the biggest culprit (Kiernan 1994). As Box 5.1 indicates, there is scope for intervention at various points in the causal spectrum to affect smoking.

So, part of the reason that there are difficulties in building a consensus about health promotion is that powerful companies are well organised to present their point of view.

Box 5.1 Two ways to cultivate cancer (South West Thames Regional Health Authority Leaflet 1993)

1. SMOKE.
2. SUBSIDISE:
Take more than £900 million a year from taxpayers in the European Community.
Pour in subsidies to Community tobacco growers at the rate of £1700 a minute.
Let Nature—and the Common Agricultural Policy—take its course.

Wide definitions of health and grey areas

Furthermore, if the definition of health is widened beyond physical conditions and applied to emotional and social well-being, 'health' can come to blur into grey areas. There is even greater scope for variation and disagreement about the nature of 'social or emotional well-being' than there is about 'physical well-being'. Deviant behaviour may be treated as evidence of an illness because it is felt to be burdensome or embarrassing to others.

CONSENSUS: HEALTH PROMOTION TO CUT RISING HEALTH CARE COSTS

On the face of it, a society would need to have a higher level of value consensus if it is committed to promoting health rather than just to responding to pain and the immediate threat of death. This is true if it is genuinely committed to acting on all the causes that have an impact on health across the causal spectrum. That would require that a society look at itself in a root and branch way. In fact, there is consensus only about one thing. Health care expenditure is escalating and it is not clear what the benefits are of this escalation. The most powerful reason for the recent importance of health promotion is that those who pick up the bills want to control cost. This is the motor driving the extension towards nurse prescribing and the movement towards giving midwives a more central position in maternity care. Lay people are expected to do more for themselves for the same reason. The determination to cut costs feeds on long-standing criticisms of reactive, hospital-dominated health care. It coincides with the long-held belief that a shift is needed towards building up community-based services where health and social care agencies work together. It coincides with the long-held view that health workers need to work with clients to enable them to live ordinary lives in the community with whatever health conditions they happen to have (O'Keefe et al 1992).

Political consensus on changing lifestyle

The move towards health promotion, and the identification of health promotion with changing the lifestyles of individuals, has been prominent in Britain for about two decades. Health promotion takes as its starting point the health problems of a population. Several values are highlighted but the key value is cost-effectiveness. Nurses' time is expensive, and its use needs to be justified to a variety of audiences. Any way that nurses can use their time in health promotion that reduces the call on publicly funded services can be expected to be applauded. This *may* coincide with what is clinically most effective as the best interest of the client requires; it *may* coincide with what is acceptable to the user as personhood demands; or it may not. As Graham (1990) has shown, the finance-led shift toward health promotion with a focus on personal lifestyle has gained popularity with governments across the political divide. The move towards focusing on healthy lifestyle as the core of health promotion and community-based care in the context of cheeseparing funding may trap some people in unhealthy lives. This is the lot of many carers. They may be overworked and unable to pursue their own lives and maintain a social network because of lack of respite care and other help (Brotchie & Hills 1991). These circumstances may shape the fact that they take little physical exercise and take comfort in alcohol.

HEALTH PROMOTION AND THE NURSE'S ROLE

There are three concepts needed to begin to understand value issues in relation to health promotion:

- best interest
- the greatest good for the greatest number
- personhood.

Most nurses have chosen this occupation because they want to work with people and they expect to work with them one by one, doing the best they can with each. This is partly why student nurses itch to start their hands-on work and sometimes find the time spent in library and lecture hall an agonising delay. What is best for the population taken as a whole is very much seen as a background issue which does not stir the blood in quite the same way. Professional nursing has overwhelmingly emphasised best interest and personhood applied to individuals as the moral principles governing its activities in the past. The turn to health promotion brings questions of what is best for the population as a whole (i.e. for the greatest good of the greatest number) centre stage. Health promotion makes interaction between professional and user much more policy-led.

PROFESSIONAL NURSING AND INTERESTS

Professional nursing revolves around the moral primacy of the health interests of individuals. The clinically autonomous doctor defines what is in the best interest of each individual. The nurse provides technical support to the doctor. Big moves are in hand to limit clinical autonomy of doctors. This is meant to save money. It is also meant to ensure that health workers are not a law unto themselves in their clinical care. What they do should be brought closer to best practice. Furthermore, the nurse could be making enormous efforts with the individuals who decide to seek care, while people who need that care more do not seek it. The guiding principle for provision shifts towards 'the greatest good for the greatest number'. This involves looking at the health interests of the population as a whole and asking how the resources available can best be used. Here the nurse's work is governed by policy, protocols, guidelines and targets that are similar to those embodied in 'The Health of the Nation' (DoH 1992). In contrast, with user-initiated contact with the health services for treatment, much health promotion involves identifying problems before they become apparent to the individuals concerned and inviting those individuals to take part in preventive activities. Regular assessment of those over age 75 in primary care is a case in point.

Best interest and reactive care

The dominant value orientation of professional health workers, including the nurse, takes the best interest of the user as of overriding importance. This has a number of components:

- focus on the individual user
- 'interest' defined as clinical need
- the user as 'sufferer'
- the user as ignorant
- the health worker, especially the doctor, as expert
- the health worker as decision-maker
- the doctor as clinically autonomous
- the nurse as technical support to the doctor
- the user as 'patient'
- reactive approach to the user.

The professional–patient encounter is patient-initiated but professionally led. The professional acts in the 'best interest' of that client. Management of the condition is meant to be based on clinical need, and health workers are expected to put aside all other feelings about that individual. This is especially important if the sufferer is criminal or has a lifestyle that the professional or a section of the community finds repugnant (Illingworth 1990). Confidentiality is necessary. This is because a sufferer's fear of disclosure of 'juicy facts' to others might deter him or her from seeking help. It would be an abuse of power for professionals to act beyond their level of knowledge or skill. Nurses and doctors have no special expertise that would license them to intervene in any other aspect of the patient's life.

Nurses are qualified to use procedures and substances that can *harm* the user. The first rule of the nurse is always to avoid harm to the client. Since the emphasis is on clinical competence, nurses must ensure that they keep up to date in knowledge base and skill. Even after 'treatment' has taken place, the client can only make a very limited judgement about how well the professional has managed the 'case'. Professionals can only be judged by those who understand the intricacies of their knowledge base and skill.

The nurse must be an advocate. This means acting against obstacles to get what the user

clinically requires not what the user thinks he or she needs. In order to ensure that health education is effective with those for whom English is a second language, best interest has led nurses to argue for interpreting services. This is to ensure that the professionals get their messages across to the user.

Best interest and health promotion

The notion of 'best interest' did little to encourage the development of the health promotion role. The reactive approach to ill health led most health workers to provide a bit of health education in the form of advice following the 'real' treatment. They might advise about diet or management of the menopause or give postoperative information about how and when to resume ordinary activities. This information could be inaccurate or distorted by commercial interests, for example of drug companies. They might additionally have preventive responsibilities in respect of antenatal care, family planning or immunisation, none of which were combined into an overall strategy for health. Their moral responsibilities include:

- treating each individual on the basis of clinical need
- maintaining standards of technical competence and safety
- protecting confidentiality
- ensuring that commercial, sexual or any other interest does not override patient interest.

Despite its shortcomings, best interest does offer pointers to moral considerations which the nurse cannot ignore. It highlights the nurse's accountability in relation to clinical standards. As Box 5.2 indicates, nurses have sometimes failed to meet their responsibilities in this regard.

Box 5.2   Cervical screening: some problems

In 1993 a number of scandals involving cervical smears indicated:

- nurses operating beyond their competence in taking cervical smears
- doctors using unacceptable practices
- nurses failing to blow the whistle on errant doctors.

Population-based health promotion: the greatest good for the greatest number

The recent emphasis on changing the health care system and on health promotion is grounded in concern about cost and effectiveness of current provision. This has led to questions of how provision might be developed to meet 'the greatest good for the greatest number'. This includes the following elements:

- limited resources and potentially limitless demand
- focus on populations
- the individual as member of risk groups
- knowing the pattern of health need
- knowing the pattern of health care cost
- knowing about effectiveness of intervention
- consideration of the whole causal spectrum
- the epidemiologist and health economist as experts
- health workers operate to policy, protocols, targets
- proactive approach to members of risk groups
- incentives to shape behaviour of professionals and clients.

Health promotion strategies have since the nineteenth century been tied to values that emphasise information-led intervention *for* the population. But information on its own may not be enough to get people to do what is in the interest of the greatest number of the population. Clients may need incentives to give greater weight to their own long-term, rather than short-term, interests and to give weight to other people's interests rather than just their own. Incentives can be positive, such as rewards tying payment of benefits to attendance at antenatal clinics, or a child's admission to school to proof of vaccination. They can be negative, such as penalties on smokers. It is considered legitimate on the basis of the 'greatest good' to try to restrict smoking, since the injury that individuals do to themselves incurs expense to society. This is measured in lost days of work and the cost of health care. Furthermore, behaviour can be restricted to protect bystanders from health damage caused, for example, by passive smoking.

Consideration of the greatest good for the greatest number is most acceptable when an individual's or organisation's condition or action has direct consequences for the health or well-being of others. This applies, for instance, to very contagious conditions that result in irreversible and serious damage, where causation is well understood, the individuals or groups at risk are identifiable and there is a high degree of confidence in the effectiveness of the intervention. Contagious disease controls involving screening at ports of entry, notification of infection and quarantine are long-standing preventive activities. More recent examples are constraints on individuals of no-smoking policies and on organisations of penalties for polluting the environment with industrial waste. These circumstances are taken to be legitimate grounds for compulsion.

The target-based role of the nurse

The nurse engages in health promotion when working to clear targets derived from an overall strategy as in 'The Health of the Nation'. The nurse is the vehicle for expertise and uses this expertise *for* the user who is viewed as a member of a given risk group within the population. The aim is to ensure that the user takes the 'correct' decisions to maintain and improve health. Training and persuasion of the client are then seen to be central to the health promotion task. Using this model, task-oriented screening, immunisation and advice-giving become the important elements of the health promotion work of many nurses attached to GP practices (see Ch. 8).

The greatest good: some problems

The emphasis on the health needs of the population as a whole in health promotion raises a number of ethical issues. It can fly in the face of what best interest requires. For instance, those in lower-risk groups are by no means risk free and may be missing out on opportunities to confront this. Also, cost–benefit calculations lead to greater importance being put on the threat of breast cancer to the 50-year-old than to the 70-year-old (Wilkinson et al 1992, Henwood 1991).

Box 5.3 Asthma: the spectrum of causation

Asthma has been described as 'the only treatable chronic condition in the western world which is growing more common, with a 13-fold increase in the number of young children admitted to hospital since 1960' (Ogden 1993). A recent national survey (Strachan et al 1994) calls this a 'major public health problem' with 14% of school-age children prescribed drug treatment in the previous year. Poorer children had a 'marked trend towards more severe, more frequent, and more sleep disturbing episodes'. The National Association of Health Authorities and Trusts (1994) recommends 'shared responsibility for management between the patient and the primary healthcare service' where 'much of the work of patient education is probably best undertaken by the practice nurse'. It presents evidence that increased use of anti-inflammatory drugs cuts GP visits and hospital admissions and 'the aim must be more economical management costs overall'. Prescription costs currently run above one-quarter of a billion pounds each year. Companies supply practices with leaflets and other teaching aids on the use of different kinds of inhalers, and sponsor nurses to go on diploma courses on asthma management (Edwards 1994). Meanwhile the Parliamentary Office of Science and Technology (1994) notes that 'the long-term trend in road traffic would be consistent with the observed trends in respiratory allergies, and vehicle exhausts are the primary cause of pollutants'. At the same time, a study funded by the Medical Research Council points to 'environmental events in early life underlying the origins of much allergy and disease' (Holgate 1994). Indicating the importance of air pollution in the home, including the house dust mite, the author argues that 'more attention needs to be given to developing primary preventive strategies for asthma rather than continuing to rely on an ever-increasing number of anti-asthma drugs and devices to administer them'.

THE WHOLE CAUSAL SPECTRUM

A population approach to health is a change from the dominant value orientation of professional health workers. The key areas and associated targets in 'The Health of the Nation' were chosen as the least expensive way of preventing conditions that are widespread and account for considerable health need and service use. Need for specific preventive measures focused on personal behaviour of individuals within specified risk groups has been identified. The rest of the causal spectrum has so far been left very much as it is. As O'Keefe & Newbury (1993) argue, its scope is potentially much wider than interaction between the health care team and an individual (Box 5.3).

Economy and standards

Mechanisms need to be in place to ensure safe practice in the context of the health worker's scope to cause harm. Much health care in future will be provided by health and social care assistants under the supervision of professionally qualified nurses. Professional nurses need to ensure that the staffing levels in the areas in which they exercise supervision ensure effectiveness not just economy. The greatest good has different implications depending on which is given prior-

ity. The nurse needs to be alert to illegitimate responsibility that could be placed on less qualified staff where resources are tight. The way into this area of ethical concern is via the notion of safety and standards. The UKCC Code provides a point of appeal as will be seen below.

The health system must always keep coming back to the spectrum of causality affecting the health of its clients. But not all models of nursing imply that it is the nurse's responsibility to be alert to the full spectrum. Indeed, as has been explained above, much health promotion, as currently organised within general practice, calls for technical skills in respect of specific procedures (taking a cervical smear) as well as communication skills to gain compliance to pre-determined target-based procedures or top-down protocols, making the nurse's work task-oriented. Nurses working to targets may treat the users as objects of policy rather than as individuals who take decisions about their own health. Informed consent may go by the board if the nurse is trying to reach targets (Tucker 1991).

PROFESSIONAL NURSING AND PERSONHOOD

The focus on interests does not encourage a learning environment in the nurse's place of work for herself or the client. This, along with evidence of the limited effectiveness of 'correct' information on its own to bring about change in behaviour, has led health promotion enthusiasts to consider values centring on personhood for working with the individual and communities. Personhood includes the following components:

- the moral primacy of the individual over the group
- the user's potential for understanding his or her health condition
- the user's right to take decisions about his or her life
- self-care and informal care as the foundation for health maintenance
- self-esteem as crucial to healthy living
- the importance of peer groups in self-esteem
- the health worker as advisor, partner, facilitator
- a focus on quality of care.

Individuals have their own concerns and priorities. They have views about what they need, the acceptability of interventions and how far outcomes are beneficial. Personhood treats people as having 'rights' because of their potential for understanding their health condition. They are not just trapped in the preferences or beliefs they happen to have. Personhood emphasises the nurse's responsibility to respect the user of services and to adopt a role of facilitation. The nurse acts in partnership *with* rather than *for* the user whenever possible. Focus on personhood treats contact between nurse and client(s) as a learning experience for both (Weare 1992). Each contact is an opportunity for health promotion, with the user able to bring issues to the agenda. This is especially true in relation to health problems for which there is no cure, where health promotion requires continuous active involvement of the service user in managing health. It also applies to hospital-at-home schemes where partnership is essential (Tatman et al 1992).

Personhood has been applied widely in mental health (Barker & Baldwin 1991) and is the underlying motif in the Department of Health and Social Services Inspectorate's handbook on mental illness (1993).

Activity 5.3

You are a member of a paediatric home care team. What steps would you take to ensure that you know what the concerns and priorities of the parent(s) are? How would this affect your way of working with them?

Activity 5.4

A dilemma in health promotion: you are concerned about informed consent but worry about target-led health promotion work where your task is to persuade. Informed consent presupposes having the relevant information and the right to opt out. You have to reach targets for whooping cough vaccination. You know that it is only fully effective if 'herd immunity' is achieved. You also know that there can be serious reactions in a small proportion of immunised children. You also know that there is inadequate compensation in the event of disability. You are supposed to encourage the parent to do what is in the interest of the population as a whole, i.e. what is required by the 'greatest good for the greatest number'. You are supposed to facilitate autonomous knowledgeable decision-making so that the parent will be able to promote the health of the child as required by 'personhood'. How do you work this through?

Responsible decision-making and imperfect knowledge

Discussing options with clients rather than persuading them to comply makes more sense, since the scientific basis and cost-effectiveness of health-promoting activities are often mixed (Calman 1994). In recognition that the knowledge base for managing health and disease is far from perfect, and that ways of managing involve different trade-offs and risks, users are being accorded more control over these decisions with professionals acting as a resource. This feeds into the right to informed consent. With proper facilitation, even children can take an active part in decisions about their health (Alderson 1990).

Unlike the focus on interests, the focus on personhood emphasises that mere patient compliance is not sufficient for many of the current health problems that prevail. Grudging compliance, as when the young woman turns up along with co-workers at her place of work to be immunised against rubella, is not going to stand up to the test if she is confronted with opportunities for risky sex. A more knowledgeable and enthusiastic commitment is required along with skills to be assertive and negotiate in sometimes unequal circumstances. She may have to build up her self-esteem.

Health and self-esteem

Nurses in the past may have been tempted to believe that health is *the* pre-eminent value held by individuals and societies. But health is just one of several values. Part of the nurse's task must be to have some idea of what the user's or group's self-esteem is bound up with. Being able to hold down a paid job or perform at a given level, having well-behaved children, looking attractive (possibly slim or young), may be of greater immediate importance than cardiovascular fitness. To prevent embarrassment caused by the behaviour of an exhausted child in a supermarket, a mother might buy sweets for the child even if she knows that this is not health-promoting. She may be trying to maintain some self-esteem, which will be eroded if she appears to others as unable to control her children. But self-esteem operates in a social context.

Oakley & Rajan (1993) identify a variety of factors that affect the mother including income, housing, number of children, sense of control and help from partner. It is not made easy for the mother to shop for healthy food if she always has to have children in tow, especially since those children will have been bombarded with advertisements for sugar- and fat-loaded and highly processed foods. It is easier for a mother who can leave the children with a baby-sitter or in a nursery when she goes to the supermarket not to give sweets to the offspring than for the harassed mother who is trying to minimise the grizzling of her child in the queue, especially since so many goodies are strategically placed at child level. It is difficult for mothers who are meant to be the key bulwark against the disease-promoting elements in the food industry to have to contend with being preached at by a nurse about what they buy.

Activity 5.5

Childhood eating patterns affect health status in later life. This can be affected by intervening at any point in the spectrum of causality. What steps could be taken for each factor listed below to make it easier for a child to choose a healthy lunch?

- the wide variety of foods full of sugars and saturated fats
- the difficult-to-understand food labels
- the absence of nutritional guidelines for cheap school meals
- habits formed at home
- advertisements in the media
- peer group pressure
- the fact that mother is rushing out to her low-paid part-time job in the morning
- lack of help from mother's partner.

Personhood and community

The empowerment of individuals and groups in their ordinary or habitual settings is the hallmark of a community-based approach to personhood. Accurate knowledge of the value people place on health is essential, given cultural diversity. Misuse of alcohol may be particularly problematic amongst those groups that consider all use of alcohol sinful (Haringey Advisory Group on Alcohol 1992). At the same time, communities change and there may be considerable diversity and conflict about values within groups with strong religious traditions as well as between them. This is borne out by the experience of women's groups (Southall Black Sisters 1989). Personhood insists that a communal perspective still sees all groups, including minority groups, as made up of individuals.

Notions of empowerment and practices of peer education are bound up with the view that self-esteem is generated and behaviour shaped in communities (Wallerstein 1993). For such reasons, the Health Education Authority's study of diet, alcohol, smoking, drugs and sexual behaviour amongst 16- to 19-year-olds recommends that interactive approaches be used with young people who persistently engage in unhealthy behaviour despite accurate knowledge of health risks (Rudat et al 1992). This also points to ordinary settings (schools, discos, workplaces)

Box 5.4   Health fax (Jackson 1993)

Community nurses worked closely with students and teachers in south London schools to devise interactive pupil-held health records. Designed to be taken to all visits to school nurse, GP or hospital, they give 11-year-olds scope to record how healthy their eating, sleeping and exercise is, whether they have someone to talk to when they have problems, what their problems are and how they want to improve their health. For each of their visits to the school nurse there is space for the pupils to write down the advice that was given as well as their own comments and those of their parents or carers.

---

as locations for health promotion rather than reliance on activities taking place in clinics (Box 5.4). (See Ch. 11.)

It is just this combination of facts, that people's conception of themselves is bound up with the way people see them and there are inequalities of health between groups, that gives a role to community development in health promotion (Box 5.5).

Personhood and the nurse

What does 'personhood' mean for the nurse? Nurses are not just the tools of their employer. They should never follow rules uncritically. They must always be accountable for their actions, and must form an ethical view about the policy, protocols, targets and instructions to which they work. This is acknowledged explicitly in the UKCC Code of ethics. They must be prepared to be advocates, which means supporting the users to achieve their goals. They are facilitators who work in partnership with users, exercising their judgement to underpin opportunistic health promotion. They must always be aware of potential conflicts between what is advanced on the basis of the greatest good for the greatest number on the one hand and the best interest of individuals on the other. They must also be aware of the potential conflict between each of these and personhood.

UKCC CODE (1992)

The ethical code governing the nursing profession in the UK brings together the ingredients

---

Box 5.5   Community development strategy: an example (Rotherham Metropolitan Borough Council 1994)

The Council, health authority, police, mosques and churches formed a healthy alliance to promote community action in Ferham. The process of developing an advice centre was designed to promote cooperation between Asian and white residents 'for the benefit of the whole community'.

---

outlined above, most particularly considerations of the best interests and personhood of individual service users. Consideration of the greatest good for the greatest number is less prominent but appears without elaboration as the requirement to act 'to serve the interests of society'. Best interest appears in reference to the nurse's responsibility to respond to users' 'need for care irrespective of their ethnic origin, religious beliefs, personal attributes, the nature of their health problems or any other factor'. The requirements to maintain safe standards of practice, to prevent harm to users and to ensure that commercial considerations do not interfere with professional judgement are grounded in best interest as well. This is clearly related to knowledge-based competence which must always be kept up to date. Personhood appears in reference to informed consent and confidentiality as well as accountability for fostering the independence of users and respecting the involvement of users and families 'in the planning and delivery of care'.

The Code has evolved with a focus on treatment rather than health promotion. There is no explicit emphasis on the health of populations. There is no strong emphasis on the socially based inequalities that groups experience. The 'greatest good' or the interests of society are acknowledged sparingly. First, confidentiality may be breached 'in the wider public interest'. Secondly, the 'environment of care' could constrain the ability of nurses to maintain the dignity of the individual, meet their clients' best interest or ensure that those they supervise are accorded due protection. With tough pressures towards cost containment, corners can be cut dangerously. The Code may need to be invoked to protect the interests of patients and colleagues.

Have regard to the environment of care and its physical, psychological and social effects on patients/clients, and also to the adequacy of resources, and make known to appropriate persons or authorities any circumstances which could place patients/clients in jeopardy or which militate against safe standards of practice. (para. 10)

Have regard to the workload of and the pressures on professional colleagues and subordinates and take appropriate action if these are seen to be such as to constitute abuse of the individual practitioner and/or to jeopardise safe standards of practice. (para. 11)

(UKCC 1992)

Beyerstein (1993) argues that professional codes should be seen as changeable rather than as authoritative guides fixed in stone. They are helpful in a variety of ways:

- expressing the present consensus on what is deemed important
- binding members together
- holding them to account
- carrying out disciplinary procedures
- settling conflict
- indicating to professionals from other disciplines what they can expect.

With health care changing so rapidly the Code will have to be developed to be of real assistance to nurses who are engaged in the specific health promotion tasks so far required in 'The Health of the Nation'. Even greater demands for development arise from the broader health promotion role nurses take on as they support, facilitate and work in partnership with individuals living in the community with long-term disease and disability. The WHO ethics target at the beginning of this chapter directs attention to the wider canvas that is needed to address the questions that nurses must face as individual professionals, members of multidisciplinary teams and citizens.

THE WHO ETHICS TARGET

The WHO European strategy brings together the pursuit of what is good for the population with community-based personhood. The WHO strategy corrects the individualist tendencies of best interest and personhood by locating them in the context of an overriding concern to reduce

inequalities in health. It does this by taking seriously the full causal spectrum affecting people's health. Health-promoting public policy that shapes lifestyle is treated as requiring a more thoroughgoing commitment by the general public than was ever thought necessary by previous generations of reformers committed to the prevention of disease and disability. This commitment is meant to be based on understanding so that health promotion is *by* the people not just *for* the people.

The strategy's new ethics target calls for the setting up of mechanisms for ethically based decision-making about health policy and health research as well as health care practice. The target calls for wide-ranging and open discussion of the 'interests of individual people, groups in the community, and the public at large'. Health workers and others need to be able 'to speak independently from government, industry and professional ... interests.' (Box 5.6).

The principles advanced are more robust than those found in the UKCC Code. Based on international agreements such as the United Nation's 'Universal Declaration of Human Rights' (1948), they combine concerns about basic material needs with a deep commitment to the language of personhood. Rights apply to all 'without distinction of any kind such as race, colour, sex, language, religion, political or other opinion, national or social origin, birth or other status'. Each human being is accorded those rights required for the free development of personality and for the exercise of freedoms. Deliberate nourishing of the competence and confidence to understand the society and take responsible decisions is required. Basic material needs are treated as necessary for human development. Hence the Declaration calls for:

Box 5.6 Requirements of the WHO ethics target

- The education and training of health professionals in ethics
- Measures to increase knowledge of ethical considerations among the public, politicians and decision-makers
- An ethical code of practice for health professionals

the right to a standard of living adequate for ... health and well-being ... including food, clothing, housing and medical care and necessary social services, and the right to security in the event of unemployment, sickness, disability, widowhood, old age or other lack of livelihood in circumstances beyond his control.

CONCLUSION

The Chief Medical Officer has identified as one of six strategic aims essential for the development of the nation's health 'to provide a highly professional team of staff, with clear values and high ethical standards' (DoH 1993). A diverse and rapidly changing society has to grasp the challenge of knowledgeable decision-making about values in health promotion. It needs to include all stake-holders including nurses and users. The WHO strategy's framework calls for widening the participation in decision-making of all sections of the population at large, as well as institutional stake-holders. The society is seen as needing to be more democratic and the population as requiring resources and opportunities to learn about and understand how health status is affected by the full spectrum of causation. The implications for nursing are clear. The moral responsibilities of the nurse are never exhausted in carrying out specific tasks and procedures. The nurse is better placed to meet her moral responsibilities if she is a reflective and self-critical facilitator.

REFERENCES

Alderson P 1990 Choosing for children. Oxford University Press, Oxford

Audit Commision 1992 Homeward bound. HMSO, London

Barker P, Baldwin S (eds) 1991 Ethical issues in mental health. Chapman & Hall, London

Beyerstein D 1993 The functions and limitations of professional codes of ethics. In: Winkler E, Coombs J (eds) Applied ethics. Blackwell, Oxford

Brotchie J, Hills D 1991 Equal shares in caring: towards equality in health. Socialist Health Association, London

Calman K C 1994 Screening in the National Health Service. DoH, London

Chadwick R, Tadd W 1992 Ethics and nursing practice. Macmillan, Basingstoke

Department of Health 1992 The health of the nation: a strategy for health in England. Cm 1986. HMSO, London

Department of Health 1993 On the state of the public health 1992. HMSO, London

Department of Health and Social Services Inspectorate 1993 Mental illness: key area handbook. HMSO, London

Downie R S, Fyfe C, Tannahill A 1990 Health promotion: models and values. Oxford Medical Publications, Oxford

Douglas M 1970 Purity and danger. Pelican, London

Dunning M, Needham G (eds) 1993 But will it work doctor? King's Fund, London

Durkheim E 1984 The division of labour in society. Macmillan, Basingstoke

Economist 1994 Battle of the bulge. The Economist 20 August

Edwards M 1994 Educating schools about asthma. Community Outlook 4(5): 28–29

Graham H 1990 Behaving well: women's health behaviour in context. In: Roberts H (ed) Women's health counts. Routledge, London

Haringey Advisory Group on Alcohol 1992 Alcohol and invisible communities: needs and attitudes of Cypriot and Turkish groups. HAGA, London

Henwood M 1991 No sense of urgency: age discrimination in health care. Critical Public Health 2: 4–14

Holgate S 1994 What's causing the worldwide rise in asthma? Medical Research Council News 63: 20–23

Illingworth P 1990 AIDS and the good society. Routledge, London

Jackson C 1993 Fax of life. Health Visitor Journal 66: 293–294

Kiernan V 1994 US backs stricter limits on dioxins. New Scientist, 17 September

National Association of Health Authorities and Trusts 1994 Asthma care: the challenge ahead. Nahat Update No. 3 January

Oakley A, Rajan L 1993 What did your baby eat yesterday? European Journal of Public Health 3: 18–27

Ogden J 1993 Asthma campaign aims to cut deaths. Health Visitor Journal 11(66): 399

O'Keefe E, Newbury J 1993 Divided London: towards a European public health approach. University of North London Press, London

O'Keefe E, Ottewill R, Wall A 1992 Community health: issues in management. Business Education Publishers, Sunderland

Parliamentary Office of Science and Technology 1994 Breathing in our cities. House of Commons, London

Rich A 1981 Compulsory heterosexuality and lesbian experience. Only Women Press, London

Rotherham Metropolitan Borough Council 1994 Community development: a way of working. Rotherham Metropolitan Borough Council, Rotherham

Rudat K, Ryan H, Speed M 1992 Today's young adults: 16–19-year-olds look at diet, alcohol, smoking, drugs and sexual behaviour. Health Education Authority, London

South West Thames Regional Health Authority Leaflet 1993 Two ways to cultivate cancer. South West Thames Regional Health Authority, London

Southall Black Sisters 1989 Against the grain. Southall Black Sisters, London

Strachan D, Anderson H, Limb E, O' Neil A, Wells N 1994 A

national survey of asthma prevalence, treatment and severity in Great Britain. Archives of Disease in Childhood 70: 174–178

Tatman M, Woodroffe C, Kelly P, Harris R 1992 Paediatric home care in Tower Hamlets: a working partnership with parents. Quality in Health Care 1(2): 98–103

Tucker R 1991 Persuading clients to attend. Practice Nursing January: 13–14

United Kingdom Central Council for Nursing, Midwifery and Health Visiting 1992 Code of professional conduct for the nurse, midwife and health visitor. UKCC, London

United Nations 1948 Universal declaration of human rights. In: Brownlie I (ed) 1981 Basic documents on human rights.
Clarendon Press, Oxford

Wallerstein N 1993 Empowerment and health: the theory and practice of community change. Community Development Journal 28: 218–227

Weare K 1992 The contribution of education to health promotion. In: Bunton R, Macdonald G (eds) Health promotion. Routledge, London

Wilkinson C, Peter T, Harvey I, Stott N 1992 Risk targetting in cervical screening: a new look at an old pattern. British Journal of General Practice 42: 435–438

World Health Organization 1993 Targets for health for all: the health policy for Europe, updated edn. WHO, Regional Office for Europe, Copenhagen

Practising health promotion

SECTION CONTENTS

6. Information and health promotion 69

7. Communication for health promotion 81

8. Groups and teams 95

9. Education for health 109

10. A life-cycle approach to health promotion 125

This section moves on to the day-to-day activity of carrying out the task of health promotion. It begins by looking at needs and sources, followed by the important topics of communication, working in groups and teams, and health education. The section ends by recommending a life-cycle approach, targetting health promotion to each of the age groups in the population.

CHAPTER CONTENTS

Introduction   69

Health promotion and resource allocation   69

Needs assessment and health promotion   70

Levels of health promotion activity   70
Client-based information   71
Describing health and disease in populations   71

Sources of health information   72
Mortality   73
Analysis of mortality data   73
Morbidity measures   75
Service utilisation data   76
Surveys of health status   76

Related information of interest to health
promotion   77
Census data   77
Population projections   79
Applying national data to local populations   79

Accessing information   80

Conclusion   80

References   80

6

Information and health promotion

Christina Victor

By the year 2000, health information systems in all Member States should actively support the formulation, implementation, monitoring and evaluation of health for all policies.

(Target 35: Health information and support, WHO 1993)

INTRODUCTION

The role and scope of health promotion, as this book illustrates, is potentially limitless. Changes in lifestyle and cardiovascular and cancer risk reduction (e.g. stopping smoking, increasing exercise), encouraging the uptake of routine screening and vaccination services, screening for early disease onset and promoting improvements in the environment such as improved housing or play space for children are just a few of the more obvious areas where health promotion has an important role to play. There are also the different levels at which such activities may be undertaken. Those concerned with environmental improvements may be working locally with a tenants' group to improve the availability of play space or at a national level by lobbying parliament and departments of state.

HEALTH PROMOTION AND RESOURCE ALLOCATION

Resources for health care if not finite are certainly limited (Ham 1993). There are clearly issues of resource allocation to be addressed at a variety of levels. The amount of money available for health care as compared with other types of government expenditure such as defence or education must be established. Once that hard decision has been made, then the allocation of funding between different geographical areas and different components of the health care system must be established. For example, funding must be allocated between a variety of different services such as primary and secondary care, between specialities (e.g. mental health or health promotion) and between client groups (older people or young adults). Within the field of health promotion then, decisions must be made about how money and staffing should be allocated between competing claims.

An essential element of the decision-making process is information. Accurate reliable up-to-date information is clearly a key requirement of the policy-making process which allocates health care resources. Failure to provide data indicating the effectiveness of health promotion interventions may result in such activities being downgraded in terms of priority for funding. There is also a need for good information about health promotion to be made available to the general population so that clients and community groups may also become advocates for health promotion. Failure to do so may mean that people do not fully appreciate the value of health promotion compared, for example, to acute hi-tech medical interventions which attract considerable press coverage.

NEEDS ASSESSMENT AND HEALTH PROMOTION

Clearly, a key task for health promotion managers is to decide where their efforts are best placed. One way of doing this is via 'needs assessment' (see St Ledger et al 1992). At its most restricted, needs assessment attempts to determine what the health care requirements or needs are within a defined population. Such exercises may be undertaken for the whole population, local communities or primary care practices. Alternatively, needs assessment may focus upon the requirements of specific client groups. The practice or caseload profiles undertaken by nurses are one example of a population-based needs assessment.

Identification of the need for chiropody amongst older people is an example of a client-group-based approach.

'Need' is a term which is frequently used in ordinary conversation. However, we are using 'need' in this context as a technical public health term. Within a public health framework it is usual to distinguish between four main types of need:

- needs determined or defined by expert or professional groups (these are termed normative needs)
- needs identified by patients, users or carers (these are termed felt needs)
- expressed needs (what users, carers or patients ask for or demand)
- needs identified by making comparisons between groups or areas, or against an established standard (these are termed comparative needs).

These four different types of need do not necessarily overlap. What professional groups identify as 'needs' does not necessarily correspond to what users identify or translate into actual demands.

Regardless of the definition of need for health promotion under consideration there is an obvious and very fundamental requirement for accurate and relevant information on which to base the needs assessment. In this chapter we consider the types of readily available population- and health-based information. Before considering the merits and drawbacks of these data sources it is first necessary to consider the different levels at which those involved in health promotion may use information.

LEVELS OF HEALTH PROMOTION ACTIVITY

As has already been indicated in this book, the

Activity 6.1

Think of health promotion examples of the four main types of need.

nurse who is involved in health promotion will be active in a variety of different spheres. In this chapter we are concerned with highlighting the need for information related to health promotion. In order to practise effective health promotion the nurse, or other health professional, will require appropriate information. Depending upon the type of work being undertaken the health pro-moter will require to collect and use different types of information. We may distinguish between three main types of information which will used by the health promoter:

- individual / client-based information
- data relating to the health status of the community, locality or practice population
- data concerned with health-related aspects of the community such as poverty, housing or environment.

Client-based information

Whatever activity the health promoter is engaged in, there will be a need to maintain records relating to the work undertaken. In many cases these records will relate to work with individual clients. In working with, for example, women who wish to give up smoking, questions will be asked by the health promoter about the motivation of clients to give up smoking, the duration of their smoking and various other related issues. In the records the advice given will be entered and the result (or outcome) achieved noted (e.g. cessation or reduction of smoking).

When dealing with particular client groups, such as people with HIV / AIDS or the parents of a disabled child, the health promoter may find that the clients are a very useful source of knowledge and advice about their condition. The health promoter should be wary of too openly wearing the label of 'expert' and should always listen to clients' opinions about their condition with an open mind.

Most, but not all, of those engaged in health promotion activity are employees of organisations such as the NHS. Regardless of their employing authority, health promoters are likely to have to provide information about their activity to their managers. For example, health visitors may be asked to make regular returns describing the number of clients seen each week, where the clients were seen (i.e. home or clinic) and the type of client seen (pre-school child, new-born or older person). They may also be asked to indicate the kind of work which they undertook with the clients seen. It is aggregation of these routine administrative records that forms much of the readily available information, both locally and nationally, about the activities of health promotion departments and other elements of the health care service. Specially commissioned studies or surveys may be based in part upon client records or case-notes. It is therefore imperative that health promoters, and other health professionals, maintain good up-to-date and accurate client records.

For example, calculating uptake of immunisation rates for a clinic or practice or the uptake of cervical cytology from clinic / staff records can be problematic if the records are not rigorously maintained. Failure of staff to exclude children or women who have moved out of the clinic or practice catchment area may result in an artificial lowering of the actual uptake rates (see Beardow et al 1989). When decisions about resource allocation are based upon inaccurate data then problems in service delivery are bound to arise.

Describing health and disease in populations

Before considering the sources of health and other relevant data available for communities it is first necessary to describe some key terms used in the presentation of such data. Health promoters will need to understand these terms when trying to access and interpret data. Two key concepts in describing health and disease in populations are incidence and prevalence.

Incidence

Incidence is the number of new cases of a specific disease occurring within a defined population during a given time period. For example, the incidence rate for dementia may be:

$$\frac{\text{Number of new cases of dementia in 1 year}}{\text{Total population aged 65+}} \times 1000$$

Although typically used to describe the number of new cases of a disease, it is easy to see that the notion of incidence is applicable to health promotion as it could also be used to describe the number of new smokers generated annually or the number of new cases of AIDS.

Prevalence

Prevalence is the number of cases of a specific disease (e.g. dementia) in a defined population at a specific point in time. The prevalence rate for dementia may be calculated as follows:

$$\frac{\text{Number of cases of dementia}}{\text{Total population aged 65+}} \times 1000$$

Incidence and prevalence rates may be used to describe aspects of lifestyle relevant to health promotion and in assessing the impact of health promotion interventions. For example, we may calculate the number of new smokers (incidence rate) as well as the number of smokers (prevalence) in particular areas or populations. We could try to describe the effectiveness of a health promotion campaign amongst school children by examining the difference in prevalence of smoking before and after the intervention.

Incidence rates are extremely useful measures for those concerned with health planning as they indicate how many new cases of a disease (or particular form of behaviour such as smoking) we might expect over a particular time period (e.g. 1 year). Changes in incidence rates show whether a particular disease or problem is increasing or decreasing in size. We may infer that decreasing incidence rates are an indication of the success of health promotion/disease prevention strategies or therapeutic interventions. For example, a decrease in the number of teenage pregnancies, suicide or HIV may all be indicative of changes in behaviour resulting from the activities of health promotion.

Defining incident and prevalent cases

Both incidence and prevalence are based upon the assumption that we may unambiguously classify the population or individuals into those with the disease/behaviour and those without. For many conditions or aspects of behaviour which are of interest to health promoters this is problematic. It is particularly problematic for chronic conditions such as dementia or physical disability where there is a continuum ranging from no impairment to total impairment. Where the line is drawn (the case-definition threshold) will greatly influence the size of the identified problem.

Activity 6.2

Think of some aspects of health promotion. For each topic, how easy is it for you to classify the people involved into cases and non-cases?

Defining what constitutes specific types of behaviour is problematic in health promotion just as in the study of many other diseases. Such problems are especially acute when attempting to define the extent of certain behaviours in our population such as dietary habits or the number of units of alcohol it is 'safe' to consume on a regular basis or how much exercise individuals should take. How should a smoker be defined? Such questions are not simply the 'academic' concern of the researcher but are important for health promoters and others who use the data. For example, if a nurse working in general practice were trying to calculate the number of sexually active teenagers in the practice then this would be highly influenced by the definition of 'sexually active'. Would this mean only those undertaking regular (however this was defined) intercourse or would the definition be expanded to include all who had ever had intercourse? Such semantic differences may greatly influence the estimated size of the local problem.

SOURCES OF HEALTH INFORMATION

Information about the health and lifestyle of the

population is available but there are limitations and flaws in most of the easily available sources. Unfortunately, for a variety of reasons, we do not have perfect information about the health of our population. Consequently we have to use 'imperfect' sources. Knowledge of the limitations in the collection, presentation and dissemination of information is an essential element in the development of intelligent health promotion planning. This section is designed to indicate the main sources of information which are available and to indicate to users the limitations of these sources, so that the data may be used and interpreted appropriately. We often have no other recourse but to use these data but it is important that we are aware of their inherent limitations.

Mortality

Information about the number and cause of deaths is available for the UK from the nineteenth century onwards. Registration of death is compulsory and a doctor is required to certify the cause of death. Data about deaths are, therefore, almost certainly a complete source of information. The information which is recorded on the death certificate includes:

- date and place of death
- name of deceased
- sex of deceased
- place of birth
- date of birth
- occupation
- usual address.

These variables define the parameters by which we may investigate mortality statistics. For example, as we can see in Chapter 12, we can look at mortality by social class but not by ethnic origin. The medical practitioner certifying the death is required to record the 'immediate' cause of death and then any underlying disease or condition which has resulted in the death. The precision with which cause of death is identified varies considerably and is generally much less accurate for older people, where multiple pathology may be involved, than for those in younger age groups. It is also likely that some causes of death

which carry a considerable social stigma, such as AIDS or suicide, are under-reported. This is important as such under-reporting may result in health promoters underestimating the size of such problems within their specific locality.

Analysis of mortality data

Death registration data are collated and analysed by the Office of Population Censuses and Surveys (OPCS). Death (or mortality) statistics are published annually and are presented in a variety of forms including the total number of deaths, geographical variations and causes of death. Table 12.1 (p. 158) is an example of the type of readily available mortality data which health promotion workers can use to establish priorities for their work and which form the general health context within which to place their work. It describes age- and sex-specific death rates for men and women in England and Wales in 1991. Routinely published mortality data are available for the major administrative areas such as counties, regions and health districts/FHSA areas. However, data are not always easily accessible for less formally defined geographical areas such as practice populations or clinic areas.

Mortality rates

When interpreting mortality data there are a number of factors to be taken into consideration. Simply presenting the number of deaths within a given area is a highly simplistic form of analysis—it is usual to calculate mortality rates which express the number of deaths as a proportion of the population (see Box 6.1).

The crude death rate is a very blunt instrument when describing the health status of a population because it is highly dependent upon the age structure of the population. As we will see in Chapter 12, the majority of deaths in a population are amongst those aged 65+. Therefore, when comparing crude death rates between populations we must be certain to confirm that any observed differences do not simply reflect variations in age structure.

Given this important limitation it is usual to

Box 6.1   Calculation of mortality rates

A. Crude death rate =

$$\frac{\text{Total deaths in population (numerator)}}{\text{Total population (denominator)}} \times 1000$$

B. Age-specific death rate =

$$\frac{\text{Deaths in women aged 65–74}}{\text{Total women aged 65–74}} \times 10\,000$$

C. Age- and cause-specific death rate =

$$\frac{\begin{array}{c}\text{Deaths from breast cancer for women}\\ \text{aged 65–74}\end{array}}{\text{Total women aged 65–74}} \times 100\,000$$

D. Perinatal mortality rate =

$$\frac{\text{Stillbirths and deaths within 7 days of birth}}{\text{Total live and still births}} \times 1000$$

E. Infant mortality rate =

$$\frac{\begin{array}{c}\text{Deaths of live-born children within}\\ \text{12 months of birth}\end{array}}{\text{Total live births}} \times 1000$$

---

calculate more specific indicators. *Age-specific death rates* describe the chances of dying in specific narrow age groups. If the age bands are sufficiently narrow, e.g. 5 or 10 years, age-specific rates may be compared between populations with little risk of the biases inherent in the crude death rate. The age-specific death rate for women aged 65–74 years is defined in Box 6.1; the formula might be used, for example, to calculate the death rate per 10 000 women in that age group in England in 1992.

Age- and cause-specific death rates are a simple extension of the above. The numerator now refers to deaths from a specific cause or group of causes (e.g. breast cancer) among the stated age group (e.g. women aged 65–74); the denominator is unchanged. The method of calculating the age-specific death rate from breast cancer among women aged 65–74 years in a defined population (e.g. of England) in a given year (e.g. 1992) is given in Box 6.1.

Special mortality rates are defined for infants. The two most commonly used are the *perinatal mortality rate* and the *infant mortality rate* (see Box 6.1).

Standardising mortality rates

As noted earlier, crude mortality rates are of only limited use when comparing the mortality experience of different populations. Consequently we often calculate the standardised mortality ratio (SMR). The SMR makes a comparison between mortality (from a specific disease or all causes) in a designated group (e.g. a social class) and a standard (or reference) population (usually England and Wales).

The SMR involves calculating the number of deaths we would expect in, for example, Kensington, Chelsea and Westminster (KCW) Health District if national mortality rates applied. The observed number of deaths is then divided by the expected number to calculate the SMR.

An SMR of less than 100 indicates a mortality experience better than the reference population whilst an SMR of 100+ indicates a worse mortality experience than expected. For example, in 1993 KCW in inner London had an overall SMR of 93. At first glance this would seem to suggest that the district had 'better' health than the nation as a whole and there were no particular local health problems. However, more detailed analysis reveals a more complex problem. First, the SMR for the 42 wards within KCW ranges from 43 to 153. Clearly even within an apparently unproblematic district there are pockets of local health problems.

Identification of geographical inequalities in health status remains an important task for those interested in health promotion. Disaggregation of the overall KCW SMR into age/sex- and cause-specific components highlights further important local issues. The age- and sex-specific SMRs highlight the high SMR of 115 for girls aged 1–14 and men aged 15–64 (SMR of 127). The cause-specific SMRs highlight lung cancer for women (SMR of 143) and suicide (SMR of 165). Such detailed mortality data provide health promotion workers with evidence of which geographical areas, client groups or health problems can be identified as specific local problems, thus enabling them to develop an appropriate strategy.

Standardised rates may be calculated for health indicators other than mortality. In a study of the health status of homeless people living in bed and breakfast accommodation, a standardised disability index was computed to enable comparisons to be made between populations of widely differing age compositions (Victor 1992). In this piece of research, 33% of the population of North West Thames Regional Health Authority were aged 16–34 compared with 72% of the homeless group. The overall prevalence of long-standing illness was 48% in North West Thames and 43% in the homeless group. When the data were converted into a standardised ratio, setting North West Thames as 100, then the homeless group was 153. This example highlights the importance of making sure that the two groups or areas being compared are similar in terms of social profile. Failure to do so may lead to erroneous conclusions being drawn and perhaps inadequate service provision being made.

Activity 6.3

You are developing a health promotion service for people with rheumatoid arthritis (or any other chronic disease) in your area. Why would mortality data be a poor indication of the number of people with this condition in your district? In what other ways might health promoters find out about the extent of the condition in their locality?

Mortality as a proxy for morbidity

We routinely use mortality statistics as a proxy, or indirect measure, for morbidity (or the amount of ill health within the population). By doing this we assume that the patterns of death observed within a population mirror those for morbidity. However, only in very limited circumstances are mortality statistics a valid proxy for morbidity statistics.

For example, death rates are:

- excellent proxies for morbidity from lung cancer and pancreatic cancer
- reasonable proxies for morbidity from coronary heart disease and breast cancer
- poor proxies for morbidity from asthma and chronic bronchitis
- hopeless proxies for morbidity from the

common cold, whooping cough, rheumatoid arthritis, multiple sclerosis and hernias.

The paucity of true morbidity measures has led many health service planners and those responsible for resource allocation to use mortality statistics because of their ready availability. In so far as justification is produced, this is on the lines that when mortality is high then so, generally, is morbidity. Data from KCW indicate that high SMR wards have very high rates of physical and mental health problems (Victor & Lamping 1994). However, mortality statistics are of very limited use in attempting to evaluate the need for and effectiveness of health promotion. For example, implementation of a routine screening system may take some time to have an impact on the number of deaths from a specific disease. Introducing screening systems, if suitable tests were available, for testicular or prostate cancer would not start to reduce mortality from the disease for some time. Observing the effects of health promotion strategies may require extremely long-term follow-up and research.

Morbidity measures

Morbidity statistics are concerned with the amount and types of illness that occur in the community. Most routinely collected morbidity data suffer from serious shortcomings. Much data originates in the administrative data collected by the NHS and is very largely concerned with the activity of various services rather than with monitoring their effectiveness or the results of their activities.

The main routinely available morbidity statistics are as follows:

- statutory notifications of infectious diseases
- notification of episodes of sexually transmitted diseases (STD)
- notification of 'prescribed' and other industrial disease and accidents
- notification of congenital malformations
- registration of handicapped persons
- cancer registration.

As this list indicates, these data are very limited

and are highly dependent upon accurate identification and notification by medical practitioners. Users also need to read very carefully the headings and categories used in these routinely available data. Some of the main points which need to be noted are as follows. First, there is underreporting by medical practitioners. This varies between these different conditions and specific areas of the country and may vary over time as people become more (or less) aware of the implications of specific conditions. Secondly, not all these data relate to individuals—some (like the STD notifications) relate to clinic attendances *not* individuals. Consequently their usefulness in determining locally based health promotion needs are strictly limited.

In England and Wales the number of notified cases of food poisoning has increased markedly over recent years. We could interpret this as a 'real' increase in the prevalence of the disease. Alternatively, it may reflect increased notification rates by GPs either because of their, or their patients', increased awareness of the condition. Consequently, interpreting a change in the number of notified cases of a condition is problematic. Furthermore, not all cases of a disease necessarily end up being included in the statistics. Cancer registrations do not always include every known case of a particular type of cancer.

Service utilisation data

Another, although limited, source of health information is concerned with the utilisation of health services. Data are available about contacts with services, first admissions to mental hospitals and prescriptions. However, these are only very crude and very indirect measures of health status and are much too general to be of much use to those interested in health promotion. Similarly,

data about the number and types of health service staff working within specific geographical areas are of little general use for health promotion.

However, data about the number of particular procedures undertaken such as abortions may provide an indirect indicator which may be of use when developing a health promotion agenda. We might speculate that an area with a very high rate of abortions might suggest a need for more appropriate and accessible health promotion advice. A high number of abortions to young women may indicate deficiencies in the availability of services for young people. However, there are readily apparent limits to the uses to which the interpretation of these data may be put.

Surveys of health status

Limited data about the overall health of the national population are available from several sources. However, the scope of these data are limited. We may distinguish between data collected regularly and those of a one-off nature.

The prevalence of chronic disability and physical ill health within the population is a major issue for health promotion, as promoting quality of life is probably a key concern. Data about the prevalence of disability is available from several sources. The 1991 census included a question about the number of individuals within households with 'long term limiting illness'. This is a very broad indicator of the prevalence of chronic health problems within the population. At both local and national level it correlates very well with data about mortality. As these data are available for small areas, this measure may be a good way of identifying particular localities or districts which are experiencing health problems and, indirectly, are the areas most 'in need' of health promotion interventions. However, as with mortality data, comparisons which are made between areas need to take into account their different age profiles.

The General Household Survey (GHS), an annual social survey undertaken by OPCS, also collects data about the prevalence of both acute and chronic health problems, although, because of sampling problems, data are not available for areas smaller than health or statistical regions. However, it is possible to apply these data to local populations and estimate the pattern of ill health within clinic or practice populations. A specially commissioned government survey also reviewed the prevalence of disability amongst adults and children in both the community and institutional settings. However, such one-off surveys do tend to become dated. Surveys which examine a topic in detail can be of great local use as they provide information to estimate the number of people within a population who might experience particular conditions such as stroke or arthritis.

It is instructive to realise that even data about some of the key issues of concern to health promotion are only covered by government surveys in an ad hoc fashion. Of more use to those interested in health promotion are the data collected by the GHS about smoking habits, alcohol consumption and exercise. Unfortunately these data are not published for geographical areas smaller than regions. Also, the GHS only includes within its sample those adults resident in the community. Excluded from the study are those resident in institutions (e.g. nursing and residential homes, prisons, etc.). This may (or may not) limit the usefulness of the data it provides to the health promoter.

The disability survey, GHS and the 1991 census all collected information about the prevalence of chronic health problems but produced differing answers. This results from the differing questions and samples used by these surveys and highlights the importance of researchers carefully examining the origin of survey data before they use them in needs assessment (or indeed other) types of exercises.

One response to the limitations inherent in many routinely available health data has been the development of local (either DHA- or RHA-based) health surveys. Such surveys can be tailored to the local community and can focus much more on health promotion issues than can routine surveys. For example, such surveys may identify how many smokers wish to give up, or look at why women do not attend for cervical screening. Clearly some aspects of lifestyle are fairly straightforward to measure (e.g. smoking)

Activity 6.5

You have become involved in setting up specialist services for adults with asthma (or children with HIV/AIDS). What sort of data would you look for in order to establish the likely demand for this service? What data sources would you consult? Who might you want to involve in the project?

---

whilst other equally important areas are more problematic (e.g. diet). Such surveys are useful but they are costly and the way the data will be used needs to be carefully considered before they are undertaken. Naturally the rules of good survey design are of paramount importance and such projects are not to be undertaken lightly and certainly not without an action plan of how they are going to be used. However, such surveys can very usefully highlight particular local problems and be used as effective arguments for the targeting of local health promotion interventions.

RELATED INFORMATION OF INTEREST TO HEALTH PROMOTION

The most basic pieces of information for any form of debate about the need for health promotion relate to the size and characteristics of the population. Data about the overall size of the population and the size of particular subgroups (e.g. pre-school-age children) are essential for calculating incidence and prevalence rates (see pp. 71–72) and applying them to the local situation.

Census data

Several important features of the population may influence the requirements for health promotion. A population which included a large number of children might require inputs about vaccination and child development. A large concentration of older people might merit more attention being

---

Activity 6.6

What characteristics of the population may influence the health promotion requirements of a specific population (e.g. a primary care practice)?

paid to issues of hypothermia and falls. Populations with large numbers of ethnic minority community members may require a different focus. The clear point is that fairly simple data about the key characteristics of the population can inform the development of health promotion strategy and initiatives which are appropriate to that population.

Basic data about the size and characteristics of the population are available from the census which is undertaken every 10 years. In England and Wales the first complete census was undertaken in 1801. Since then there has been a full census every 10 years, with the exception of 1941. The census is conducted by the Office of Population Censuses and Surveys (OPCS).

What data are collected in the census?

The precise information that is collected varies from census to census but it usually includes age, sex, marital status, place of birth, occupation, number of children, usual place of residence and length of present residence. The 1991 census included details of ethnic origin and an indicator of chronic health problems. In addition the head of the household has to provide details of the residence including its type, tenure, accommodation and facilities. Some information which would obviously be useful in determining the need for health promotion, such as wealth or the number of homeless people in an area, is not collected. Direct measures of income or 'social position' are not explicitly collected either. However, data about car ownership, an indirect measure of social group, is collected. Information about the number of adults in employment, and those unemployed, is collected as are details about the types of jobs held by the employed and retired. It is these data which form the basis of the social class classification data provided by the census (see Ch. 12). Data about housing status are available but they are of limited scope. No routine data are readily available about the incidence and prevalence of poverty.

The availability of census data

Census information is provided in a variety of

Activity 6.7

What are the limitations imposed by the fact that a census is undertaken every 10 years?

---

different formats. Published tables provide information about specific topics (e.g. pensioners, ethnic minorities) or about specific geographical areas (e.g. Great Britain, regions or inner London). These are available in most reference libraries and can form the basis of useful population profiles. However, only limited amounts of the wide spectrum of potential data are routinely published. Raw data on computer disks for analysis are also provided which enable local workers to build up more detailed profiles of their local areas. Typically, public health departments provide such detailed analyses in their public health reports. The report produced in 1994 by KCW is typical of this activity and provides profiles of the localities into which the agency is divided and the constituent wards.

Because the census only takes place every decade, information which is routinely used by those undertaking needs assessment work can become out-of-date. Whilst there are estimates of the way the size and age–sex composition of the population is changing between censuses (see below) there are no ways of routinely reviewing the accuracy of data about the social characteristics of the population. For example, over a 10-year period there may be important changes in the marital or ethnic status of the population as a result of migration or social change. It is largely impossible to estimate the extent of such changes, although some of these unrecorded changes would be very important for the provision of health promotion activities if information were available. For example, a large influx of homeless people would not be obvious from routine data but would be of crucial importance in determining the needs of a local population for health promotion.

Estimates of population between censuses

The size and demographic characteristics of the

population in non-census years is estimated by deducting deaths and emigrants from numbers recorded in the census and adding births and immigrants. At the same time the age distribution of the people remaining is adjusted. These are known as *inter-censal estimates*. Unfortunately errors occur which are compounded by the passage of time. The main sources of error in the inter-censal estimates arise through inadequate recording of immigration and emigration both in numbers and in respect of age and sex. Furthermore, there is no method of recording the amount of internal migration (changes of residence within the country). Thus the greater the time that has elapsed since a census, the less the precision of the estimate, especially estimates relating to small areas within the country. Revised estimates of population are not usually provided for small areas such as electoral wards. Furthermore, such estimates do not identify changes in the size and characteristics of minority communities. A change in the nature of the ethnic population of a district would be of considerable importance. For example, the replacement of a community of those from the Caribbean by refugees from Somalia would radically alter the health promotion needs of the population. The fact that such changes are not part of routine population estimates creates problems for the health promoter interested in putting together a profile of, for example, the population served by a specific clinic.

Population projections

For planning purposes it is often essential to have some idea of the likely size and composition of the population in years to come. The essential difference between population estimates and population projections is that an *estimate* is based on knowledge of the births, deaths and migration that have happened, and a *projection* is based upon what is thought likely to happen. Therefore assumptions are made about trends in mortality, birth rates and migration. These projections are likely to be less reliable the further forward they are made because the assumption of birth and death rates remaining unchanged is likely to be

increasingly inaccurate. Like population estimates, population projections are not made for small areas such as wards because of statistical unreliability. The combined effect of such factors is that health professionals working in small localities or areas may often be basing their activities on inaccurate population data. This limitation should be noted when presenting population profiles based upon out-of-date census data.

Applying national data to local populations

As we have seen, there are a variety of readily available health indicators and, in combination with census data, we may use these to build up a profile of the health of local populations and the potential for local health promotion initiatives. We may apply national data to local populations in order to describe the extent of particular problems. For example, Table 6.1 illustrates how national data about the prevalence of dementia have been used to estimate the number of people with this disease in KCW, an inner London DHA. Using a similar methodology, it would be possible to estimate the number of heavy drinkers or smokers in a local population or client group. Application of national data about specific aspects of health and disease can certainly bring home the size of the problem to local health promoters and others interested in the health of the population.

Table 6.1 Dementia: estimated number of people aged over 60 years suffering from dementia in Kensington, Chelsea and Westminster Commissioning Agency

Age group	Prevalence (%)	Total number suffering from dementia
60–64	0.5	73
65–69	1.1	143
70–74	3.9	429
75–79	6.7	643
80–84	13.5	900
85–89	22.8	788
90+	34.1	440
60–90+		3416

ACCESSING INFORMATION

Although our information base about the health of the population is far from complete, this chapter has indicated that there are a variety of data sources available which may be of use to the health promoter. As well as knowing what is available it is important to know where to get the information and how best to use the available data. There are a variety of different sources of access to the data including: public health departments and annual reports, health authority purchasing plans, local authority community care plans, local authority planning departments, local libraries (for copies of national reports) and voluntary agencies.

This vast, and probably incomplete, array of places which may be of use to the health promoter seeking information indicates that it is probably best to work as part of a multidisciplinary team when trying to use and interpret these data. It is not necessary for everyone to be an expert in the retrieval and interpretation of the data. Rather it is important to know colleagues who do understand the sources and to be able to understand their explanations (and be sympathetic when they cannot provide every piece of information you want!).

CONCLUSION

Health promotion is an activity of considerable importance at both local and national level. The recent health strategy, 'The Health of the Nation' (DoH 1992), has served to highlight how little readily available data there are about the health and health habits of our population. The establishment of specific targets within this strategy will probably serve as an impetus to improve the range and quality of the available data. However, for all but a few topics we continue to have to adapt existing data to fit the purposes for which we wish to use them. Producing meaningful local health profiles will continue to be a frustrating experience for all concerned! It is not necessary for every person interested in health promotion to be an 'information expert'. Rather it is important for health promotion workers to know where to get data and help with their interpretation.

REFERENCES

Beardow R, Oerton J, Victor C R 1989 Evaluation of cervical cytology screening programme in an inner city health district. Bristish Medical Journal 299: 98–100
Department of Health 1992 The health of the nation: a strategy for health in England. Cm 1986. HMSO, London
Ham C 1993 Health policy in Britain, 3rd edn. Macmillan, Basingstoke
St Ledger S, Schneider H, Walsworth-Bell J P 1992 Assessing health needs using the life cycle framework. Open University Press, Milton Keynes

Victor C R 1992 Health status of the temporarily homeless population and residents of North West Thames Regions. British Medical Journal 305: 387–391
Victor C R, Lamping D 1994 Is mortality a good proxy for morbidity. Paper presented at the Faculty of Public Health Medicine Summer Conference
World Health Organization 1993 Health for all targets: the health policy for Europe, updated edn. WHO, Regional Office for Europe, Copenhagen

CHAPTER CONTENTS

What is communication? 81

Counselling and communication 83
  Therapeutic communication 83

Language and listening 84
  Linguistic minorities 84
  Active listening 84
  Questions: their variations and effects 86
  Some special areas of communicating 86

Written communication 87
  Records and record-keeping 87
  Report writing 88

Nonverbal aspects of communication 88
  Vocal expressions 89
  The use of space 89
  Touch 90
  Body orientation 90
  Movement and posture 90
  Gestures 91
  Facial expression 91
  Eye contact 91

Conclusion 92

References 92

Further reading 92

7

Communication for health promotion

Diana Forster

By the year 2000, education and training of health and other personnel in all Member States should actively contribute to the achievement of health for all.

(Target 36: Developing human resources for health, WHO 1993)

WHAT IS COMMUNICATION?

Communication forms the basis of all human interaction. It underpins every attempt made to promote the health and well-being of other people, thus helping to achieve the World Health Organization's Target 36 (WHO 1993) which heads this chapter. Its success depends upon the other person or group of people understanding and making sense of the message intended. This chapter aims to relate communication issues to the promotion of health in a society with a rich variety of languages, religions, customs and cultures set in the wider, world environment.

How can health workers ensure that they communicate effectively with the various people and communities they work with? Understanding some of the processes and skills involved will help communication to be more effective. This in turn will give clients a greater sense of partnership and a feeling that they are sharing in making decisions about their health and its promotion.

Elements of communication

Five elements are needed for successful communication to take place:

- a communicator
- a message
- a receiver
- complete understanding by that receiver
- feedback to the communicator.

Skills

Skills need to be practised; it is not enough merely to read about them. For examples of workbooks see Burnard (1992) and Kelcher (1992), and readers are encouraged to find out what courses on communication might be available and appropriate for them. The ability to work with and on behalf of other people depends to a large extent on our communication skills, so these are worth developing. Increasing our knowledge and insight into ourselves, and reflecting upon the sort of people we are and how this relates to our work are vital aspects of developing our relationships with others.

Everyday conversations give many opportunities for practising and learning skills and some opportunities for observing them. It is important to monitor improvements, and giving feedback to oneself is an effective way of doing this (see Box 7.1).

Box 7.1   Principles of giving feedback to yourself (Nicolson & Bayne 1990)

- Comment on behaviour, and try to be fairly specific, e.g. 'I seemed very relaxed—I think it was the way I sat and my use of silence.'
- Include positive comments.
- Criticise behaviour that could be changed and try to say what you might do differently: one or two things at a time only.
- Be brief: three or four comments at the most.

Self-knowledge and self-evaluation are essential skills in improving competencies relating to communication (Burnard 1992).

In health promotion, communication skills may be used:

- to accomplish specific and general goals with patients, clients and the wider, world-wide community
- in assessing and understanding patients, clients, their families and relatives
- in planning, carrying out and evaluating health promotion activities personally, locally and nationally.

Communication skills may be used to help people as shown in Figure 7.1.

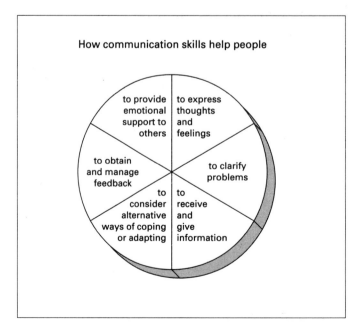

Figure 7.1   How communication skills may help people.

COUNSELLING AND COMMUNICATION

Counselling has been defined in many ways, from encompassing specialist psychological help on the one hand, to a set of qualities and skills for communicating effectively on the other.

Although nurse–client communication may demonstrate skills associated with counselling and the organisation of talk and body movement, it may not always be used for the benefit of the client or patient. Health carers may use their skills to control interactions, for example by standing up and moving away when, from the other's point of view, a discussion still needs to continue. Communication for health promotion should be therapeutic, i.e. used to enhance health.

Therapeutic communication

Therapeutic communication is an important aspect of the helping, counselling relationship. It is suggested that helpers need to communicate three basic qualities if a helping relationship is to be successful (Rogers 1983). These are:

- empathy
- warmth
- genuineness.

Empathy

Empathy is the ability to understand another person's experience, almost owning it. It involves being sensitive to another individual's changing feelings and being in touch with that person. In fact, a health worker cannot actually experience the same physical pain, emotional distress or uncertainty and fear which a client may face, but he or she can attempt to grasp the meaning of those feelings, perceiving the situation as accurately as possible from the client's language and terms, and using the same tone of voice—sad if the client is sad, or fearful if the client is fearful. (Bradley & Edinberg 1990).

Sometimes hospital nurses may distance themselves emotionally from patients so that they can cope with their own feelings of anxiety, which are generated by working constantly with the sick and dying. This demonstrates the opposite of empathy. The ability to establish and communicate feelings of empathy is an important step along the way towards understanding the needs of patients so that their health and well-being may be promoted and put before the feelings of carers. The carers themselves of course will need their own support group or someone to empathise with them in coping with their needs.

The highest expression of empathy is accepting others and being non-judgemental. Rogers (1980) tells the story of a psychologist who was researching people's visual and perceptual history, including difficulties with seeing and reading. He simply listened to the subjects with interest and so gathered his data. A number of subjects came back to thank him for his help. This surprised him, as in his opinion he had given them no help at all. He thus recognised that interested, non-evaluative listening has much therapeutic value.

Sympathy is not the same as empathy; indeed a sympathetic carer may be overwhelmed with feeling sorry for the patient and become ineffective and upset as a result.

Because of the uniqueness of each individual's feelings and reactions, clients may doubt a health professional's ability to really understand their deep feelings. For instance, an elderly bereaved man may believe that a young female nurse cannot possibly understand what it means for him to have suffered the death of his wife. But the young professional can ask him to help her understand his feelings, and then listen carefully to his response. This shows her willingness to be involved and to be committed to care about, accept, hear and understand as much as possible about the client's experience (Faulkner 1992).

Warmth

The second feature of helping identified by Rogers (1983) is 'unconditional positive regard', which is also described as acceptance or warmth. Clients need to know that the helper accepts them for what they are, whatever feelings there may be about what clients have or have not done. The helper accepts the clients' rights to decide their own lives for themselves, without judging them in any way.

Genuineness

The third feature is genuineness, or authenticity. This is characterised by a directness and openness in the helpers' communication, saying what they really mean and showing honest feelings. This approach in turn encourages clients to be open and honest also, helping them to express their thoughts, concerns, hopes and fears.

LANGUAGE AND LISTENING

Successful verbal communication depends upon the listener or reader of the message understanding its meaning. In order to promote health there needs to be an effective channel of communication—a common channel or shared language.

Linguistic minorities

The language of the majority of the United Kingdom population is English—all NHS staff speak it and for most of them it is their only language. Most clients' leaflets and letters are written in English, and most directions, signs and posters are in English. Yet many people from linguistic minority communities have only a limited command of English, perhaps because their own community satisfies all their communication needs, or they have had no opportunity to become bilingual. Careful use of communication skills can help health care workers to liaise closely with trained bilingual co-workers, appropriate interpreters and advocates in promoting the health of non-English-speaking clients. It is important that sentences are kept short and simple when working with an interpreter; for example 'What did the other doctor say?' is much easier to translate than 'I'm wondering about what the other doctor told you and whether he said anything congruent or very similar to our findings?' The health care worker should also pause frequently so that the interpreter only has one or two ideas to translate at a time (Nunnally & Moy 1989). The use of a check list relating to sensitive areas such as diet, hygiene practices, religion, death and bereavement can guide nurses in effective information gathering and health

care teaching. Communication may be considered as an activity of living which needs to be explored in relation to linguistic minorities. This approach should form the basis of a partnership between client and carer; patients and clients who can communicate effectively are more likely to express their own preferred health care goals.

The Stepney Nursing Development Unit, in London, employs a Bengali linkworker who, together with a health worker, runs a child health clinic in a Bengali women's group. Gooch (1993) explains that this was set up to meet the needs of women and their children who live in the ward which has the highest deprivation indices and is furthest from GP and trust health care premises. Communication skills are vital for health promotion in circumstances like these.

Active listening

Listening to someone effectively involves much more than just hearing. It is an active process in which the whole mind is concentrated on attending to what is being said and communicated. It is the basis of all effective communication one-to-one and requires hard work on the part of the listener. It is difficult not to talk or think about what to say next, not to worry about one's own feelings or what is happening in the background or somewhere else, but just to concentrate.

Activity 7.1

Ask yourself:
- Do I listen to what people say, instead of thinking of my responses while others talk?
- Do I ask clarifying questions when I do not understand?
- Do I paraphrase what people say to me to make sure I get the full impact?
- Do I hear beyond the words and recognise other people's feelings or states of mind?

Listening—nonverbal skills

Certain counselling skills which help to convey a caring relationship include 'SOLER', an acronym coined by Egan (1990). The letters stand for:

- **S**quare—sitting squarely in relation to the client, not turning away
- **O**pen—maintaining an open posture without crossing arms or legs
- **L**ean—leaning slightly towards the client rather than away
- **E**ye contact—maintaining regular eye contact
- **R**elax—sitting calmly and still.

Active listening, essential to discovering the client's needs and values, includes letting the speaker know he has been heard, which the SOLER approach encourages. Listening with attention and commitment conveys respect for the client. It also emphasises a willingness to establish a shared approach to promoting the client's health.

Listening to the patient is a key factor in assessment and diagnosis, yet the medical practitioner's failure to listen is one of the most common complaints that patients make.

Encouraging someone to talk

Exploring ideas and feelings by talking about them can be facilitated by the listener smiling or nodding when appropriate, leaning forward, making short verbal interventions—'mm', 'aha' or 'I see'—and generally showing attentiveness.

Individuals who know that they are dying, or who are experiencing serious illness such as HIV-related symptoms, may find it valuable to talk about their thoughts and feelings concerning death. However, listeners need to take their lead from the person who is experiencing the illness, and not force a discussion about death on someone who is dying (Anderson & Wilkie 1992).

While helping a patient to examine his feelings the listener should encourage a balance between the expression and exploration of feelings on the one hand, and a downward spiral towards depression on the other. If this balance is not maintained the patient may be left with feelings which are difficult to handle. He needs to be sensitively rescued from the depressed mood after being given time to express all he wishes to, by gently moving on to discuss other aspects of his care for example, without diminishing the importance of his concerns (Faulkner 1992).

Silence

The capacity to be comfortable with silence is an important listening skill. Clients may need time to think about their responses, organise their thoughts and decide how to put their worries, hopes, feelings and concerns into words. Shared silence can be a powerful component of communication; it can be tempting to rush in and speak when all that is really required is to be with the other person, concentrating on him and providing silent empathy.

Reflecting

Reflecting back to a client what has just been said gives a clear indication that the message, including feelings such as anger or sadness, has been heard and understood. A phrase, idea or significant word may be picked out and repeated. For instance, if a client says 'It's the children I'm bothered about', the listener responds 'children …?'.

Clarifying

This term is used to describe another ploy which helps make clear to the client what he is trying to put into words, and it allows the listener to check that the message has been correctly understood. For example: 'Are you trying to tell me that you're afraid your father is not going to get better? Is that what you feel?'

Paraphrasing

Paraphrasing is similar to reflection except that its emphasis is on capturing the meaning of the communication and putting it into the listener's own words. This process of rewording enables the client to correct the rephrasing if necessary, and to be reassured that the listener really does understand the message communicated. Bradley & Edinberg (1990) include the following example of paraphrasing:

'I don't believe all this garbage about smoking. I've smoked a pack a day for 35 years with no problems.'

Response: 'You're not convinced about the dangers of smoking because they haven't affected you.'

An unacceptable response to this statement might be: 'You won't believe that smoking is dangerous until you have a heart attack!'

Summarising

Summarising is the skill of outlining the main points said and implied in a discussion up to that point. It can help focus thoughts and feelings, and should present the relevant facts, perhaps providing the opportunity to reflect further on certain issues or to move forward to new ones.

Example: 'Well, we have discussed the stages of gradually weaning James on to family meals; now shall we talk about the amount of milk he will still need?'

Questions: their variations and effects

Health professional–client interaction generally involves a considerable amount of questioning, typically on the part of the health professional. There are several ways in which a practitioner can improve the quality of questions asked:

- Questions should be phrased simply, without medical jargon.
- Questions should be short—that is, phrased concisely.
- Only one question should be asked at a time.
- Questions should not be phrased in an accusing manner—such as: 'Why didn't you attend the breast screening clinic?'
- Questions should avoid suggesting anything that influences the client's answer. Such a leading question might be: 'You have cut down on the amount you drink, haven't you? (adapted from DiMatteo 1991).

Open-ended questions

These are questions which do not have one correct answer or a one-word answer. They invite clients to describe their feelings, concerns and issues to be discussed in their own words. They encourage the client to talk, and answers may contain unexpected but relevant, useful information as well the expression of ideas and opinions.

Example: 'How have you been feeling since we last talked?'

Closed questions

These limit the other person's options for responding and usually produce a one-word, factual answer such as 'yes' or 'no'. They are useful in gathering information and clarifying particular issues. However, closed questions fail to help clients explore their own thoughts and ideas, and they place the main responsibility for the interaction on the questioner.

Example: 'How many cigarettes do you smoke a day?'

Some special areas of communicating

Hearing impairment

Loss of hearing can cause problems in communication with others, together with frustration, anxiety and feelings of isolation.

In their work with deaf clients, Nunnally & Moy (1989) noted that similar considerations apply as in work with non-English-speaking clients. Interpreters should be fluent in signing as well as knowledgeable about the daily life experiences and typical issues faced by deaf people. Because of educational difficulties, many deaf people, though intelligent, have poor reading and writing skills. Devlin (1992) reports the findings of a research midwifery team. These emphasised the importance of midwives finding out the deaf mother's own method of communication and understanding its uses and limitations. The main methods are:

- writing pad
- hearing aids
- lip-reading
- finger spelling
- sign language
- using an interpreter.

The research team, led by an award-winning

midwife, developed and sold packs containing information on:

- anatomy and physiology of the ear
- hearing loss
- communication methods
- deaf awareness
- care before, during and after birth
- parentcraft teaching
- evaluating care
- genetic counselling
- identification and screening for hearing loss in the newborn
- a list of further reading.

Profits from the sale of the information packs was partly used to provide equipment in hospital for deaf mothers. A text telephone—'minicom'—was bought for the delivery suite. This device enables deaf parents to telephone the unit by typing a message, instead of speaking, and reading the reply on their own minicom screen instead of listening.

Language and learning difficulties

Morton (1993) discusses the importance of the carer's use of language in her behaviour support team which provides a specialist service to people with learning difficulties and severe challenging behaviour. In helping clients to make decisions and personal choices, the carer's language should match the client's level of linguistic ability. Long sentences carrying complex messages can impede rather than enable such a client's decision-making.

Jargon

Barriers to communication may exist even when people speak the same language. Health care workers sometimes have difficulty explaining things in plain, jargon-free words that clients can understand.

All professional groups develop their own language. Because medical terms are familiar to health care workers it is easy for them to assume that other people also understand them. DiMatteo (1991) provides examples of misunderstandings in health care settings (see Box 7.2).

Box 7.2 Jargon: examples of attempts by patients to understand 'Medspeak', the language of the medical profession (DiMatteo 1991)

One patient said she was taking 'peanut butter balls' (phenobarbitol) for a seizure disorder. Another said his child had 'sick-as-hell anaemia' (sickle cell anaemia). These attempts to make sense of what they have been told show how patients make guesses rather than asking questions to clarify what has been communicated—or mis-communicated. Another patient said she had been referred to a 'groinocologist' instead of a gynaecologist, and a man with deep-vein thrombosis reported that he had 'internal flea-bites'.

Communicating with children

Explanations, requests and general conversations with children need to be carried out in simple, straightforward language, appropriate to their level of understanding. Where possible, the child should be included in any communication between parents and health carers (see Ch. 10).

WRITTEN COMMUNICATION
Records and record-keeping

The UKCC's 1993 summary of the principles underpinning records and record-keeping includes:

- 'the record is directed primarily to serving the interests of the patient or client to whom it relates and enabling the provision of care, the prevention of disease and the promotion of health' (Section 41. 1)
- 'the record is clear and unambiguous' (Section 41. 4)
- 'the record provides a safe and effective means of communication between members of the health care team and supports continuity of care' (Section 41. 6).

The UKCC guidelines emphasise that effective record-keeping by nurses, midwives and health visitors is a means of communicating with others and describing what has been observed or done. Properly made and maintained records will aid the involvement of patients or clients in their own care, thus helping to promote their health.

Patient- or client-held records

The UKCC is in favour of patients and clients being given custody of their own health care records when this is appropriate. This empowers clients, and can enhance open, honest and trusting communication between client and professional.

Patient or client access to records

Since November 1991, patients and clients have had the right of access to manual records about themselves. This has brought such records into line with computer-held records which have been required to be accessible since 1984 (with exceptions if mental or physical health might be endangered or if a third party might be identified). All practitioners who create records or make entries in them need therefore to give careful consideration to their use of clear, unambiguous language, 'and recognise the positive advantages of greater trust and confidence of patients and clients in the professions that can result from this development' (UKCC 1993).

Report writing

Before writing a report there are two questions to ask:

Box 7.3   Report writing (Kelcher 1992)

- The beginning should provide an introduction and include background information.
- The middle should give the main points and describe findings.
- The conclusion should provide a summary, review key points and make recommendations.

Check list

Have I:
—used headings to help people understand what I am writing?
—used facts and figures and kept to the point?
—said what I wanted to say?
—proofread the final draft?
—used short words rather than long, e.g. 'use' rather than 'utilise'?
—kept sentences short?

- why am I writing this report—what do I want to happen as a result?
- who am I writing it for?

Reports should have a clear beginning, a middle and a conclusion (see Box 7.3).

NONVERBAL ASPECTS OF COMMUNICATION

Language alone is not enough to enable us to communicate fully with others, we also need to use and understand body language, or nonverbal communication. Nonverbal communication adds weight to the words we speak, or conveys messages without the addition of words. It is concerned with:

- vocal expressions—aspects of speech other than words, such as loudness and pitch
- the way we use space, including touch and body orientation
- movements, gestures and expressions.

Nonverbal communication serves a number of functions, including:

- Giving and receiving feedback. For example, knowing what the results of our communication are can be assessed partly by cues such as a puzzled expression or a nod of the head.
- Communicating emotions and attitudes. Feelings are conveyed by facial expressions and body language, often more than by what is said.
- Synchronising conversation. The flow of conversation is maintained by one person 'catching the other's eye', glancing away, providing feedback by head nods and indicating a wish to speak.
- Supplementing speech. Speakers may stress

Activity 7.2

Watch a variety of television programmes. Observe some of the actors and speakers (sometimes with the sound turned down), and note aspects of their body language. Which nonverbal communication was helpful in conveying the message intended? (Kelcher 1992)

---

certain words, vary the tone, pitch and speed of speech or otherwise supplement the conversation nonverbally. They may even contradict the verbal message by providing different nonverbal messages (Niven 1989).

Vocal expressions

Many features of speech are related to our emotions. Such features include:

- loudness
- pitch
- speed
- voice quality
- smoothness of speech.

Anxious people tend to talk faster than normal, and at a higher pitch. A depressed person usually talks slowly and at a lower pitch. Speaking quickly may also indicate anger, surprise and animation, while slow speech can mean sadness, boredom or disgust. Pauses in our speech provide punctuation, while stress and pitch show whether a question is being asked, and provide emphasis.

The use of space

We each have our own personal space, which may be likened to a bubble surrounding us and protecting us against invasion from outside. It can feel threatening when personal space is invaded, for instance by someone standing too close. In a situation where people have to stand closer to one another than they would wish, such as on crowded public transport, then they tend to cope with it by avoiding eye contact with those around them.

In the promotion of health through caring for others, it is often not possible to avoid invading a client's personal 'bubble'. Part of the experience of being ill includes the expectation that health carers will be allowed into this area. Asking permission before carrying out an act which will invade the personal, intimate space normally reserved for special, loved ones indicates understanding of a patient's feelings (Porritt 1990). Health professionals can attempt

to reduce anxiety when close contact with a patient becomes necessary, such as when doing a physical assessment, by ensuring that privacy is provided.

Nurses should also guard against unwittingly placing increased distance, indicating distaste or disgust, between themselves and people who are handicapped or disfigured in some way, or whose appearance is otherwise unusual. Fear of catching a contagious disease, and fear of AIDS, may also lead to health promoters maintaining a greater distance and avoiding opportunities to provide health education. Smells and odours can also become barriers to health promotion. Research suggests that a diseased person suffering from malodour is likely to be reacted to with negative feelings (Friedman & DiMatteo 1989). Nurses may sometimes increase the distance between themselves and patients who produce unpleasant odours due to their illness, medication, diet or treatment. Patients may notice this reaction and feel embarrassed or unworthy, and not listen to advice or helpful support even if it is offered.

In a society enriched by the wealth of many cultures, religions and ethnic groups, the world of difference in their traditions, expectations and needs has to be considered if health workers are to genuinely promote health. Because people do not consciously recognise their own use of personal space, they have difficulty understanding a different cultural pattern.

Problems may arise when individuals from different cultures cannot agree on a comfortable interpersonal distance—one person is unable to get close enough because the other keeps moving back, with a kind of dance taking place. Americans, Canadians and British require the most personal space, while Latin Americans and Arabs need the least.

Health professionals should be aware of cultural and individual differences in the norms for physical proximity. For example, speaking too close to someone may seem intrusive, while speaking too far away appears cold and impersonal. An understanding of personal space by nurses can facilitate the assessment process and improve nurse–client interaction.

Touch

Touch can be used to communicate reassurance, comfort and caring, and may therefore be a powerful form of interaction. Touch can communicate feelings between people who care about one another when words would not be adequate. Touch is considered magical and healing in some societies. Certain health care workers are beginning to combine laying on of hands (touch) and prayer with other forms of treatment.

The many cultural differences in the use of touch include for example some cultures normally shaking hands in greeting while others hug and kiss each other. Mediterranean peoples are usually more physically expressive than northern European ones and the cultures derived from them such as those of Australia, Canada and the United States. For some people a pat on the arm may be an effective way of making contact, especially if it is carried out in a wholly natural manner, but for others it could be resented and interpreted as being patronising or intrusive (Brenner 1982).

Because of its possible sexual connotations, and some religious and cultural customs, there are many taboos about touch. Certain groups of devoutly religious people may not want anyone from outside their faith to touch the body of a relative or friend after death, for example, in some cases because that would be believed to disturb the soul.

The health carer and promoter can avoid further distress in such bereaved people by respecting their wishes. Illness often forces patients into a dependent state, unable to regulate the close contact and touching which may be necessary between them and their carers. Two main aspects of touch are identified by Bradley & Edinberg (1990):

- procedural touch
- caring touch.

When speech, hearing or sight are limited, as sometimes happens in elderly people, the skilful use of touch can enhance the patients' awareness that they are cared for. Such patients can also be helped, again through the use of touch, to learn to carry out certain health activities for themselves—perhaps eating or washing—and thus feel less helpless and dependent (Macleod Clark 1991). The first of these would be an example of caring touch and the second of procedural touch.

Touch should happen spontaneously if it is to convey empathy, and should be soothing and gentle for it to be therapeutic. The back rub, a hand on the shoulder or the squeeze of a hand can all encourage closeness and communication between health worker and client. However, as Faulkner (1992) suggests, health professionals who in their normal lives touch only a few very close people should not feel guilty because they are uncomfortable with using touch as part of their professional behaviour.

Body orientation

Where we sit or stand in relation to others generally signals attitudes such as our willingness to cooperate, to dominate, to be friendly and helpful, and our relative status. Sitting on the same level as a client can suggest the intention of being an equal partner in discussion and dialogue, whereas standing or sitting at a greater height generally indicates dominance or higher status. We need to develop an awareness of posture, personal space and positioning so that we may appear relaxed and non-threatening to clients who are possibly bed- or chair-bound. It is important to talk to people if possible at a level which is comfortable for them, and facing them directly.

Movement and posture

The way people walk, sit and stand can indicate their emotions and attitudes. For instance, some-

---

Activity 7.3

How big a part does touching and being touched play in your life? If dissatisfied with your touch behaviour, set yourself goals for improvement and monitor and evaluate your progress.

one sitting with head in hands in a drooping posture may be depressed or despairing, while a person walking along with a rapid swing of the arms and head held high is probably feeling confident and cheerful. Health professionals can read a whole set of attitudes from a client's movement and posture.

Gestures

Gestures and body movements are learned from the culture we grow up in, and can add substantial emphasis to a verbal message. Head nods are a special kind of gesture and can convey interest, agreement and encouragement without the need for words. Hands are also used by many people to add expression to what is being said, or to convey messages without words. For example, a clenched fist is an angry gesture, while hands held out with palms upward suggests openness. Certain cultures use their hands in gesturing far more freely than others.

Facial expression

Our faces are the main factor in our identity. We are recognised and distinguished one from another mostly by our faces. The face is also the most expressive physical aspect of each person, and plays an important part in nonverbal communication. Changes in eyes, mouth and other facial features are often indicators of the person's emotional state. Displeasure, worry or confusion may be displayed by a frown, questioning or disbelief by raised eyebrows, and happiness by a smile. Emotions may also be displayed by physiological responses such as blushing or perspiring.

Some studies show that people tend to 'mirror' the facial expression of the person they are communicating with; in an empathetic response the listener's expression may be sad, thoughtful or joyful, matching that of the speaker. Fear and pain are emotions which health carers often see in their clients' and patients' faces. The ability to 'read' facial cues is an important one for health promoters, as clients may sometimes not want to reveal their pain or worry, because they do not

wish to take up the time of a busy professional, or to appear 'weak'.

Eye contact

One of the most studied aspects of nonverbal communication is eye contact. Research shows that if we look at someone while they are talking to us they will continue to talk, as they interpret our gaze as interest in what they are saying. We often seek eye contact when talking to help us get feedback on how the other person is responding. Maintaining good eye contact (frequent contact without staring) can help clients feel that their problems are of interest and concern, and they may then disclose more. In turn, clients can send many messages with their eyes. Often if they are stressed because of uncertainty related to their health they may totally avoid eye contact with nurses. Avoidance of eye contact can also express feelings of shame, guilt, fear or low self-worth. It may also indicate pain and discomfort or even hostility towards the carer. Someone who has something difficult to say will often look away from the listener.

In normal society, individuals are not encouraged to disclose personal matters, and so it may be easier for a client not to look at a health professional while discussing intimate details. Nurses could respond with empathy after such disclosures by acknowledging the difficulty, perhaps by saying, 'I know that it must have been hard for you to tell me all that, but it helps me to understand' (Faulkner 1992). Eye contact may then be regained.

There are many varied cultural differences in normal eye contact patterns, which need to be remembered by health promoters talking to

---

Activity 7.4

Talk to a partner for about 1 minute. Ask the partner then to look away from you after 15 seconds as you continue talking. For the rest of the activity get the person to look anywhere else but at you while he is still listening. Reverse your roles, and then discuss how it feels to have lack of eye contact.

people with backgrounds different from their own. Middle Eastern and Latin clients will tend to expect more eye contact than western European ones for example. Some Asian and American Indian cultures use less eye contact than Europeans and, among these groups, it can be regarded as disrespectful to look into someone's eyes.

It can feel most uncomfortable and perhaps threatening to be stared at by someone else. One example of staring sometimes occurs during medical rounds in hospital, which patients can find dehumanising (Bradley & Edinberg 1990). The team of medical and nursing staff may spend considerable amounts of time staring at a patient, discussing his condition but not communicating directly with him.

Difficulties can also arise when health workers are developing relationships with people who are physically handicapped or disfigured in some way. They should not stare of course, but the strategy of maintaining constant eye contact to avoid looking elsewhere may seem rigid and obvious to the client, perhaps making him feel embarrassed and unworthy.

CONCLUSION

Communication is an essential part of health promotion in all settings. Communication skills help the health worker to understand the world of clients, patients and their families. They in turn can then be empowered to live more resourcefully, managing their own health and lifestyles. Helping people to recognise their own health needs, and to raise their competence in doing what they think is important for them and their community, depends on high levels of communication skills. It is through communication that helping relationships are formed, problems identified and discussed, and information about physical, mental and community health conveyed.

REFERENCES

Anderson C, Wilkie P (eds) 1992 Reflective helping in HIV and AIDS. Open University Press, Milton Keynes
Bradley J C, Edinberg M A 1990 Communication in the nursing context, 3rd edn. Appleton & Lange, Norwalk CT
Brenner D 1982 The effective psychotherapist. Pergamon, Oxford
Burnard P 1992 Know yourself! Self awareness activities for nurses. Scutari, London
Devlin R 1992 Breaking the sound barrier. Nursing Times 88(46): 26–28
DiMatteo M R 1991 The psychology of health, illness and medical care: an individual perspective. Brooks/Grove, Pacific Grove CA
Egan G 1990 The skilled helper, 4th edn. Brooks Cole, California
Faulkner A 1992 Effective interaction with patients. Churchill Livingstone, Edinburgh
Friedman H S, DiMatteo M R 1989 Health psychology. Prentice-Hall, Englewood Cliffs NJ
Gooch S 1993 Healthy options. Nursing Times 89(8): 41–43
Kelcher M 1992 Better communication skills for work. BBC Books, London
Macleod Clark J 1991 Communicating with elderly people.

In: Redfern S J (ed) Nursing elderly people, 2nd edn. Churchill Livingstone, Edinburgh
Morton S 1993 Behavioural challenge. Nursing Times 89(10): 54–56
Nicolson P, Bayne R 1990 Applied psychology for social workers, 2nd edn. Macmillan, London
Niven N 1989 Health psychology: an introduction for nurses and other health care professionals. Churchill Livingstone, Edinburgh
Nunnally E, Moy C 1989 Communication basics for human service professionals, Sage, Newbury Park CA
Porritt L 1990 Interaction strategies: an introduction for health professionals, 2nd edn. Churchill Livingstone, Edinburgh
Rogers C R 1980 A way of being. Houghton Mifflin, Boston
Rogers C R 1983 Freedom to learn for the eighties. Merrill, Columbus OH
United Kingdom Central Council for Nursing, Midwifery and Health Visiting (UKCC) 1993 Standards for records and record keeping. UKCC, London
World Health Organization 1993 Health for all targets: the health policy for Europe, updated edn. WHO, Regional Office for Europe, Copenhagen

FURTHER READING

Burnard P 1992 Communicate! A communication skills guide for health care workers. Edward Arnold, London

Ellis R B 1992 The nurse as communicator. In: Kenworthy N, Snowley G, Gilling C (eds) Common foundation studies in nursing. Churchill Livingstone, Edinburgh

Ewles L, Simnett I 1992 Promoting health: a practical guide, 2nd edn. Scutari, London

Faulkner A 1992 Effective interaction with patients. Churchill Livingstone, Edinburgh

Porritt L 1990 Interaction strategies: an introduction for health professionals, 2nd edn. Churchill Livingstone, Edinburgh

Tschudin V 1982 Counselling skills for nurses. Baillière Tindall, London

CHAPTER CONTENTS

Introduction 95

**Life context and the primary health care
    approach 96**

Definition 96

Groupwork skills 96
    Skills development 96
    Self-awareness 97

Group characteristics 97
    Group processes 98

Leadership 100
    Leadership style 101
    Groupthink 101

Teamwork 102
    Teamwork in primary health care 103
    Team building 104
    Collective approaches to health 105

Self-help groups 105
    Research 107

References 107

8

Groups and teams

Diana Forster

*By the year 2000, primary health care in all
Member States should meet the basic health
needs of the population by providing a wide
range of health-promotive, curative,
rehabilitative and supportive services, and by
actively supporting self-help activities of
individuals, families and groups.*

(Target 28: Primary health care, WHO 1993)

INTRODUCTION

As individual people we develop our personalities, relationships and ways of coping with the world, within the various groups to which we belong. These may include:

- parents
- family
- nursery
- school
- friends
- co-workers
- other social networks.

Groups help to form links between individuals and the wider social system. Skills of working with groups in many varied settings can be enhanced and developed. These skills are essential tools for health promoters, enabling them to share their own knowledge and skills and to help others make realistic health choices which reflect their wants and needs. Such skills are also relevant for health promoters acting as advocates for others and for developing effective teamwork. The focus of groupwork should be upon empowering others, viewing them as partners in health promotion.

Nurses have a unique contribution to make in the health promotion movement. They can liaise with:

- housing officers
- environmental health officers
- voluntary organisations (e.g. Age Concern, Shelter)
- pressure groups (e.g. Public Health Alliance)
- local neighbourhood groups or patient groups

and many others. Concepts of health incorporated in new nursing curricula recognise that people live in a changing world of health care, and that positive health behaviour is easier in a supportive environment (see Ch. 13). Nurses will therefore be working increasingly with groups from other disciplines.

This chapter will outline some basic group and team concepts, characteristics, processes and dynamics in relation to the promotion of individual and community health.

LIFE CONTEXT AND THE PRIMARY HEALTH CARE APPROACH

There is a need for a shift in focus from concentrating only on personal behaviour which may affect people's health, for example cigarette smoking, towards the consideration of external factors which are also capable of influencing health. This approach is based on the key principles which were set out in the Declaration of Alma Ata (WHO 1978) (Box 8.1). Health promotion includes health education for individuals and groups, but it also attempts to produce environmental and legislative changes which can help to improve health. Current housing policies, for example, deny many mothers access to the homes they need for themselves and their children (Graham 1993). Collective efforts in community settings can empower people to have control over wider aspects of their lives than merely attempting to change their own behaviour, such as smoking, which may be their only way of coping with their environment.

Box 8.1   Key principles in the Declaration of Alma Ata (RCN 1992)

- Accessibility: health care which is provided close to where people live and work
- Acceptability: health care which is appropriate and provided in ways which people find acceptable
- Equity: all people have an equal right to health and health care
- Self-determination: people have the right and the responsibility to make their own health choices
- Community involvement: people have the right and the responsibility to participate individually and collectively in the planning and implementation of their health care
- A focus on health: primary health care concentrates on the promotion of health as well as on the care of people who are sick, frail or disabled
- A multisectoral approach: housing, food policies, environmental policies and social services have an important part to play

---

DEFINITION

The term 'group' may be defined in a variety of ways, relating to its function, to the kinds of people who belong to it, to their reasons for joining and whether membership is voluntary or not. Lassiter (1992) suggests 'it is a collection of interacting individuals who have a common purpose or purposes. Each member influences and is in turn influenced by every other member to some extent'.

GROUPWORK SKILLS

Groups play an important part in our daily lives. All health workers will have experienced group life, whether at home, at work, during leisure or in other community settings. Nurses often participate in groups and teams when planning care and other health-focused action with clients. This knowledge and experience helps us to understand the processes which operate in group dynamics, to be considered later, and forms the basis of the development of groupwork skills.

Skills development

Nurses and other health promoters may be frequently required to develop and run various kinds of groups in different settings. Group facili- tation training is increasingly becoming part of basic and continuing nurse education, and is available in many colleges and university depart- ments. Burnard (1992) describes three types of verbal interventions which may be used while conducting groups of various kinds. These focus on three separate aspects of time—recent past, present and future—and are headed:

- Clarifying recent talk
- Developing current talk
- Initiating further talk.

Clarifying recent talk

Clarifying recent talk helps the group to clearly understand what the discussion is focusing upon. Burnard (1992) suggests the following methods of achieving this:

- summarising the discussion so far and identifying the main issues
- drawing together various discussion points into a cohesive whole
- disagreeing, by putting forward a reasoned alternative which may lead to further discussion.

Developing current talk

Developing current talk to encourage further discussion requires the use of client-centred coun- selling skills, such as:

- reflection—repeating the last few words spoken or paraphrasing the last few statements made
- checking for understanding—rephrasing what has been said and asking if the meaning has been correctly interpreted
- support—agreeing with statements made and encouraging more discussion.

Initiating further talk

Initiating further talk is helpful when the group seems ready to move the discussion into new areas, and requires group development skills, including:

- proposing a new topic for discussion or a plan of action for the group to consider
- using open questions to stimulate discussion
- disclosing the facilitator's own thoughts, feelings or experiences which may encourage others to share their thoughts in a similar way (Burnard 1992).

Self-awareness

Skills of working with groups may be developed through an increase in self-awareness—getting to know ourselves better. One example of a group activity designed to enlarge self-awareness and promote more open communication, which is used in many training groups, is known as the Johari window (Fig. 8.1). It is a model named after the two American teachers who designed it—Joseph Luft and Harry Ingham (Luft 1970). The window represents four types of behaviour. Window pane A represents our behaviour in the public area of knowledge; those aspects of ourselves we and others are aware of, such as our sense of humour or liking for certain kinds of people. Pane B is the blind area; the aspects of ourselves which others see but we do not know about—for example our behaviour or moodiness, perhaps when we are nervous or embarrassed. Pane C represents our private selves which are hidden from other people—our unshared hopes, plans and anxieties for instance. Finally, window pane D is the unconscious, unknown part of us which neither we nor others know about. In training groups using this model, group mem- bers can use self-disclosure, sharing thoughts and feelings, and ask for feedback from others to enlarge the public areas and reduce the hidden, blind and unknown areas. Self-development through increased self-awareness can enhance skills in working with groups, helping us to reflect upon our own thoughts and feelings.

GROUP CHARACTERISTICS

Groups can be divided into two categories:

- primary groups
- secondary groups.

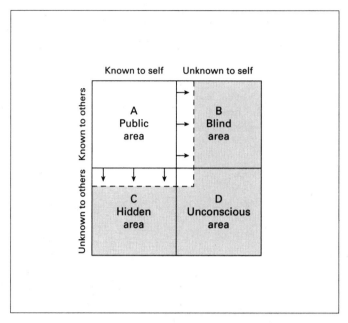

Figure 8.1 The Johari window

A primary group is one in which members come face to face, such as in a family, a group of friends, or in the more formal set-up of a school or college class or a primary health care team meeting. Secondary groups are those in which members do not necessarily meet face to face, but share common characteristics, such as being pregnant women or school nurses.

People can gain from attending a group meeting such as that of a self-help group, carer's support group or other community group by:

- making new relationships
- meeting others who share similar experiences and thus feeling less alone
- learning coping strategies through discussion in a supportive setting
- sharing views, ideas and emotions, and feeling valued through contributing suggestions

---

Activity 8.1

List three primary groups and three secondary groups to which you belong.

- feeling able to express fears and worries in a safe environment.

Group processes

Processes consist of the means by which the group goes about achieving its tasks, and what influences it while doing so. The effects of seating arrangements and other vital aspects of the physical environment are discussed in the chapter on teaching and learning (see Ch. 9).

Establishing and achieving group goals

Group members should all have a part to play in developing group goals and making decisions. If they do not, their level of commitment suffers and they may become unwilling to take responsibility for achieving goals (Box 8.2). Jackson (1983) studied the effects of having nursing and clerical personnel in a hospital outpatient clinic take more part in making decisions about the daily organisation of the clinic. Managers and superiors traditionally ran the clinic without discussion with other members of staff. After regular group meetings for all staff were intro-

> **Box 8.2 Questions which help to achieve group goals (adapted from Grasha 1989)**
>
> - What goals are we trying to reach with this project or task?
> - What are several different methods we could use to accomplish our goals?
> - What do we need to think about doing?
> - What would help to get more of us to take part in achieving our goals?
> - What skills and interests can each of us contribute towards reaching our goals?
> - Can we break our goals into smaller steps and identify a timescale for each one?

> **Box 8.3 Examples of violating group norms**
>
> - Stepping to the front of a queue for tickets instead of joining the end of it
> - Wearing very smart clothes to a party when everyone else is dressed informally
> - Talking all the time in a discussion so that no-one else has a chance to contribute

duced, participants were found to have higher levels of job satisfaction and more understanding of their roles. There was less conflict with managers and between other staff members. Communication between colleagues became more effective. A higher standard of well-being for staff was therefore reached through greater participation (Grasha 1989).

The benefits of encouraging all group members to take part in setting goals and making decisions are also apparent in self-help groups and in multidisciplinary teams, which will be considered later. Examples suggest that group goals should be relevant both to the needs of the group as a whole and to its individual members.

The effects of group norms on behaviour

A group norm is a shared idea about standards for group members' behaviour, attitudes and perceptions (see Box 8.3).

Group norms have three main functions:

- task function
- maintenance function
- influencing members' perceptions and interpretation of reality (Lassiter 1992).

The task function ensures that the group concentrates on its tasks and returns to working towards goals if discussions or activities have been sidetracked. In carrying out the maintenance function, group members support each other, for example by:

- seeking new ideas for resolving issues of concern

- listening to each person's contributions
- setting and modifying group goals.

People are most productive when their psychological and social well-being is supported. Group members can help to reduce one another's worries and tensions; concern shown by others helps people to talk about their thoughts and feelings and to resolve conflicts. One example of this is a group set up for users of mental health services (Gell 1990): the Nottingham Patient Council Support Group (NPCSG).

The aims of the NPCSG were:

- to create more awareness and control by users of the services
- to create user-only meetings in wards, day units and community mental health centres, and to support such groups in taking up issues raised by them
- to influence the planning and management of mental health services
- to educate workers both locally and nationally about the need for user involvement.

Gell (1990) highlights some of the many successful outcomes achieved by the NPCSG, which included an improvement in the condition and delivery time of food in one hospital following users' complaints and suggestions. Similarly, Whittaker (1990) discusses the successful involvement of people with learning difficulties in meetings affecting their own daily lives. People with learning difficulties can chair conferences and lead multidisciplinary workshops relevant to their needs.

The third function of group norms refers to the pressure they exert on members of the group. This is illustrated in a well-known series of psychological experiments described by Asch (1955).

He studied groups where all except one of the members were briefed beforehand to say that what was clearly the shorter of two lines was in their view the longer one. The unbriefed members would begin to doubt the evidence of their own eyes and would in many cases agree with the rest of the group.

The powerful effects of group norms can be useful in many aspects of health promotion, such as in helping people to conform to agreed targets of losing superfluous weight when they wish to.

Meeting needs for inclusion, control and affection

These three needs—for inclusion, for control and for affection—have been identified as important in influencing the way people interact with one another in a group (Schutz 1982).

Inclusion is the personal need people feel for keeping in contact with others and becoming involved in effective relationships with them. The need for control is associated with power and authority in our lives. People want and need directions and guidance from others, including health workers, but also want the ability to control their own lives and be self-empowered. Affection involves our preferences for close, intimate relationships. Quality of life may be enhanced by a feeling of 'belonging' in a group or community. Helping other people in a group to meet their needs for inclusion, control and affection helps them to make health choices, and cope with health challenges. Families who are affected by potential or actual sickle cell disease, for example, need support, information, genetic counselling and the chance to form partnerships with health professionals and lay groups in the communities where they live and work.

The effects of group roles on behaviour

A widely accepted list of eight roles which are desirable if a group or team is to be fully effective has been developed by Belbin (1981). He concluded from his research that teams of people who thought and behaved alike were rarely as successful and creative as teams which included people with a variety of different characteristics. For a team to be effective it has to have the right mix of personality styles to ensure that certain functions are performed in the team. The roles he identified are:

- The chairperson or leader. He or she coordinates, focuses and balances the efforts of the group, helping it to be effective in what it sets out to achieve.
- The shaper. This is the task leader, outgoing and dominant, whose strength lies in drive and passion for the task—the 'slave-driver' who sets team objectives.
- The plant. This is the most creative and intellectual member of the group; it is he or she who is the main source of original ideas and proposals.
- The monitor–evaluator. This person's contribution is the careful analysis and checking out of ideas and proposals, with the ability to point out the flaws in an argument and to evaluate the group's progress.
- The resource-investigator. This is the popular, communicative group member who is sociable, extroverted and relaxed. He or she will liaise with other people and agencies.
- The company worker. The company worker is the practical organiser who turns ideas into manageable tasks, and who is an efficient administrator.
- The team worker. This group member supports the others by listening, encouraging, harmonising and understanding.
- The finisher. This person's perseverance ensures that tasks are completed and deadlines are met by the group.

A balanced team is needed for effective and harmonious groupwork. Health promoters in group settings may be aware of the gaps if all roles do not appear to be represented. They may then be able to combine roles to help the group to be more effective, for example in managing time or encouraging ideas.

LEADERSHIP

Leadership is a process of providing guidance and direction to a group through the use of interpersonal influence. Effective leaders are felt by the group to have influence because of their knowledge and ability, their access to information and resources needed by the group and their status in the community or organisation. Leaders can help to inspire a trusting climate in their group by developing:

- open and honest communication
- acceptance of others
- the sharing of common goals
- respect for the opinions of others on how to achieve the goals of the group.

Leadership style

A democratic, or participative, style of leadership provides support and encouragement to group members so that they are likely to explore all aspects of decision-making and planning in reaching whatever goals they have set themselves.

Nurses and other promoters of health may use varied leadership styles according to their assessment of the group's needs. When groups request information and wish to develop skills, the leader can be most helpful by telling people what needs to be done and how to do it, before encouraging them to participate. Parents, for instance, are being increasingly involved in their children's care in hospital.

Since the Platt Report (1959) emphasised the importance of parents being encouraged to remain with their children, family-centred care has developed in paediatric hospitals and units. Parents are ideally viewed as partners, taking part in planning, carrying out and evaluating their children's care. They become part of the group of carers whose leadership changes according to the specific activities being undertaken. Parents may become the leaders when explaining or demonstrating their child's preferences in some aspects of care. They may also share a leading part in setting up support groups for siblings, such as those described by Stone (1993) for siblings of children with cancer.

When groups wish to work at tasks together, the leader will be more effective if she concen-

Activity 8.2

Draw up a list of leadership activities that you have observed recently. What styles of leadership were identifiable? Assess whether these were appropriate in each situation.

trates on developing relationships and communication as well as task-related activities. Groups of people who wish to work independently, who show initiative and the ability to take responsibility, need a participative leader who is not directive but acts as a facilitator, using skills discussed earlier.

Macmillan & Pringle (1993) consider the skills required in the management of change by practice managers in primary health care. They explain: 'good leaders are not authoritarian, nor are they shrinking violets. They believe in forging consensus and then helping everybody to share in the implementation. They delegate, with support, and with reasonable expectations of an individual's capabilities. They value people for what they can do and help them to recognize and tackle those areas they find difficult.'

Groupthink

Groups tend to develop their own norms and ideas, to which the members are usually expected to conform. If members are encouraged to discuss and share ideas and information openly, then groups generally make better choices about courses of action. When norms for such open communication are missing, group members may begin to think alike and agree with one another, not listening to essential information which may be available. They may ignore or refuse to gather any opinions from outside their group. Such groups are in danger of becoming too cohesive and 'cosy', insulated from outside influences. The conscience of each member tends to be ignored in favour of group harmony. No conflict is allowed to spoil the cosiness; doubts are ignored. Decisions are then made without systematically considering all possible options and implications. This is the process of 'groupthink' (Janis 1972).

Sometimes groupthink occurs when a group is under stress because a decision is needed urgently, or because the group is dominated by a very directive leader. Groupthink can occur in well-established, long-lived teams in health care settings when members have grown used to working with one another. A cosy, amicable atmosphere is the norm at such meetings, where disagreement and conflict may be avoided and questioning and change are resisted (Garrett 1992).

TEAMWORK

A team may be defined as a small group of people who relate to each other and contribute to a common goal.

The promotion of health through the delivery of health care services and through local, national and world-wide policies depends largely upon effective and efficient decisions being made by relevant groups and teams. It requires a conscious effort to develop teamwork and a continuous effort to maintain it. A successful team depends not only on the qualities of its individual members but also upon how they work together. The potential for new ways of delivering primary health care, for instance, has never been greater, and teamwork is the key to effective health promotion within primary health care. However, many issues still cause concern and need to be resolved, such as problems of accountability—there is a tension between cultivating a team spirit and having different sources of financial control.

Once people are involved in a team, the ideas and aims of others have to be considered. In health care settings it is easy to lose sight of the fact that the team exists for the benefit of the clients and their needs (Garrett 1992). The director of team activity is ideally viewed as the patient

or client, with the team leader facilitating the activity. Ross (1986) states: 'fundamental to the concept of teamwork is ... division of labour, coordination and task-sharing, each member making a different contribution, but one of equal value, towards the common goal of patient care.'

Task-sharing requires team members to understand one another's roles. The junior nurse may spend more time with patients than do senior medical personnel, and therefore be able to contribute valuable insight into patients' feelings, needs and behaviour. Nursing staff are likely to be in the best position to coordinate the input of other team members. However, Davies (1994) stresses the importance of involving all team members in planning and implementing changes and carefully evaluating team care.

Teamwork is a skill which can be learned, and if a productive working relationship is established then the benefits include:

- improved standards of care for clients and patients
- higher levels of job satisfaction for staff
- increased morale for the team as a whole
- mutual support for team members in their work.

A senior nurse who was responsible for infection control recognised the need for a nutritional support team in the hospital where she worked (Clark 1994). A study was carried out to examine levels of care for patients receiving total parenteral nutrition (TPN) in the hospital. Findings showed that it was difficult for nurses to develop clinical expertise because patients receiving TPN were scattered throughout the hospital. The sepsis rate was higher than anticipated, except for patients in the intensive care unit where most staff were specially trained in TPN procedures. A TPN special interest group was set up within the hospital to try to reduce sepsis and other complications. This was a multidisciplinary team which included:

- a senior nurse—infection control
- a consultant microbiologist
- a consultant biochemist
- a consultant physician
- a pharmacist

Activity 8.3

Identify one team to which you belong, and consider this question: What are my own personal goals within this team for the next year?

- a dietitian
- an anaesthetist
- link nurses
  —an intensive care unit sister
  —a surgical ward sister
  —a medical ward enrolled nurse.

This team devised specific TPN protocols and guidelines which were available at ward and unit level. In-service education was also established to promote knowledge, ensure compliance with the protocols and standardise care (Clark 1994). The patients' health and well-being were therefore promoted through the avoidance of sepsis.

Teamwork in primary health care

Good teamwork is the essence of effective primary health care. The Harding committee defined the primary health care team (PHCT) as 'an independent group of medical practitioners, secretaries and/or receptionists, health visitors, district nurses and midwives who share a common purpose and responsibility, each member clearly understanding his/her function and those of other members so that all pool skills and knowledge to provide an effective primary health care service' (DHSS 1981).

However, there has been much debate about what is really meant by the term 'primary health care team', and how such teams should function. The varying roles of the team members need to be carefully assessed in deciding upon an appropriate skill mix. For example, district nurses and district enrolled nurses may be supported by health care assistants or nursing auxiliaries who could carry out routine hygiene care, while qualified staff concentrate on using their full range of skills, including health promotion activities.

The PHCT is considered to be the most appropriate forum for health promotion because of its regular contact with the general public. At least once a year 75% of the population visit their general practitioner, and 90% do so within 5 years (Cant & Killoran 1993). There should therefore be the chance for a multidisciplinary team to offer a range of health-promoting options. Users of the service may be regarded as partners and as an extension of the PHCT itself. The people in the

best position to judge the quality of community care services are those who use them, and quality assurance checks should involve representative groups of such users.

Issues identified in the Cumberledge report (DHSS 1986) such as accountability, integration of services and the relevance of particular training and core skills continue to be vital aspects needing to be constantly addressed.

Community multidisciplinary teams

Primary health care teams can share in multidisciplinary approaches to health care in the community, where people from different professions and agencies work together forming alliances.

In one health authority a team approach to providing community care for people with late-stage HIV infection has been developed. The hospice movement, working with PHCTs and liaising with HIV social workers, clinical psychologists and many other health professionals and volunteers, aims to provide the best possible physical, social, psychological and spiritual aspects of care. Patients and carers are helped to prepare for death in whatever way they wish, while optimum control of pain and symptoms is provided. In this example the team includes three clinical nurse specialists in palliative care, two doctors, an occupational therapist and a dietitian. Patients and the people closest to them are central to clinical care and communication. They are invited to attend multidisciplinary meetings when their own cases are being considered. Medical back-up is shared between the GP and the team. Patients are encouraged to help plan their care and treatment in order to achieve the best possible quality of life until their death (Edwards 1992).

Community mental health teams and centres

Mental health teams working in the community have a special role in promoting health and preventing unnecessary hospital admissions for those with mental health problems. People returning from hospital, and those with chronic and disabling mental health conditions are also supported by such teams. In some areas, specialist mental health teams for older people, children or for families have been developed. However, there has been mounting public concern that people with severe mental health problems are not receiving adequate care in the community. Ford & Repper (1994) describe the 'assertive outreach' approach successfully adopted in four district teams. Case managers did not take rejection from clients at face value when services were refused, but persisted indefinitely in maintaining contact and responsibility for clients who could be at risk of neglect, self-injury or of harming others. As well as team support, mental health nurses will need training, clinical supervision and lower caseloads in order to exercise their increased responsibility for the delivery of mental health care services.

Community teams for people with learning difficulties also exist to provide specialist skills for those who need them.

Patient advisory groups

Some primary health care teams have patient-advisory groups, where users of the services provided can support the practice team with advice and comments on their service provision, and perhaps contribute lay skills and resources. If users are consulted about producing a practice leaflet for example, they may be able to contribute useful ideas and possibly the skills and expertise to publish the leaflet.

Screening targets may be more successfully achieved by involving relevant users. The uptake of one cervical screening programme was doubled after the standard letter of invitation was reworded by one of the women participants (Pritchard & Pritchard 1992).

Team building

Team building activities are undertaken by many primary health care teams. If team building is to be successful, all members taking part should feel comfortable with the idea of working more closely and harmoniously together. Effective working relationships should be positive and open (Pritchard & Pritchard 1992). There needs to

be a spirit of equity which does not allow professional rivalries and 'pecking orders' to influence teamwork. A good team needs to have clear objectives, developed by all its members. Each person will then feel committed to owning and achieving the objectives. For this to happen, regular meetings need to be held for all team members.

The informal basis for team care is often maintained by day-to-day contact between members, either face to face or through messages and telephone calls. However, this contact is not sufficient for the development of shared objectives and a shared vision (Robison & Wiles 1993). Vision for a PHCT might be: 'to work effectively as a team and in partnership with the practice population and other agencies to provide a targeted programme of health promotion aimed at developing the health and well-being of the local community' (Poulton & West 1993).

Wiltshire Family Health Services Authority set up a research study to examine the benefits to patients arising from a high level of team work in primary health care (Robison & Wiles 1993). At practices where PHCT meetings were held, staff viewed them as crucial to team development. Researchers found that many health and social care professionals attended the meetings, besides the health visitors, midwives and district nurses who were defined as 'core' members for this study. They included community psychiatric nurses, Macmillan nurses, counsellors and school nurses. Opportunities were created for collaboration, and access to a wide range of skills, resources and knowledge which benefited patients was provided by inviting relevant health personnel to meetings. Learning about one another's roles was identified as an important step in developing teamwork. One practice nurse said: 'I understand the job of other members of staff much more since we've had PHCT meetings and people have given their job description in full.' Practice managers, receptionists, and health visitors were most likely to feel that others did not understand their roles. Only one of the 20 GP practices in the study had discussed and agreed upon a written goal for the PHCT. This team carried out an audit, identifying the needs of the practice population and working out the best way of providing an effective service.

The study concluded that individual patient care should not be discussed routinely at meetings, but that protocols and policies, and the development of a shared vision and shared objectives should be the main considerations (Robison & Wiles 1993).

Although professionals in health and social services may work closely together on shared tasks in a cohesive team, their management structures and the legal framework in which they operate are usually very different. Their values and beliefs may also be different. In addressing issues like these, a GP and a management consultant have devised a workbook which presents a programme of 13 learning and practical exercises for PHCTs to work through with little or no outside help (Pritchard & Pritchard 1992). Their emphasis is always on key issues facing these teams, including for example:

- the nature and purpose of teamwork
- team goals and tasks
- roles within the team
- patients as team members
- evaluating the effectiveness of the team.

The key message of team building is to ask the right questions in the right order (see Box 8.4).

Community oriented primary health care (COPC)

COPC aims to increase health gains through synthesising the strengths of primary health care, with its focus on populations, health promotion and anticipatory care. It is a model developed by

---

Box 8.4 Key questions for team building (Pritchard & Pritchard 1992)

- What are our goals? What is the task? Does it need teamwork?
- What are our various roles in the team? Who will carry out the task?
- What are the agreed procedures for successful teamwork? How do we carry out and evaluate the team tasks?
- Are our interpersonal relationships as good as possible? Is team effectiveness threatened by unresolved conflict?

---

the King's Fund, designed to help PHCTs acquire skills and respond better to the needs of the local population (Plamping 1994).

Collective approaches to health

A community is more than the sum of its individuals; its strength can be in its unity. By working together people can make sense of their lives through sharing experiences, learning from each other and gaining self-confidence (Billingham 1993).

Examples of collective approaches to health include groups facilitated by health visitors and other promoters of health in the community (Drennan 1988), community health groups in which people address health issues outside the medical remit, such as safety standards in council housing (Watt & Rodmell 1993), and self-help groups.

SELF-HELP GROUPS

These are usually set up by people who have similar problems and who aim to share information, experiences or perhaps ways of coping. There are, for instance, many self-help organisations for weight control, including the well-known 'Weight Watchers' whose approach is based on group meetings which offer social support, nutritional information and behavioural techniques such as self-monitoring of food intake.

Self-help groups range from long-established organisations such as Weight Watchers to small, newly formed associations of people with rare or little-known chronic diseases and disabilities.

Research from nine countries of Europe and North America, reviewed at a workshop convened by the International Information Centre on Self-help and Health, covered reports from groups for those with:

- diabetes
- rheumatism
- chronic skin disease
- cancer
- sarcoidosis
- hypertension

Activity 8.4

Can you identify any self-help groups which meet in your locality? Find out from the local Community Health Council, Council for Voluntary Services or Social Services department which groups exist.

- blood diseases
- Huntington's disease
- learning difficulties

and many other conditions (Branckaerts & Richardson 1992).

Groups also include those for people with various kinds of addiction, such as gambling, drinking, smoking and the abuse of drugs, solvents and other substances. Sufferers themselves or their relatives, friends and carers may start or join groups which can significantly contribute to health promotion by being concerned with:

- the social and health needs of members
- broader policies for health care and its provision.

Groups often initiate research and sometimes develop extensive resources which may include specialist literature and information packs. They may also lobby for improvements in the provision of aspects of health care locally and nationally, as in the example in Box 8.5.

Support may be given within groups, which reduces stigma and provides information and coping strategies. Loneliness and a sense of isolation can be overcome through shared activities.

Box 8.5   United Kingdom Advocacy Network (UKAN) (Read & Wallcraft 1992)

UKAN is a confederation of user-led patients' councils, advocacy projects and user forums in England, Scotland, Wales and Northern Ireland. It is funded by the King's Fund, the Mental Health Foundation and Research and Development in Psychiatry.

UKAN has a national management committee and 10 regional networks. Policy is decided by an annual meeting at which all the member groups are represented.

Emotional and social support can be offered at every stage, from prevention to day-to-day health care and rehabilitation. Self-help groups are particularly appropriate for people adjusting to chronic conditions likely to involve changes in lifestyle and body image. For example, a patient waiting to undergo ostomy surgery (i.e. surgery that results in an ileostomy or other stoma being formed) may be visited in hospital, and at home after surgery, by a group member who is living proof that life with a stoma can still include the social, sporting, family, leisure and work activities enjoyed before. There is as much need here for psychological support as for the 'which ostomy bag is best' approach. This type of lay, self-help support complements nurses' and other professionals' health teaching, care and treatment.

Sometimes, however, self-help groups can have a negative impact on members by:

- isolating them from the wider community
- creating high expectations which are unrealistic and cannot be fulfilled
- presenting a narrow approach to problem solving and failing to consider alternative strategies (Branckaerts & Richardson 1992).

Who joins self-help groups? Evidence suggests that joiners tend to be middle class, educated, female, elderly and not usually from ethnic minorities or rural areas (Richardson 1991). Obstacles preventing people from taking part include lack of transport, money or a baby-sitter. Another obstacle is not knowing that a group exists. These barriers need to be addressed when health workers are identifying local needs or planning group activities. Health workers can provide support to existing groups and make them available to more people by:

- telling patients, clients and carers about relevant self-help groups available locally and nationally
- offering practical advice to groups about publicity and premises
- acting as a resource to provide specialist information or as a facilitator within a group
- offering support to group leaders and founders

- encouraging local professionals to help in establishing and supporting groups—as in the following example.

An Afro-Caribbean mental health project

In the late 1980s, some community groups in Manchester became concerned about the high level of psychiatric diagnosis and admissions to local hospitals of young black people. A study of local psychiatric hospitals showed that although Afro-Caribbean people comprised about 6% of the immigrant population in central Manchester their admission to psychiatric hospitals varied between 25% and 40% of all admissions (Ferguson & Lal 1992).

The Afro-Caribbean mental health group was formed by concerned representatives of professional workers, local community groups and local residents. Public meetings were held where information was shared, and local black users of the psychiatric services described their experiences of being diagnosed and treated for mental illness. The Afro-Caribbean mental health project was set up in 1989, with funding from various non-statutory agencies for staff and running costs. This ongoing project has set out to question whether the kinds of diagnostic tools used to measure levels of behaviour in order to determine mental illness are appropriate for the Afro-Caribbean population. Training sessions are provided within the project for nurses, multidisciplinary teams, social workers and community groups in an attempt to encourage health and local authority mental health services to become more accessible, appropriate and sensitive to the needs of the Afro-Caribbean community. Self-help groups play an important part as they are supported by outreach workers who act as advocates for individual users of the mental health services, their families and their community groups (Ferguson & Lal 1992).

Research

Nurses and other health professionals have an important role to play in researching self-help groups, so that questions about their effectiveness in promoting health and well-being and other relevant issues may be addressed.

A 6-month study was designed in an inner city area of Birmingham to assess the effects of a self-help group for diabetic patients and their relatives (Jennings et al 1987). The results showed a significant improvement in diabetic knowledge and in diabetic control which was still maintained 12 months after the self-help group had finished.

A study to explore carers' reasons for joining a support group and the benefits they perceived of attending the group is described by Morton & Mackenzie (1994). The main benefits identified were mutual and social support, which included:

- being amongst people in similar situations who will listen
- sharing advice with carers of people with different illnesses
- gaining respect from people who understand
- knowing that you're not alone
- the opportunity to meet people and 'have a chat'
- the opportunity to 'get out'.

What is the future of self-help groups? Lay participation in health promotion reflects the developing partnership between health professionals and non-professionals. The growing interest in health in its broadest sense will perhaps lead to the promotion of new self-help groups concerned with reorienting health services towards promoting health more generally, placing health issues firmly in the context of healthy public policy and taking a holistic view of health needs.

REFERENCES

Asch S E 1955 Opinions and social pressure. Scientific American 193: 31–35
Belbin R M 1981 Management teams. Heinemann, London

Billingham K 1993 Partners with the community. Partners in health (supplement). Primary Health Care 3(6): 2–3
Branckaerts J, Richardson a 1992 Self-help groups: their

impact and potential. In: Kaplun A (ed) Health promotion and chronic illness. WHO Regional Publications, European Series, 44

Burnard P 1992 Developing skills as a group facilitator. In: Horne E M, Cowan T (eds) Effective communication: some nursing perspectives, 2nd edn. Wolfe Publishing, London

Cant S, Killoran A 1993 Team tactics: a study of nurse collaboration in general practice. Health Education Journal 52(4): 203–208

Clark L 1994 Safety first. Nursing Times 90(5): 64–68

Davies S M 1994 An evaluation of nurse-led team care within a rehabilitation ward for elderly people. Journal of Clinical Nursing 3(1): 25–33

Department of Health and Social Security 1981 The primary health care team. Report of a Joint Working Group of the Standing Nursing and Midwifery Advisory Committee (the Harding Report). HMSO, London

Department of Health and Social Security 1986 Neighbourhood nursing—a focus for health care. Report of the Community Nursing Review. HMSO, London

Drennan V 1988 Health visitors and groups. Politics and practice. Heinemann Nursing, Oxford

Edwards D 1992 A team spirit. Primary Heath Care 2(6): 16–18

Ferguson G, Lal P 1992 Afro-Caribbean mental health project—Manchester. In: Lynch B, Perry R (eds) Experiences of community care. Longman, UK

Ford R, Repper J 1994 Taking responsibility for care. Nursing Times 90(31): 54–57

Garrett G 1992 Teamwork: an equal partnership? In: Horne E M, Cowan T (eds) Effective communication: some nursing perspectives, 2nd edn. Wolfe Publishing, London

Gell C 1990 User group involvement. In: Winn L (ed) Power to the people: the key to responsive services in health social care. King's Fund Centre, London

Graham H 1993 Hardship and health in women's lives. Harvester Wheatsheaf, Hertfordshire

Grasha A F 1989 Practical applications of psychology, 3rd edn. Little Brown, Boston

Jackson S E 1983 Participation in decision making as a strategy for reducing job-related strain. Journal of Applied Psychology 68: 3–19

Janis I L 1972 Victims of groupthink. Houghton Mifflin, Boston

Jennings P E, Morgan H C, Barnett A H 1987 Improved diabetes control and knowledge during a diabetes self-help group. Diabetes Education 13(4): 390–393

Lassiter P G 1992 Working with groups in the community. In: Stanhope M, Lancester J (eds) Community health nursing. Process and practice for promoting health, 3rd edn. Mosby Year Book, St Louis

Luft J 1970 Group processes: an introduction to group dynamics. Mayfield, Palo Alto

Macmillan L, Pringle M 1993 Practice managers and practice management. In: Pringle M (ed) Change and teamwork in primary care. BMJ Publishing Group, London

Morton A, Mackenzie A 1994 An exploratory study of the consumers' views of carer support groups. Journal of Clinical Nursing 3: 63–64

Plamping D 1994 Promoting community oriented primary health care. Nursing Times 90(35): 44

Platt H 1959 The welfare of children in hospital. Report of the Committee on Child Health Services. HMSO, London

Poulton B C, West M A 1993 Effective multidisciplinary teamwork in primary health care. Journal of Advanced Nursing 19(6): 918–925

Pritchard P, Pritchard J 1992 Developing teamwork in primary health care. A practical workbook. Oxford University Press, Oxford

Read R, Wallcraft J 1992 Guidelines for empowering users of mental health services. COHSE and Mind Publications, London

Richardson A 1991 Health promotion through self-help: the contribution of self-help groups. In: Badura B, Kickbush I (eds) Health promotion research: towards a new social epidemiology. World Health Organization, Regional Office for Europe, Copenhagen

Robison J, Wiles R 1993 Building teamwork: the value of the multidisciplinary meeting. Primary Care Management 3(11): 9–11

Ross F M 1986 Nursing old people in the community. In: Redfern S (ed) Nursing elderly people. Churchill Livingstone, Edinburgh

Royal College of Nursing 1992 Powerhouse for change: report of the task force on community nursing. RCN, London

Schutz W 1982 Profound simplicity. Bantam Books, New York

Stone M 1993 Lending an ear to the unheard: the role of support groups for siblings of children with cancer. Child Health 1(2): 54–58

Watt A, Rodmell S 1993 Community involvement in health promotion: progress or panacea? In: Beattie A, Gott M, Jones L, Sidell M (eds) Health and wellbeing: a reader. Macmillan, Basingstoke

Whittaker A 1990 Involving people with learning difficulties in meetings. In: Winn L (ed) Power to the people: the key to responsive services in health and social care. King's Fund Centre, London

World Health Organization 1978 Alma Ata declaration. WHO, Geneva

World Health Organization 1993 Health for all targets: the health policy for Europe, updated edn. WHO, Regional Office for Europe, Copenhagen

CHAPTER CONTENTS

Health education as 'freeing' 109

Types of learning 111
Cognitive learning 111
Affective learning 111
Psychomotor skill learning 113
Learning styles 113
A holistic approach 113
Empowerment 114

Motivation to learn 114
Maslow's hierarchy of needs 114
Learning from experience 115
The community development approach 116

Getting the message across 117
Process 118
Assessing needs 118
Planning 118
Implementation 119
Evaluation 122

References 122

Further reading 123

9

Education for health

Diana Forster

By the year 2000, accessible and effective education and training in health promotion should be available in all Member States, in order to improve public and professional competence in promoting health and increasing health awareness in other sectors.

(Target 15: Health competence, WHO 1993)

Health education is concerned with health as a quality of life. It is associated with five main components:

- social health—the ability to interact well with people and the environment; having satisfying interpersonal relationships
- mental health—the ability to learn; one's intellectual capabilities
- emotional health—the ability to control emotions so that one feels comfortable expressing them when appropriate and does express them appropriately; the ability not to express emotions when it is inappropriate to do so
- spiritual health—a belief in some unifying force; for some that will be nature, for others it will be scientific laws, and for others it will be a godlike force
- physical health—the ability to perform daily tasks without undue fatigue; biological integrity of the individual (Greenberg 1992).

HEALTH EDUCATION AS 'FREEING'

These five aspects of health need to be balanced and integrated with each other for a high level of 'wellness' to be present. The goal of health education may be defined as freeing people so that they may make health-related decisions based on their own needs and interests, as long as such decisions do not adversely affect others. The concept of health education as freeing is based on the assumption that people may be trapped and enslaved by factors such as low self-esteem, poor decision-making skills, a lack of social support and a sense of powerlessness. Other reasons for this lack of control are low levels of health-related knowledge and understanding and undeveloped problem-solving skills. Health education then, should be designed to remove these enslaving factors, helping people to understand the motives behind their behaviour more, feel better about themselves, clarify their values and thus feel freer to make informed decisions (Greenberg 1992).

The recent changes in NHS policy which are discussed in Chapter 3, the advent of Project 2000 in nursing education and the increasing public expectations about health have all contributed to the need for a greater emphasis on health education. Principles of adult education, such as:

- that clients work from their own experience
- that clients are able to choose how and what they learn

are fundamental to health education today, with its focus on helping people make choices for themselves.

The European target heading this chapter may be achieved by:

- making existing knowledge about health better known
- emphasising a wider range of lifestyle issues, including self-esteem, personal skills and social support

---

Activity 9.1

Identify some examples of groups and activities available in your home, college or work locality which would encourage people to develop decision-making, interpersonal and coping skills—for instance sports, social, educational and counselling activities and self-help groups.

- giving training and education in health promotion to all health professionals
- training other groups and disciplines to increase awareness of health promotion opportunities
- providing an effective infrastructure and adequate resources for implementing and coordinating health education programmes (WHO 1993).

Until recently, many health education programmes have provided information to people in the hope that they will change their behaviour in the light of knowledge about risks to their health. Now, more health education addresses the importance of self-esteem, personal skills and social support in developing healthy lifestyles. However, the particular needs, concerns and living patterns of children, young people, women, older people, those with physical, mental and learning disabilities and people from ethnic minority groups are not always considered in the health education material produced. Within a health promotion framework, the central aim of health education should be to build health competence among the whole population. Programmes are required which will empower people, helping them to develop and use their physical, mental and emotional capacities as much as possible. This can be achieved by strengthening decision-making skills, developing interpersonal relationships and improving coping strategies. People's options are thus widened, giving them more control over their lives.

Health educators need to be able to work with clients in various settings (see Ch. 11), communicating to people the process of making health-related decisions rather than telling them what their decisions ought to be. This approach is certainly more democratic than programming people like computers to behave in ways thought to be healthy, and then evaluating them on whether they carried out the recommendations (Greenberg 1992).

This chapter will introduce some theories of how people learn and are motivated to do so, and consider a sample of health education interventions which may be applied to individuals and groups.

TYPES OF LEARNING

Three types of learning have been described by learning theorists:

- cognitive
- affective
- psychomotor.

Cognitive learning

Cognitive learning is the process of thinking, knowing, and working with information which has been acquired. Also included within this domain are the processes of critical, creative and reflective thinking, decision-making and problem-solving.

For example, a health education programme developed with outpatients at a clinic for people with chronic mental illness focused on increasing cognitive knowledge about how:

- to maintain health and fitness
- to use and apply information about safety
- to prevent common health problems
- to gain access to health services which were required (Byrne et al 1994).

In any learning activity, the nature of the material to be learned should be considered as well as the abilities and characteristics of the learners themselves. For instance, older people affected by HIV or AIDS, or just wanting to know more about them, may require different efforts made to communicate with them than with younger people. They should be offered a choice of media to use for learning, perhaps being supplied with taped and videoed information as well as leaflets. One Asian HIV project produces information on music cassettes, often performed by older, traditional Asian musicians (Kaufmann 1993). The material should be organised in such a way that people are encouraged to learn and it is possible to assess whether the desired learning has taken place.

An important consideration is the level of learning planned. Bloom (1969) developed an ordered list or taxonomy of the various levels at which learning can happen, from the simplest to the most complex (see Box 9.1). These levels

> **Box 9.1 Levels of cognitive learning (adapted from Bloom 1969)**
>
> - Knowledge—simple knowledge of facts, concepts, terms, theories, etc.
> - Comprehension—an understanding of the meaning of this knowledge
> - Application—the ability to use this knowledge and comprehension in new situations
> - Analysis—the ability to separate out material into its different parts and to see relationships between ideas
> - Synthesis—the ability to form new patterns of thoughts and ideas and organise them into a meaningful 'whole'
> - Evaluation—judging or comparing ideas and concepts

of learning are useful to consider when planning health education interventions. For example, a nurse preparing a teaching plan should decide what the client *must* know and be able to do, and what it would be *helpful* for the client to know and be able to do. This distinction gives clues about what the level of learning should be. As the level of learning becomes more complex, then methods of learning need to involve the client more actively in applying and analysing the content.

Methods appropriate for developing cognitive information include lectures and lecturettes, reading assignments with study guides, audio-visual aids, interactive computer-supported learning, quizzes and self-paced programmed learning.

Affective learning

This is the aspect of learning which includes values (see Ch. 5) attitudes, beliefs and emotions (see Box 9.2).

Adults bring to their learning a store of established attitudes, thought patterns and fixed ways of doing things. This can help them to adapt to new situations. On the other hand, it may make it difficult for them to readjust attitudes, for instance to their own changing bodily functions and body image following sickness or injury (see Box 9.3). Health-related behaviour, such as changing eating or drinking habits and patterns,

---

Box 9.2 Attitudes and beliefs

An attitude may be defined as a predisposition to think, feel and act in a certain way towards some aspect of one's environment, including other people. Attitudes are learned, not innate, and may be changed as a result of knowledge and understanding, although attitudes are relatively enduring and not easily changed.

An attitude has three fundamental components:

- Cognitive—this is associated with the person's belief of what is true about the objects, people or events towards which the attitude is addressed
- Affective—this element refers to the feelings and emotions associated with a belief, which are called 'values'
- Behavioural—this component is the expression of a person's attitudes in their behaviour—a tendency towards action, which may indicate positive or negative tendencies.

Box 9.3 Altered self-image: the special kinds of problems faced by patients who are severely burned (Friedman & DiMatteo 1989)

Young women who lose their physical attractiveness because of severe burns tend to assume that they have also lost their sexual desirability. In spite of assurances from husbands or boyfriends, these women may be overwhelmed by the feeling that they are no longer attractive. Their response is to withdraw. Withdrawal from social contacts and close social relationships prevents such patients from re-establishing their identity.

---

is also dependent upon attitudes. Research shows, for example, that merely increasing people's knowledge about nutrition does not lead to changes in eating behaviour. Attitude change depends upon information being interpreted as relevant and favourable to the people concerned before they will act upon it. It is important for health educators to realise that they cannot 'instil' confidence or 'motivate' people. However, they can help participants themselves to build their own confidence and develop their willingness to change aspects of their behaviour which they think is relevant to them. The adolescent girl who wishes to change her diet requires control over which foods are available to her, as well as

support from family and friends. There also have to be the opportunities to put the new behaviour into practice (Stockley 1993). Changing people's attitudes towards healthy eating should be part of an approach which helps them to be self-empowered, through having relevant knowledge of both diet and how to influence government and local policies. Graham (1993) reports that mothers in her study found that smoking was a hard habit to break, although they knew about the health-related problems for themselves and their children. Living and caring in disadvantaged circumstances, such as inadequate housing and being in debt, meant that smokers clung to the support they felt their habit provided, and they graphically described smoking as a way of coping 'when life's a drag'.

The emotional state of learners will influence how they learn, and can help the learning process or, conversely, interfere with successful learning. Taking learners' emotional needs into consideration involves helping them to acknowledge and explore their own feelings. A relationship based on respect, empathy and genuineness, as discussed in Chapter 7, helps to develop an atmosphere of mutual trust and equality between teacher or facilitator and learner, making health choices more accessible. Educators need to be sensitive to the nature and magnitude of the behavioural changes that people may be expected to attempt. The changes in sexual behaviour some clients may need to make in order to avoid risking HIV infection can be very demanding and difficult for them. Information alone is not enough. The rapid changes towards safer sexual practices among gay men in large cities throughout the western world became possible only partly through increased understanding of the risks of unsafe sexual practices. A supportive social environment as part of community-based health promotion initiatives was necessary for individuals to change their behaviour (Anderson & Wilkie 1992).

Methods of teaching which may be successful in the affective domain include role play and group discussion and interaction, so that attitudes and beliefs can be explored in relation to other people, and feelings may be shared in a supportive environment (see Ch. 8).

Psychomotor skill learning

Skills may be learned and developed through practice once the necessary tasks and movements have been taught, as for example:

- breast self-examination
- self-injection
- self-catheterisation
- techniques of applying a dressing by carers
- safe use of condoms.

Suitable methods of teaching in this domain include demonstration (in person or on film), individual supervised practice and coaching (see Box 9.4).

Learning styles

Each of us has a preferred learning style. Those with an 'internal' style will prefer to discover

---

> **Activity 9.2**
>
> Consider your own most recent learning experiences. What styles of learning do you think are most successful for you?

---

information for themselves, discuss it with the health facilitator and others in their group or family and then make decisions or judgements themselves. Those with an 'external' style will probably wish to rely on information being given and will seek praise and positive feedback. Some people prefer to read, watch videos or be told factual information; some will want to work alone and some with other people. When designing health education programmes with smokers who wish to stop, plans will need to reflect whether clients would be most successful by stopping immediately, or by cutting down gradually, perhaps by smoking one cigarette less each day (Clarke 1992).

A holistic approach

A holistic approach to health education includes all three types of learning discussed—cognitive, affective and psychomotor. Emotional, social and spiritual aspects of health are as important as physical ones. Health education should be tailored carefully to the personal experience and social and cultural background of clients or groups. For instance, a day hospital activity programme for mentally ill clients living in the community incorporated holistic wellness, self-assessment skills, personal goals, and self-care. Clients were encouraged to set reasonable personal goals for each wellness topic, including:

- nutrition
- sexuality
- fitness
- consumer health
- managing harmful habits
- stress management.

This helped them to manage more successfully in the community, empowering them to make

---

> **Box 9.4   Breast self-examination (Stein 1987)**
>
> A programme developed for breast self-examination in Florida is described as follows:
>
> The woman learner, undressed to the waist, lies on a treatment table in a private room. She learns to use the flat part of her three middle fingertips moving them in three small half-circles applying light, medium and deep pressure at each spot. She then practises exercises on two specialised breast models. The first is to develop finger sensitivity for the feel of normal breast nodularity and the second is to experience the sensation of benign and malignant simulated lumps. She then transfers these skills to her own breast tissue. A third breast model is then selected which matches the woman's own breast firmness and nodularity and which contains simulated benign and malignant lumps. The woman then practises on the matched model and her own breast tissue which helps her to develop palpation skills to detect the differences between her own nodularity and a discrete lump. Feedback is an important component of this programme. The trainer observes all the procedures practised and makes corrective suggestions as needed. The woman then takes the matched model home with her and is encouraged to carry out breast self-examination each month.

choices and take responsibility for their health and lifestyle (Byrne et al 1994).

Empowerment

No-one can give power to another person but we can help people to retain and regain their own power. The Patients' Charter (DoH 1991), for instance, established the principle that every woman should have a named midwife, and that the mother and baby should be at the centre of all planning and provision of maternity care. The woman should be an active partner with health workers in making decisions affecting her care. Empowerment then, is an interactive process which helps others by sharing knowledge, expertise and resources. AIDS programmes for example need to take into account the social context of people's lives. When targeting specific groups of people it is important to look at and assist them with other health needs, for example by teaching self-treatment for common ailments. Basic sex education may be the first step towards building their self-confidence and understanding of AIDS and sexually transmitted diseases.

Through empowerment, people are more likely to become masters of their own health by being encouraged:

- to express their feelings
- to identify and set realistic goals for themselves as individuals, groups and communities
- to increase their knowledge and awareness of health issues
- to choose whether, and how, to develop life-skills which promote health (see Box 9.5)
- to seek to influence and change their environment.

This approach fits in with nursing's focus on:

- health as a basic resource for everyday living
- identifying and building on clients' strengths
- adapting programmes to fit a variety of needs
- joint decision-making with clients.

Health education in relation to such a concept of empowerment is very different from education which is designed to change behaviour so that patients become compliant and conform to treat-

---

> **Box 9.5 Examples of life-skills (adapted from Hopson & Scally 1980)**
>
> - Effective communication
> - Making and managing relationships
> - Managing conflict
> - Being assertive
> - Working in groups
> - Influencing others
> - Managing stress
> - Coping with life-changes

ment goals imposed upon them. It is, however, linked to Greenberg's (1992) notion of education as 'freeing' discussed earlier. Cribb (1993) raises the classic concern of possible manipulation:

Am I using the language and skills of 'self-empowerment' to try to make someone change their behaviour? Is that my real objective though it may be hidden (even from myself)? Am I treating someone with respect and encouraging their participation because this allows more subtle and possibly more effective forms of manipulation?

Empowered nurses

Studies show that if health education is to be facilitated in the hospital setting, nurses need to feel valued, supported, autonomous and empowered members of the ward team. This is more likely to happen in a climate of democratic ward management with primary or team nursing highlighted (Wilson-Barnett & Latter 1993). Such developments for health workers in the community can take place in multidisciplinary team-building and group activities (see Ch. 8). These activities help teams with an appropriate mix of professional skills to provide high-quality, cost-effective primary health care. Multidisciplinary audit empowers teams to set professional standards which they can use to evaluate their performance.

MOTIVATION TO LEARN

Maslow's hierarchy of needs

An important consideration for health educators was formulated by Maslow (1970), a psychologist who suggests that we are all driven by five motives. He ranks these areas of basic human need into a hierarchy as follows:

1. physiological needs
2. safety needs
3. belongingness and love needs
4. esteem needs
5. self-actualisation needs.

The most basic, physiological drives for necessities like food, water, sleep and oxygen provide the strongest motivation. For most people these must be satisfied before seeking to meet needs for safety from physical or psychological harm, at Maslow's second level. People with unmet safety needs may perceive the world as overwhelming, hostile or threatening, while those whose safety needs are met are likely to view their world as trustworthy and to be more self-directed and interested in others.

Emotional needs then come into consideration—the most fundamental of these is to feel loved and wanted and part of a group. Unmet love and belongingness needs lead to feelings of desolation, alienation and rejection. Not until this level of need is satisfied does a person seek to acquire self-esteem and the feeling of being valued by others (see Ch. 5). This is also the level at which people desire recognition of effort, independence, prestige and the ability to demonstrate competence. The highest level of fulfilment is self-actualisation, which includes self-expression, self-understanding and a sense of fulfilment of possible abilities and talents. This is similar to the concept of a fully empowered person. Generally, needs are satisfied and personal growth is facilitated by other people, through support, reassurance, acceptance, protection, love, willingness to listen, gentleness and kindness (Maslow 1970).

When applied to health education, Maslow's hierarchy would suggest that the more basic needs, including hunger, thirst, sexual needs, sleep and relaxation, must be met before learning can take place. However, such claims have been exposed to forceful criticisms. Tennant (1988) argues that this is patently untrue. If it were so, people who suffered deprivation of physiological and safety needs would not move on to learn and develop, while those raised in comparative luxury would become more creative and original

personalities. Facts do not bear this out; people do not feel compelled to attend to safety needs before pursuing love and belongingness, and danger can spur people on. Research does, however, indicate that satisfactory learning is not likely to happen without sufficient motivation to learn. People learn best when:

- they feel secure and can try out things in safety
- their needs are being met in ways that they can see are relevant and appropriate
- they know what they have to do; especially when they have been involved in setting their own goals
- they are actively involved and engaged
- they know how well they are doing
- they see and experience that they are welcomed and respected as individuals in their own right (Daines et al 1992).

Taking account of these aspects of motivating people to learn helps to reduce their levels of stress. The person undergoing any change process, such as learning, is likely to feel stress and confusion. A certain amount of anxiety can increase motivation to learn, but too much may cause fatigue, loss of concentration, feelings of resentment and other possible barriers to learning (Edelman & Mandle 1994).

Learning from experience

It is meaningless to talk about learning in isolation from experience. Learning can only take place if the experience of the learner becomes part of the process (Boud et al 1993). As little time as possible should be spent on passive tasks such as reading and listening, and as much as possible on active participation, or experiential learning. Macleod Clark & Dines (1993) found that encouraging patients to participate fully in programmes to help them stop smoking was a hallmark of success. Results were better than when patients merely received advice.

Learning always relates to what has gone before. New ideas and new experiences link to previous experience and, through this, sense may be made of what is learned (Boud et al 1993). How people go about the task of learning depends upon how they have responded in the past. Earlier experiences may have encouraged taking the risks of responding to new opportunities, or on the other hand may have had an inhibiting effect. If expressing their own interests and learning needs has not been encouraged before, and their own knowledge, expertise and opinions have not been taken into account, then people may find experiential learning more challenging. Time then needs to be devoted early in the learning scheme to introducing and discussing different styles of learning and teaching and encouraging people to express concerns, emotions and ideas.

Reflection

Experience alone is not enough to ensure that learning takes place. New experience has to be made sense of by reflecting and thinking about past experience. Reflection may be carried out individually, when someone thinks through the process of integrating old and new experiences and looking ahead to future events. One useful tool which Burnard (1992) suggests is the use of a learning diary. Reflecting on what we do involves consciously noticing thoughts, feelings and changing attitudes as new skills are carried out. The diary can aid reflection on the process of change and review progress in 'learning through doing'. Such a diary of course remains private to the individual learner. Reflection may also be a group process, when sense is made of experiences through group discussion. For reflection as a

---

Activity 9.3

Plan a reflective process for yourself:

- Preparation—anticipate an activity in which you will be taking part and think in advance about what you might learn from the experience.
- Experience—engage in the activity, noticing your behaviour, thoughts and feelings, other people and the environment you are in. This is reflection in action.
- Reflective process—return in your thoughts to the experience, attending to feelings particularly, and re-evaluate the experience, planning how to apply your new perspectives in future.

---

group activity to be successful, the group leader is required to act as a facilitator. Skills of group facilitation are discussed in Chapter 8. In a reflective group, the facilitator encourages members to explore the meanings and explanations of experiences for themselves, without imposing her own views and interpretations. This reflection on past experiences helps people to plan for future events, for example changing social activities to reduce alcohol consumption. It also focuses attention on the emotional aspects of people's experiences, and therefore fits into the affective domain of learning discussed earlier.

The community development approach

At the level of promoting community involvement in health, Brearley (1990) notes that people have not always been encouraged to think and choose for themselves. Many World Health Organization initiatives for community participation have been ineffective, partly because people are so used to solutions being imposed upon them by experts that they are reluctant to become actively involved themselves. One example of people becoming active participants in health education initiatives is described by Barker (1994). He visited the Collaborative Support Programs of New Jersey (CSPNJ) in the north-east USA. The state is slightly smaller than Scotland but has almost 1 million more inhabitants, with a population of about 6 million. CSPNJ is a consumer-run, non-profit-making mental health agency representing over 89 000 adults with a serious mental illness who previously used, or are currently using, mental health services. CSPNJ has become a national leader in the development of consumer programmes. Health education aspects include:

- advocacy training
- practical coping skills
- symptom management
- peer support skills.

This focus on identifying and developing personal strengths and abilities—the core elements of empowerment—fit into wider health promotion activities which include supported housing schemes. Barker (1994) explains that each person's experience of mental illness is regarded as a tool and a skill which can be developed. The underpinning belief is that people with mental illness should have the opportunity to live, work, learn and socialise in homes and communities of their own choice.

Health-oriented health education programmes should be planned according to opportunities identified within a community (Downie et al 1990). These programmes may be designed for individuals or collections of people within the community. Such an approach avoids the possible negative focus of trying to persuade people to stop smoking, reduce their alcohol intake or make other changes in lifestyle to avoid becoming sick sometime in the future, which is not usually effective, as discussed earlier. Taking measures to improve one's health usually involves effort (e.g. exercise) or giving up some pleasurable activity such as smoking or eating sweet food. It is hard to forego short-term satisfaction to prevent long-term consequences which may never happen. A holistic, life-context format for health education is more likely to be sensitive to the needs of particular individuals in their community setting. Rotherham community development strategy described in Chapter 5 (Box 5.5, p. 62) is an example of this.

The community development approach is concerned with helping people to re-examine critically the society they are in, to understand ways in which various political and administrative systems work, and to acquire skills in self-organisation and more specific skills relevant to self-chosen topics. This approach to health promotion planning dovetails specific preventive services such as screening and immunisation and health protection measures, for instance promoting adequate housing, with health education programmes. Such planning may occur at the level of a relatively large community like a Scottish health board area or an English health district, or on the scale of smaller geographical patches (Downie et al 1990). Health education programmes planned in this context avoid the tendency for many separate initiatives devoted to single topics, such as preventing dental disease or heart disease, springing up in isolation from one another and having little impact on the community as a whole.

The positive focus goes beyond 'medical' risk factors in an individual's lifestyle towards a holistic view of health and its determinants, as shown in the New Jersey mental health initiatives discussed earlier. People's own health concerns are based on wider issues than just preventing disease. They may feel unable to concentrate on changing health-related behaviour because of external factors which include:

- poverty
- poor housing
- social stress
- lack of access to leisure and leisure facilities

and a general lack of power over their lives, as Graham (1993) found in the study discussed earlier.

People in the study group knew about the main health problems caused by their smoking, and understood a great deal about the effects of health-damaging behaviour. No difference was found in knowledge between the ethnic minorities and the white majority. The circumstances of people's daily lives are thus once more shown to be highly relevant concerns in health education. 'Health promotion works through effective community action. At the heart of this process are communities having their own power and having control of their own initiatives. ... Health promotion supports personal and social development through providing information, education for health and helping develop the skills which they need to make healthy choices.' (Ashton & Seymour 1988).

GETTING THE MESSAGE ACROSS

General principles for teaching and learning in health education include the consideration of:

- the aims of the intervention (the WHY)
- the audience (the WHO)
- the content (the WHAT)
- the learning method (the HOW)
- the learning environment (the WHERE).

Process

The steps of the teaching process—assess, plan, implement and evaluate—are similar to those of the nursing process; both are circular, with ongoing assessment and evaluation constantly redirecting the planning and teaching.

Assessing needs

The decision to carry out some form of health education, as previously discussed, rests on the identification of a *need* to do so. A need may be identified for people with diabetes to be enabled to prevent complications by maintaining as near normal blood glucose levels as possible. This would involve balancing their diet with insulin or tablets and making adjustments for the effects of exercise, stress and illness. Planning to meet such an educational need would require the health professional to be an educator, motivator and supporter, helping clients to undertake good self-care, in the key setting of a health centre or hospital.

A midwife might identify the need for a discussion group where:

- prospective parents could explore their anxieties about labour and birth
- realistic expectations of labour and birth could be promoted
- information about pain relief, hospital procedures and the course of labour and birth may be provided (Braun & Schonveld 1993).

A health visitor may use local statistics to identify the need to reduce unacceptably high rates of road traffic accidents in children. This would perhaps lead to an attempt to raise the consciousness of local families by taking a community action, non-victim-blaming approach to improving road safety. The safe management of traffic, particularly concerning speed regulation, is as vital as training adults and children how to cross roads.

Planning

Having identified needs, the key to the success of any health teaching activity is effective planning and preparation. To begin with, overall aims should be established. Aims are general statements which indicate the overall purpose of an individual session, course or programme. They are usually expressed in general terms, for example:

- to improve understanding, general skills or physical coordination
- to modify attitudes, beliefs or standards
- to impart information, knowledge or ideas
- to stimulate action
- to encourage changes in behaviour (Daines et al 1992).

Clients, patients or groups should be involved as much as possible in deciding upon aims, or goal-setting as it is sometimes called. Participants can then identify their own health and well-being needs and share responsibility for the successful outcome of learning activities. In a study described by Brearley (1990), patients who took part in writing goal-planning statements with their nurses made greater progress than control patients. However, further research may be needed to find out whether goals are more appropriate if patients participate in setting them, if the patients are more motivated because they are involved, if nurses are more motivated to help these patients achieve their goals or whether the results depend upon all these factors.

A patient who has recently experienced a cerebrovascular accident may not be able initially to be actively involved in setting goals. As the condition improves, however, involvement can increase, with nurses providing information and encouragement in setting goals relevant to the patient's expressed needs.

Objectives

Aims can be further broken down into specific objectives. 'An objective is a description of a performance you want learners to exhibit before you consider them competent' (Mager 1990). An objective describes an intended result of health teaching rather than the processes of teaching and learning. Objectives should be realistic, achievable and able to be measured and evaluated. They may be designed according to the three types of learning discussed earlier.

Cognitive objectives are those to do with increasing the learner's knowledge. Those in the affective domain are concerned with how people feel: their attitudes, beliefs, values and emotions. The self-empowerment approach to objectives involves helping people to think critically about their values and beliefs and to examine and perhaps challenge their own attitudes. For instance, the attitude of some women towards protecting themselves from contracting HIV and taking a positive approach to safer sex can be affected by fears of being rejected or humiliated by their partner.

Psychomotor objectives are related to learning skills and ways of carrying out actions, such as administering a child's eyedrops or changing a dressing. Skills are also required in coping with new situations including childbirth, bereavement or unemployment. Ley (1988) discusses objectives for the exact medication-related behaviour which a patient would need to exhibit if using the medication properly—see Box 9.6.

A simple written plan outlining the medication regime may help patients to achieve these objec-tives. Gooch (1990) developed a useful plan which includes the use of symbols for patients who cannot read.

Strategies for accomplishing aims and objectives

When deciding how to facilitate learning, the health educator should choose methods and materials appropriate for achieving the selected aims and objectives, such as the medication plan discussed above. A session plan is the teacher's practical working document and contains a selection from:

- date and time of session
- venue and room
- type of group and what they already know
- number in group; seating plan
- topic
- aims and objectives
- learning resources, e.g. overhead projector, flip chart, whiteboard, blackboard, slides, nursing equipment
- arrangement of environment
- session timing, content and methods
- evaluation.

A community approach, such as to the promo-tion of healthier eating, would need to coordinate and manage action at local and national levels. Possible strategic aims for such an approach are suggested by Stockley (1993)—see Box 9.7.

Implementation

Methods

An imaginative combination of methods is likely

Box 9.6 Objectives example: main categories of behaviour for patient to take medication for maximum benefit (Hermann et al 1978)

- To know how to take the drug:
  —to take a specific dose
  —to take a dose in a specific manner (e.g. with meals)
  —to take a dose at a specific time
- To know how to store the drug:
  —to store it properly
  —to recognise the time at which the medicine becomes subpotent
- To know how the drug is expected to help:
  —to recall the basic facts about the complaint
  —to recognise the desired effect and act upon its absence
- To recognise problems caused by the drug:
  —to recognise unwanted effects if they do occur
  —to recall that certain effects can only be detected by clinical examination or tests
  —to recall circumstances indicating a need for change of treatment and act if they occur
- To verify components of the medicine
- To act if overdosage occurs

Box 9.7 Possible strategic aims for national and local alliances (adapted from Stockley 1993)

To ensure that by the year 2005 people are more knowledgeable, better motivated, and more able to acquire and maintain healthy eating patterns, by enjoying a variety of foods; consuming the amount needed to achieve and maintain a healthy body weight; and consuming amounts of fat, fibre, starch, salt and sugar which are recommended for health.

to be more effective than any one used alone; a variety will help to maintain people's interest and motivation. Learning will be helped by clients taking part in a range of activities through listening, looking, talking and doing.

Talks, lectures and presentations

Talks and lectures are an efficient way of presenting health-related information and ideas within a specific period of time, to a number of people. The audience should be challenged to choose, judge and manipulate ideas rather than just listen passively, so that they may be actively involved in the learning process. Careful preparation is required so that clarity and interest are maintained in both the material and its presentation. It is generally best to give a talk from notes written on paper or cards (Ewles & Simnett 1992).

A straightforward, logical approach may be based on:

- an opening
- a set of key points
- a summary.

Participative activities should be built into the presentation using well-prepared learning resources and visual aids. A common mistake is to attempt too much. Ewles & Simnett (1992) emphasise that three or four key points are enough in one teaching session—teaching more does not mean that people learn more, but that they forget more.

Introducing the talk. The opening should gain and hold attention from the start, motivating learners to stay interested, and briefly explaining the aims of the presentation. Suggestions for starters include:

- a relevant anecdote
- a thought-provoking question
- a reference to, or a request for, listeners' experiences
- a picture or other visual image.

Key points. Arranged in logical order, these should begin with a brief explanation of what is to follow. Key points should have signposts to indicate structure and direction, e.g. 'I'd like to

talk about the measles, mumps and rubella immunisation: firstly, at what age it is usually offered; secondly, why it is of benefit; and thirdly, some practical points about what to expect when it is given; and then we can discuss any points you raise.'

Linking sentences help to join parts of the talk together, and main points may be emphasised by repeating them in a different way or going over them again. Participation can be encouraged by planning a buzz group, brainstorm, small-group discussion followed by a reporting-back session, a video or other audiovisual aids. A time for questions should also be allowed for. These group activities are considered more fully later.

The last few minutes of the session can be used:

- to summarise the main points
- to help people consolidate and value what they have achieved
- to motivate them to continue with their learning
- to find out what participants thought about the session—perhaps by distributing a questionnaire.

Demonstration

People learn best from a combination of seeing, hearing and doing. When teaching someone to perform a skill, the activity should be broken down into basic steps or movements, and as each step is carried out the demonstrator should clearly explain the actions. The stages should be:

1. State the activity involved and its purpose or outcomes.
2. Arouse and maintain the learners' interest.
3. Reveal the main steps of the activity and identify likely problem areas.
4. Inspire confidence in learners so that they themselves will be willing to try.
5. Enable learners to undertake individual practice afterwards and receive feedback about their performance. (Daines et al 1992).

Verbal and nonverbal communication skills are most important in ensuring that the process being taught is clearly heard and thoroughly understood (see Ch. 7). Interpersonal skills are also needed so that confidence can be inspired in the learners, and questions and points of uncertainty dealt with. It is necessary to check that people understand each stage of the activity and how it fits into the whole demonstration. Finally, a discussion which gives encouragement to people to try for themselves leads into:

Individual practice, support and supervision. The amount of practice needed varies with the complexity of the task, and the capabilities, physical limitations and past experiences of the learner. Most children love to practise, but adults may lose interest and motivation if they are not immediately successful and if the skill requires a great deal of practice. If there is a high degree of precision needed, more frequent rest periods are required. Learning to give oneself an injection or to perform self-catheterisation will probably take many practice periods. During practice, feedback about the correctness of the performance is crucial so that modifications can be made (refer back to Box 9.4, p. 113).

Learning in groups

A working knowledge of group process is helpful for the teacher, leader or facilitator (see Ch. 8).

The principles of learning discussed in this chapter apply whether an educational activity is planned for an individual or a group. Being part of a group satisfies people's need for feeling safe and favourably regarded, and for giving and receiving attention. Attitudes may be reconsidered and modified in a supportive atmosphere and new skills can be developed and practised. More varied and more stimulating ideas can be produced in a group than by individuals working alone. Teaching plans should provide opportunities for group members to learn and develop through their interaction with each other. Larger

---

Activity 9.4

Plan a learning programme for a client, patient or friend designed to teach him or her a particular skill.

---

groups may be divided into smaller units of six to eight people, which generally allows interaction between all members to happen. In a diabetic clinic, for example, clients may learn about food exchanges and how to administer an injection of insulin. It is common for teaching in health care settings to be directed to families or small groups of clients or patients.

Groupwork with learning-disabled adults. Groupwork is not commonly used with people with severe learning disabilities. However, Rushton (1994) carried out a research study to find out if an existing project to present socio-sexual education, using groupwork, to learning-disabled adults was in fact effective. The overall aims of the workshops studied were:

- to improve the social functioning of the participants
- to increase the amount of socio-sexual knowledge of the participants
- to increase the participants' knowledge of appropriate socio-sexual behaviour.

The study's findings were that social functioning skills did improve as a result of participating in the workshops, while the control group showed no change over the same period. Skills relating to friendships, conversation, listening and relating to others showed the greatest improvement. Gains in socio-sexual knowledge and to a lesser extent in socio-sexual behaviour were also demonstrated.

Getting the environment right in group settings. To facilitate a free flow of ideas, chairs should be arranged in an informal way—a close U-shape or a circle with gaps to allow movement in and out. Everyone should be able to see everyone else in the group easily and be able to converse with them without having to change position. The temperature and lighting of the room should be checked to be certain that neither is uncomfortable or distracting.

Materials on aspects of health such as videos, leaflets, tapes and slides may be used to stimulate group discussion. All equipment should be carefully checked beforehand to make sure it is in working order. The group size should be limited to about six to eight people for effective interaction to take place in a learning situation. Larger groups may be divided into smaller ones for discussions to be held, or for other activities such as:

- Buzz groups—pairs or trios discuss a short question or topic briefly—a useful way to involve people which can be fun and 'punchy'.
- Role play—short, spontaneous acting out of situations; group members play specific roles, but may of course opt out if they wish. Plenty of time should be allowed for debriefing afterwards.
- Brainstorming—leader asks for a list of ideas, proposals and suggestions related to a particular theme to be called out and recorded on a flip chart. This provides the basis for discussion to follow. Every contribution has equal value, people are encouraged to produce ideas quickly and no comments or judgements of contributions are made.

Evaluation

Any health education intervention needs to be evaluated so that its effect on participants may be determined. Evaluation also makes it possible to

---

Activity 9.5

Reflect upon a group activity you have recently been involved in, as either a participant or facilitator. What were the main positive, successful aspects of the group's interactions? Consider how the environment or activities might have been improved to meet members' needs more fully than they were.

---

modify aims and objectives to meet participants' needs more effectively. It can provide justification for the programme to be continued or repeated. Evaluation, as the final step in the teaching programme, also restarts the teaching process, providing direction for changes and modifications in the assessing–planning–implementing–evaluation cycle. However, evaluation is part of the ongoing learning and teaching process, not just the final point, and it should involve learners and facilitators or teachers alike. The terms 'process' or 'formative' are applied to evaluation used as a continuous check or process of feedback throughout the programme of learning. Am I talking too fast? Is the environment too distracting? Am I making my points clear? These are examples of questions which may be answered by self-evaluation as the session progresses or by requesting feedback from participants. Peer evaluation may also be helpful in pinpointing strengths and weaknesses in teaching (Whitman et al 1992). Process evaluation is used to check if objectives are being met during the learning process. Outcome evaluation is a measure of whether objectives have been met at the end of the learning process, by the use of questionnaires for example, or by observing changes in knowledge, skills and attitudes or behavioural changes. Written tests, check lists, interviews, observations and health records are examples of tools to measure outcome evaluation.

Evaluation of health education interventions helps to determine how well the objectives have been achieved, and the goal of health education research is to identify the most efficient, cost-effective and feasible way of achieving these objectives.

REFERENCES

Anderson C, Wilkie P (eds) 1992 Reflective helping in HIV and AIDS. Open University Press, Milton Keynes
Ashton J, Seymour H 1988 The new public health. Open University Press, Milton Keynes
Barker P 1994 Inspired to alternatives. Nursing Times 90(31): 59–60
Bloom B 1969 Taxonomy of educational objectives. Longman-Green, New York
Boud D, Cohen R, Walker D (eds) 1993 Using experience for

learning. The Society for Research into Higher Education & Open University Press, Milton Keynes
Braun D, Schonveld A 1993 Approaching parenthood: a resource for parent education. Health Education Authority, London
Brearley S 1990 Patient participation: the literature. Scutari, London
Burnard P 1992 Know yourself! Self awareness activities for nurses. Scutari, London

Byrne C, Brown B, Voorberg N, Schofield R 1994 Wellness education for individuals with chronic mental illness living in the community. Issues in Mental Health Nursing 15(3): 239–252

Clarke J 1992 Motivation can prolong life expectancy: a health education programme to help people give up smoking. In: Horne E M, Cowan T (eds) Effective communication: some nursing perspectives, 2nd edn. Wolfe Publishing, London

Cribb A 1993 Health promotion—a human science. In: Wilson-Barnett J, Macleod Clark J (eds) Research in health promotion and nursing. Macmillan, Basingstoke

Daines J, Daines C, Graham B 1992 Adult learning. Adult teaching. University of Nottingham, Nottingham

Department of Health 1991 The Patients' Charter. Department of Health, London

Downie R S, Fyfe C, Tannahill A 1990 Health promotion: models and values. Oxford University Press, Oxford

Edelman C L, Mandle C L 1994 Health promotion throughout the lifespan, 3rd edn. Mosby, St Louis

Ewles L, Simnett I 1992 Promoting health: a practical guide, 2nd edn. Scutari, London

Friedman H S, DiMatteo M R 1989 Health psychology. Prentice Hall, Englewood Cliffs NJ

Gooch J 1990 Medication to take home. In: Professional nurse: patient education plus. Austen Cornish, London

Graham H 1993 When life's a drag: women, smoking and disadvantage. HMSO, London

Greenberg J S 1992 Health education: learner-centred instructional strategies, 2nd edn. Brown, Iowa USA

Hermann F, Herxheimer S, Lionel N D W 1978 Package inserts for prescribed medicines: what minimum information do patients need? British Medical Journal 2: 1132–1135

Hopson B, Scally M 1980 Lifeskills teaching: education for self-empowerment. McGraw-Hill, London

Kaufmann T 1993 A crisis of silence: HIV, AIDS and older people. Age Concern, London

Ley P 1988 Communicating with patients. Croom Helm, London

Macleod Clark J, Dines A 1993 Case studies of health promotion with adults: nurses working with people who wish to stop smoking. In: Dines A, Cribb A (eds) Health promotion concepts and practice. Blackwell Scientific Publications, Oxford

Mager R F 1990 Preparing instructional objectives, 2nd edn. Kogan Page, London

Maslow A 1970 Motivation and personality. Harper & Row, New York

Rushton J 1994 Learning together. Nursing Times 90(9): 44–46

Stein G H 1987 The value of breast self-examination: myth or fact? In: Hobbs P (ed) Public education about cancer. Hans Huber, Toronto

Stockley L 1993 The promotion of healthier eating: a basis for action. Health Education Authority, London

Tennant M 1988 Psychology and adult learning. Routledge, London

Whitman N I, Graham B A, Gleit C J, Boyd M D 1992 Teaching in nursing practice. A professional model, 2nd edn. Appleton & Lange, Norwalk CT

Wilson-Barnett J, Latter S 1993 Factors influencing nurses' health education and health promotion practice in acute ward areas. In: Wilson-Barnett J, Macleod Clark J (eds) Research in health promotion and nursing. Macmillan, Basingstoke

World Health Organization 1993 Health for all targets: the health policy for Europe, updated edn. WHO Regional Office for Europe, Copenhagen

FURTHER READING

Boud D, Cohen R, Walker D (eds) 1993 Using experience for learning. The Society for Research into Higher Education & Open University Press, Milton Keynes

Dines A, Cribb A (eds) 1993 Health promotion concepts and practice. Blackwell Scientific Publications, Oxford

Ewles L, Simnett I 1992 Promoting health: a practical guide, 2nd edn. Scutari, London

Kiger A 1995 Teaching for health: the nurse as health educator, 2nd edn. Churchill Livingstone, Edinburgh

Webb P (ed) 1994 Health promotion and patient education: a professional's guide. Chapman & Hall, London

Whitehead M, Tones K 1990 Avoiding the pitfalls. Health Education Authority, London

Wilson-Barnett J, Macleod Clark J (eds) 1993 Research in health promotion and nursing. Macmillan, Basingstoke

CHAPTER CONTENTS

Introduction   125

Infancy and childhood   126
Prenatal care   126
Antenatal screening   126
Infancy   127
Surveillance   127
Childhood   127
Nutrition   128
Preventing childhood accidents   128
Promoting exercise   129

Adolescence   129
Aspects of cognitive development   130
Social and identity changes   130
Patterns of risky behaviour   131
Drug and alcohol abuse   131
Homelessness   132
Meeting growing nutritional demands   132

Health promotion in adulthood   133
Coronary heart disease and stroke   133
Mental health promotion and quality of life   134
Cancers   134
Accidents   135
HIV/AIDS and sexual health   136

Health promotion in later life   136
Patient education   137
Prevention in later life   137
Emotional and sexual needs   137
Mortality and risk factors   137
Older people and work   138
HIV, AIDS and older people   139
Ageism   139

References   139

Further reading   140

10

A life-cycle approach to health promotion

Diana Forster

By the year 2000, there should be continuous efforts in all Member States to actively promote and support healthy patterns of living through balanced nutrition, appropriate physical activity, healthy sexuality, good stress management and other aspects of positive health behaviour.

(Target 16: Healthy living, WHO 1993)

INTRODUCTION

The WHO target at the head of this chapter may best be achieved by taking a holistic approach to promoting healthy patterns of living throughout life, which is discussed in Chapter 1 and includes:

- increasing health and environmental awareness
- developing and strengthening coping skills
- promoting healthy eating patterns based on recommended nutrient standards and dietary guidelines
- promoting healthy physical and other leisure activities
- encouraging the giving and receiving of social support (WHO 1993).

However, this approach needs to be based on the foundation of health-promoting public policy (see Ch. 3). Efforts to achieve healthy settings for living in the city, at home, in the workplace and at school should underpin health promotion strategy. Such efforts require collaboration between community health and family health services (i.e. primary care) and community health and social services (i.e. community care). Health education is the process which creates the public awareness and support needed to maintain healthy settings, involving many different agencies, and to help change lifestyles and behaviours when this is desired. If professional intervention in community settings is to be successful it must be integrated with users' lifestyles and reflect their value systems, as discussed in Chapter 5. Traditionally, services have failed to reflect the diversity of needs, interests and values within the population as a whole.

The basic point of health education and health promotion is to lay the foundations for self-development in a world of complicated inter-connections. Work for health is essentially an enabling process, concerned with making choices available to people. It is a question of providing the appropriate foundations for health by removing obstacles and providing the basic means by which biological and chosen goals can be achieved (Seedhouse 1986). This chapter introduces some of the many issues relating to health promotion at different stages of life.

INFANCY AND CHILDHOOD

Prenatal care

The way in which a couple prepare themselves for conception and pregnancy can directly affect the health of the unborn infant. Pre-conceptual health promotion and pregnancy care are usually offered by the primary health care team, especially community midwives and health visitors, backed up by other health care workers. The pregnant woman should have the right to choose which professional (whether midwife, GP or other) is to be her initial point of contact with, and introduction to, the health care system. She should be able to participate, and have the ultimate say, in all decisions relating to the manner of her care, and be entitled to carry her own case-notes before and after birth (Silverton 1993). Early, ongoing monitoring and prenatal care should be available in order to promote the health of mother and baby, and detect any signs

---

> **Activity 10.1**
>
> Identify voluntary and health service groups or sessions available for preparation for childbirth in your locality. Consider whether you think these are publicised enough, and if the venues and times are likely to be appropriate for local parents-to-be.
>   How might improvements to the services on offer be brought about?

of complications. Parents can be helped to understand the nutritional needs of the pregnant woman, the benefits of appropriate exercise, and the possible adverse effects of cigarette smoking, alcohol and drugs on the fetus, to enable them to make healthy choices in preparing for the birth. The importance of avoiding certain infectious and toxic agents, such as the rubella virus early in pregnancy, sometimes associated with birth defects, needs to be emphasised. Preparation for parenthood classes and groups, where stimulating and informative discussions are held, where questions can be answered and anxieties, thoughts and feelings shared and birth plans developed, are a vital aspect of primary health promotion.

Antenatal screening

Antenatal screening, counselling and support are the right of all pregnant women. Also important is the need to develop community genetic services, involving population screening, counselling before, during or after pregnancy and the management of possible abortion for fetal abnormality. Within multi-ethnic Britain this is particularly important for women with such diseases as thalassaemia and sickle cell disease (SCD). In Britain today, SCD occurs in 1 in 400 people of Afro-Caribbean origin, and its carrier state, sickle cell trait, occurs in 1 in 10. Genetic counselling by an experienced counsellor is most important; however, Anionwu (1993) has found that despite the vast amount of knowledge about the condition available in the scientific literature, there is a lack of awareness among health professionals and therefore among families affected. This results in couples being denied the opportunity to even discuss the implications in relation to their family's health and well-being.

Women with other conditions such as epilepsy, diabetes, sensory impairment or learning disabilities are examples of those who also need specialised health promotion and care during pregnancy, childbirth and afterwards.

Newcastle's community midwifery care project

This project was an attempt to assess the impact of giving enhanced midwifery care to women at risk because of their socioeconomic situation, in an area with high levels of long-term unemployment. Midwives tackled the underlying problems relating to health, providing care and individual health education for mothers who were likely to smoke, have poor diets and take little exercise. Receiving enhanced care affected the experience of childbirth; women felt more confident and less pain relief was used. Continuity of care and accessibility of staff were central to the concept of enhanced care, with mothers emerging from giving birth with more confidence in their coping skills (Davies 1993).

Infancy

Promoting health during infancy is an important aspect of primary health care, with the community midwife and health visitor taking leading roles in partnership with parents. Healthy infant feeding, promoting breast feeding where possible and desired by the mother, and supporting the mental and physical health of the mother are vital concerns (Robertson 1991).

Surveillance

All infants and children should have access to the surveillance programme which includes:

- oversight of their physical, social and emotional development
- monitoring of developmental progress
- arranging intervention when necessary
- prevention of disease through immunisation.

Primary health care workers should be part-

ners with parents in promoting children's health and well-being, sharing health records and discussing needs and any interventions which become necessary. Children with special needs, those of travelling families and homeless people, and children of armed forces personnel may sometimes require particular efforts to ensure that the network of services is available for them.

Childhood

Perhaps more than any other stage of life, childhood has a profound impact on health. Children acquire many habits which may influence their health status throughout life, bringing benefit or harm. There is therefore great scope for health promotion, including health education. Parents and teachers, as well as health workers and carers, can be encouraged to learn how to help children make healthy life choices. Parents and teachers can role play with children significant issues such as refusing to accompany strangers, or being able to stand up to peer pressure to smoke or experiment with harmful substances. Available evidence suggests that only a small proportion of young people regularly misuse drugs; however, that number increases with age, so health education should begin in early childhood and be returned to regularly. Parents can cooperate with schools at the primary stage for instance in reinforcing appropriate parts of the National Curriculum, an example of which is given in Box 10.1.

Parental input has become more important recently as the implementation of the National Curriculum leaves less time for health education sessions. The need for carefully planned and evaluated health education is illustrated by Prendergast (1992) who found that 1 in 10 girls reported having no knowledge of the menarche before their first period, and 10% of girls begin their periods while at primary school. On the other hand, research shows that children have a wider knowledge of sexuality than is sometimes expected (Goldman & Goldman 1982). Pre-adolescents were aware of divorce, homosexuality, rape, child abuse, pornography and prostitution, partly through the wide media coverage these subjects receive.

Box 10.1 Requirements of the National Curriculum Science Order (1990)

- Pupils aged 5–7 to be 'introduced to ideas about how they keep healthy ... and to the role of drugs as medicines'.
- Pupils aged 7–11 to be 'introduced to the fact that while all medicines are drugs, not all drugs are medicines'. They should also 'begin to be aware of the harmful effect on health resulting from an abuse of tobacco, alcohol and other drugs' (National Curriculum Council 1990).

Parents can be encouraged to reinforce this information, which is usually given in the context of education about healthy living, linked with work on the human body and safety in the home and the environment generally.

Nutrition

Eating habits are usually established during childhood; parents can be encouraged to promote their child's growth and development through healthy eating. They can also be invited to join alliances which seek to provide health-promoting schools for their children, where a healthy diet is one of the policies (see Ch. 11). Health promoters may need to clear up misconceptions and myths about healthy foods, partly because of past information and food recommendations. Because a child needs protein and calcium for growth, parents were once encouraged to provide plenty of eggs, cheese, meat, whole milk and ice-cream in the diet. Research has since shown that such a high-cholesterol, high-fat diet increases the risks of atherosclerosis, so low-fat alternatives including lean meat, poultry, fish, skimmed milk and vegetable sources of protein should be offered. When children are in hospital, familiar and acceptable foods can be comforting and helpful in promoting an adequate diet. If health workers are aware of their child patients' cultural and family eating practices they can encourage healthy eating patterns.

Children need help in resisting the temptations of media advertising—particularly television. One dentist, whose children used to chorus a song advertising a chocolate bar, 'a bar a day helps you work, rest and play', taught them to sing to their friends instead: 'a bar a day helps your teeth rot away'.

Preventing childhood accidents

Each year, many children die or are injured as a result of road traffic accidents, home accidents, drowning, fires and poisoning. One of the main 'Health of the Nation' targets is to reduce the death rate for accidents among children aged under 15 by at least 33% by the year 2005 (DoH 1992). Road vehicle accidents are the main cause of death in males aged between 1 and 14 years, accounting for 18% of deaths in this age group (DoH 1994). Measures to keep children safe on the roads and inside vehicles are of paramount importance. Before school age most fatal accidents occur in the home, where children spend much of their time. Almost half of accidental deaths in the home are the result of fires. In the search for health needs, the health worker should be aware of particular risk factors, such as the fire risks for people in temporary accommodation who may have no option but to use unsafe heaters without adequate fireguards. A safety equipment loan scheme set up by health visitors and run by parents themselves is described by Wright (1994). Such projects may be seen as the first step in a safety awareness programme, strengthening working relationships among:

- local authorities
- health authorities
- voluntary and commercial agencies approached for financial help
- parents themselves.

Their common aim in forming an alliance is to promote the safety of children.

Children should be taught how to swim and where it is safe to swim, and how to enjoy bicycles, skates, swings and a variety of other recreational activities in safety, using helmets and other recommended equipment. Displays illustrating the types of safety equipment available have been developed for use in health centres, libraries, community centres and GP practices in one inner London Health Authority, and child accident prevention exhibitions are held at public

---

Activity 10.2

Arrange a visit to your local health promotion unit and ask what safety campaigns or other health promotion activities are planned for the next year.
  Consider ways in which you might help to publicise these.

> **Box 10.2 Safety initiatives planned for an inner-city health authority (Woodroffe & Williams 1994)**
>
> ● Car seats for babies to be on sale at the general hospital
> ● Contract with the local taxi company operating from the hospital to be re-negotiated to ensure that car seats are provided for babies and children
> ● The Child Accident Prevention Trust to be commissioned to provide 100 training sessions with local parents

events (Woodroffe & Williams 1994). Other initiatives planned by this authority are shown in Box 10.2.

Careful, effective health education techniques and evaluation are needed to make sure that healthy attitudes are promoted—'telling' is never sufficient. Similarly, parents and others with children in their care should be encouraged to become aware of the potential health risks in every environment, and to overcome the feeling of invulnerability—'but I didn't realise that this little tot could possibly climb on to the dressing table, stand on my jewellery box and reach the pills on top of the wardrobe'. Thanks to the advent of lead-free paints and child-proof containers, fewer children die each year from accidental poisoning. However, poisoning is one aspect of safety in the home which still needs improvement. Transcultural aspects of home safety should be carefully considered by health educators so that teaching and health promotion are targeted to specific needs (Parmar 1993).

Promoting exercise

Although today's children appear to be healthy and are taller and heavier than previous gen-

erations, they may not take enough exercise to develop strength, endurance and agility and to avoid conditions such as osteoporosis and cardiovascular disease later in life. Parents and children may need help and encouragement:

● to appreciate the physical, mental and social benefits of exercise
● to negotiate for adequate leisure facilities to be available locally, with low prices for those who need them.

Children may prefer to watch television to the extent of not leaving any time for active pursuits, and for their children's safety and security parents are obliged to drive them rather than encourage them to walk alone to their destination. Endurance exercises such as:

● swimming
● cycling
● running and jogging
● skipping
● walking and hiking

will improve cardiovascular fitness. Ideally, children should choose the activities they enjoy, and parents should be encouraged not to pressurise children to win in competitive exercise. If possible, exercise should be a part of family activities, so that habits are more likely to be continued after childhood and school are left behind. In Wessex the 'Look After Your Heart Workplace Charter' has been linked to the local school's curriculum, forming a health alliance. School children and adults join in a variety of health-promoting activities, including exercising together to music in a keep fit programme (Chalmers 1993).

ADOLESCENCE

The adolescent is in a transitional period between childhood and adulthood. Dramatic changes occur during adolescence in:

● physical characteristics
● thought processes
● personal identity
● social relationships

—in fact, in most aspects of life. The adolescent

has to pass through interrelated stages of cognitive, social, emotional and physical development. These require considerable adaptation, with cultural expectations likely to add further pressures. The purpose of adolescent health care is to support this process and to enable young people to become healthy and competent adults (DoH 1994).

Active participation and approaches that seek to raise self-esteem as well as provide factual information have been found to be the most effective ways of imparting health knowledge and promoting healthy lifestyles (see Ch. 9).

Aspects of cognitive development

Adolescence is a key time:

- for learning—especially by exploring new ideas and behaviours
- for developing values, attitudes and lifestyles
- for making decisions about health-related activities which will influence future health and well-being.

By this stage in their lives most young people have the capacity to understand abstract concepts, such as the implications for the future of what they do now. Multiple verbal directions and rules can be handled, and vocabulary becomes more extensive. Adolescents are able to understand ideas about health promotion and have the ability to identify healthy behaviours. However, they are also likely to have feelings of inviolability—nothing can happen to them—which can lead to inadvisable risks and unhealthy behaviour.

There's a lot of family disharmony. Poverty, bad housing and unemployment affect the stability of family life. Young people round here don't see much future for themselves and don't have a positive attitude about themselves. With families there are often language difficulties, for the parents at least, so they're not aware of the services that are available—it must affect young people too. There's also conflict within families—especially over sex and contraception.

(Allen 1991)

This quotation is taken from a research interview with an inner-city health visitor, and it illustrates the difficulties some young people experience in reconciling the culture of their homes with that of the society they live in.

Social and identity changes

As teenagers pass from childhood into adulthood, they face the task of developing their own sense of identity. Gradually, they try to assert their independence, partly withdrawing from the family and increasingly relating to peer groups. This may provoke conflict between adolescents and their parents, typically with disagreements over such items as dress style, musical taste, suitable friendships and activities, including sex and contraception as shown in the quotation above, and perhaps career choice. As parents recognise that adolescents are becoming independent from them sexually, socially and emotionally, their task is to achieve a balance between providing support and allowing the young people to be responsible for what they do and make decisions about themselves and their lives. This balance is particularly important in relation to sexuality, as such problems may be traumatic and emotionally damaging, as well as posing threats to health. In order to feel fulfilled, lead happy and healthy lives and feel good about themselves, young people need to be empowered to make informed decisions about the kind of sexual life they lead. This principle applies to all the potentially problematic issues of adolescence. The English National Board has recently produced guidelines which cover a wide range of health issues (ENB 1994). Health educators can help parents to promote the health of the whole family of an adolescent by inviting them to group sessions in schools or colleges where issues they choose can be addressed, and where discussions between parents of adolescents can be encouraged. Box 10.3 outlines some strategies for sexual health promotion.

The rise in unemployment among school leavers, the shortage of alternative housing and the time spent in full-time education all tend to lengthen the period of dependency upon parents. Those with life-threatening illnesses, previously

---

> **Box 10.3 Strategies for sexual health promotion**
>
> The promotion of sexual health should include:
>
> - giving young people support and information to help them form fulfilling sexual relationships
> - providing information and support in relation to contraception, and choice and control over pregnancy
> - promoting safe sexual practices
> - providing counselling, and treatment and care when necessary, for those affected by HIV/AIDS and support for carers.

---

fatal in childhood, may now survive and require continuing care into adolescence and adulthood (Woodroffe et al 1991). Parents therefore need ongoing support and health promotion initiatives to be available in the community.

Patterns of risky behaviour

Research suggests that young people are adopting patterns of risky behaviour at an earlier age than previously (Woodroffe et al 1991). This indicates a lack of empowerment and choice of lifestyle for many adolescents, possibly due to inequities discussed in Chapter 12. These risky behaviours may include smoking, drunkenness, violence, illicit drug-taking, poor dietary habits and multiple sexual partners. Also a matter for concern is that suicide and self-inflicted injury form the cause of death ranked third (following road vehicle deaths and other causes of injury and poisoning) in the age group 15–34 years, indicating a great need for counselling, support and helping people to improve their self-esteem and life chances.

Targeting health promotion

Such trends pose a challenge to health educators trying to target their services where needs are greatest. Health promotion should be available particularly to adolescents who have limited access to transport, who change their address frequently and whose first language is not English. Innovative ways are needed to overcome the 'inverse prevention law' (linked with the inverse care law discussed in Ch. 12), which states it is the healthiest and wealthiest who tend to respond best to health promotion and preventive programmes. The primary health care team can be of great value, particularly in primary and secondary prevention, offering support, guidance and counselling as well as health information. For example, in relation to alcohol-related problems, lifestyle guidance programmes may include advice about sensible drinking patterns, and counselling the young heavy drinker has been shown to be effective (Murray 1992).

Drug and alcohol abuse

Research shows that experimenting with drugs and alcohol is not always associated with emotional problems. However, it can sometimes be linked to both a lack of emotional support from parents and the lack of consistent behavioural controls (Paton & Brown 1991). The young person then strives for acceptance by a peer group which can provide support, and some adolescents believe that drug-taking is the only way they can make friends. The feelings induced by the drugs often serve to enhance feelings of confidence and self-worth. Abuse may also occur as a form of rebellion against parents who are seen as overprotective, stifling the young person's initiative and causing frustration. The euphoria that often accompanies substance abuse serves as a reinforcer—when frustrations are experienced again the user will seek to repeat the relief felt by the use of drugs or alcohol. Besides its direct effect, drug abuse also has serious implications for the transmission of HIV. Health education programmes directed at this problem are vital; they are needed to promote awareness of the links between drug use, sexual relationships, HIV and unwanted pregnancies (Paton & Brown 1991).

School-based education programmes will be most effective if they involve school nurses, health visitors, teachers and parents (see Ch. 9). Programmes for adolescents should be designed to discuss the emotional aspects of relationships and the option of postponing sexual involvement, as well as covering safe sexual practices (Burns & Wright 1993).

Box 10.4 Young people's family planning and counselling services (Allen 1991)

These should be an integral part of mainstream family planning services.

Two main types of service should be offered to young people:

- 'direct services', available at a defined base directly to young people who come there
- 'outreach services' which go out from the base to young people or those working with them.

Direct services should include:

- a clinic service with a doctor available offering contraceptive advice and supplies, post-coital contraception, pregnancy testing, pregnancy

counselling, referral for termination of pregnancy, AIDS counselling and health education of a more general nature in response to need. The opportunity to respond to the health education needs of a group who tend not to visit a GP or health centre very often should not be overlooked.

- a 'drop-in' service offering a range of health-related options, with a counsellor present and geared to local needs.

Outreach work should take place in collaboration with the local health promotion department of the health authority, the local education authority and with AIDS education officers or coordinators.

Homelessness

The number of homeless adolescents has increased, partly because benefit changes have led to much poverty in this age group. Emotional distress and physical and mental ill health can be the result. There is great scope for health promotion and health education among homeless people; they are particular examples of the need in health promotion to address all aspects of life, including the attempt to influence local policy decisions and government housing, employment and fiscal policy (see Ch. 3).

A research project has been set up in a Liverpool health centre where there are many temporary accommodation units nearby (Gaulton-Berks 1994). A health worker who is both a registered general nurse and a registered mental nurse is being funded for 3 years to provide health promotion interventions for homeless people and assess the impact of such work on homeless people and families. Adolescents in such situations need many topics to be covered, including:

- contraception
- stress management
- nutrition
- HIV
- information about health screening
- self-esteem (see Ch. 9).

In these days of a rapidly changing NHS, Gaulton-Berks (1994) asserts, the role of the nurse has never been broader. This applies to nurses in general practice and the community setting as well as to those in institutional settings. For example, Box 10.4, based on findings from a research study (Allen 1991), outlines family planning services that are dependent upon nursing input, which should be available for young people. Teenagers can be encouraged to know and understand the teachings of their culture, family and religion regarding family planning, and to make their own choices, recognising the implications and responsibilities of such choices.

Meeting growing nutritional demands

Rapid growth means that more calories are needed in adolescence than in childhood, but the diet should still be well balanced and varied. Peer pressure can lead to food fads and irregular eating patterns, although these may not be harmful to health.

Adolescents can be encouraged to explore facts about healthy eating, individually or in groups, perhaps using health promotion materials available from local health promotion units, the Health Education Authority or through special campaigns developed by health workers. They can be encouraged to lobby local shopkeepers to stock healthy foods, and consider influencing caterers where they normally buy meals to offer health-promoting menus.

General practice nurses and other primary health care workers can seek advice from a dietitian, and invest in skills training and team-building activities relating to promoting dietary support for teenagers in the community. Most adolescents do not have a weight problem, but some may be obese or suffer from eating disorders. Anorexia nervosa and bulimia are the main eating disorders, but they occur in less than 1% of adolescents (DoH 1994). Obese teenagers may be helped, if they wish, by being encouraged to explore possible reasons for being overweight, and then to decide how to lose weight and with what available support systems, such as a local self-help group and various sports activities. Because anorexia nervosa is a nutritional problem based on an emotional disturbance, referral to specialist help is usually appropriate.

With the recent policy of housing people with learning disabilities in the community, many adolescents in this category are, perhaps for the first time, facing the complexities of shopping and meal planning—all of which require decision-making skills. A health education programme designed to promote a healthy, balanced diet for those with learning disabilities who cannot read is described by Spooner & Rudge (1993). Taking an action–research approach, and with the help of other health workers, the authors designed and developed a teaching package of 120 laminated food photographs, with written guidelines for the health educator's use. This is an example of the wider range of visual aids needed to empower adolescents with learning disabilities to reach optimal levels of physical and mental health, for which a healthy balanced diet is vital.

Activity 10.3

Select a health promotion topic currently in the news (e.g. substance/drug/alcohol abuse, healthy eating, HIV/AIDS or road traffic accidents). Build up an information/resource package for use with groups of teenagers, collecting as wide a range as possible of information and promotional materials using all available sources. If other colleagues are interested in this project then take a group approach. Consider publicising and offering your package to local organisations for young people.

HEALTH PROMOTION IN ADULTHOOD

The five key areas—cardiovascular disease, mental health, cancers, accidents and sexual health—identified by 'The Health of the Nation' strategy (DoH 1992) are all examples of important priorities for health promotion in adults. These targets are endorsed by WHO (1993) as being applicable to other countries also. Multisectoral approaches are needed (see Ch. 1) to attempt to provide healthy environments free from health hazards, and to equip people with the knowledge and skills necessary for them to develop healthy life chances and influence health policies in their favour. This illustrates the limitations of the biomedical approach to the five key areas, which does not take account of social, cultural and emotional needs and values, and highlights the need for an integrated approach. The principle of partnership between users and providers of health care services is paramount in health promotion with adults, as it is with other life stages. Some examples of ways in which targets may be met in adult health promotion are discussed below. It is important that the environment is conducive to achieving the objectives. Conflict between what is recommended and what is acted upon can occur for instance when health promotion activities are carried out for the prevention of heart disease and cancer in places where staff smoke, where work environments cause undue stress or where menus are not consistent with the dietary messages being delivered.

Coronary heart disease and stroke

One of the main targets is to reduce death rates for coronary heart disease (CHD) and stroke in people under 65, by at least 40% by the year 2000 (DoH 1992). The risk factor targets are:

- smoking—to reduce the prevalence of cigarette smoking in men and women aged 16 or over to no more than 20% by the year 2000
- diet and nutrition—to reduce the average percentage of food energy derived by the population from saturated fatty acids by at least 35% by 2005

- obesity—to reduce the percentage of men and women aged 16–64 who are obese by at least 25% for men and at least 33% for women by 2005
- blood pressure—to reduce mean systolic blood pressure in the adult population by at least 5 mmHg by 2005
- alcohol—to reduce the proportion of men drinking more than 21 units of alcohol per week from 28% in 1990 to 18% by 2005 and the proportion of women drinking more than 14 units of alcohol per week from 11% in 1990 to 7% by 2005.

Evaluation of the progress so far in meeting these behaviour-related targets shows that many composite programmes have been developed focusing on 'healthy living'. These address the factors that contribute to CHD/stroke—smoking, poor diet and nutrition, obesity, high blood pressure, alcohol abuse and lack of physical ability (DoH 1993). The main contribution of the nursing professions has been to:

- increase awareness of CHD/stroke in the general public
- develop programmes of care to aid the recovery process following CHD/stroke
- evaluate the efficacy of education, promotion and treatment activities.

Evaluation suggests that it is probably unwise to attempt to change too many CHD risk factors at once, and that it is more effective to concentrate on high-risk people and those who are ready to make positive changes to their lifestyles.

Life screening services

Screening in health promotion in the secondary prevention of CHD/stroke typically involves general practice nurses and community nurses holding clinics which include:

- general lifestyle assessment
- measuring height, weight and blood pressure
- body fat analysis
- lung function testing.

These clinics may be held in health centres, in the workplace, in hospitals (helping staff as well as the public) and in private health care facilities.

Promoting health through positive messages

Health promotion information provided in association with screening includes information leaflets and videos in languages appropriate to the local community, posters and stalls in the local high street, market place or carnival and use of the local radio and newspapers. Fitness tests and well-man and well-woman clinics offer primary prevention in promoting choices of healthy lifestyles—empowering people to maintain and improve their health status.

Mental health promotion and quality of life

One of the key targets of 'The Health of the Nation' strategies for mental health is to 'improve significantly the health and social functioning of mentally ill people' (DoH 1992), and to monitor progress towards this target by means of assessing symptom state, social disability and quality of life. Simmons (1994) points out that, despite developments in mental health care, research into the causes and hence possible cures for major psychiatric illness (in particular schizophrenia) is still at a relatively early stage. For the foreseeable future, therefore, there is a need to focus on developing good practices and services which meet the needs of clients and their carers. One approach, in this example of secondary prevention, entails the appointment of a key worker for each person being discharged from a psychiatric hospital. This worker is often a community psychiatric nurse who will maintain close contact with the client, and liaise with other professionals and agencies providing mental health care in the community. In developing such services the quality of life of both clients and carers is of vital concern (Simmons 1994). Helping clients enhance their daily living skills, level of social interaction and family support can prevent relapse and readmission to hospital.

Cancers

'The Health of the Nation' targets include a reduction in the death rates for cancers of the lung and breast, and a reduction in the incidence of invasive cervical cancer and skin cancer.

Multidisciplinary teams in some centres aim to provide support to patients, relatives, carers and staff through:

- information
- clinical research
- targeted health promotion programmes
- screening programmes

with support from specialised nursing staff (DoH 1993). For screening programmes to be effective, the watchword should be 'quality assurance'. There are inequities in the take-up of screening programmes, with women living in poverty particularly likely to miss out (see Ch. 12). Public information should be freely available and clients need to be talked through the information, perhaps with greater use of outreach facilities such as mobile units.

Stop-smoking programmes

As smoking is the greatest risk factor in lung cancer and has a causal effect on many other cancers and conditions, much health promotion activity is directed at its prevention, at many different levels (see Ch. 4). From the point of view of influencing individual behaviour, a variety of programmes are developed (see Boxes 10.5 and 10.6).

The practice nurse at one GP practice was invited by a local leisure centre to provide two evening sessions on smoking cessation. An incentive was provided for smokers to give up in the form of half-price swimming sessions for clients

---

Box 10.5   A stop-smoking programme (Wood 1987)

A comprehensive smoking cessation programme should include:

- mass media public information and advice programmes
- the provision of self-help literature
- the provision of postal advice to enquirers
- telephone help lines
- GP and nurse counselling
- the provision of pharmacological support, i.e. Nicorette chewing gum
- stop-smoking clinics or groups
- stop-smoking community advice centres which embody all the elements described above.

Box 10.6   Factors which help smokers to stop

- Personal desire to succeed
- Social pressures
- Planned preparation
- Information on 'how to stop'
- Concern for the health of family or friends
- The economic considerations and aesthetic factors

---

who joined, with the slogan 'stop smoking, start stroking', which aroused much interest (DoH 1993).

Evaluating outcomes

Examples of the evaluation of outcomes include:

- breastcare nurses auditing the quality of the care delivery process
- midwives auditing the provision of smoking advice in antenatal clinics
- community nurses evaluating the effect of the Macmillan Service on patients and carers (DoH 1993).

Accidents

One of the main ways in which to meet the general objectives of the target to reduce ill health, disability and death caused by accidents is through the reduction in numbers of drunk drivers. The media convey messages that alcohol is acceptable in many ways, directly through advertising and indirectly through role models who drink while enjoying social occasions, power and commercial success. Tones & Tilford (1994) maintain that there is a need for local community programmes which have a strong interpersonal education component. They also point out that alcohol education programmes frequently produce a change in knowledge and occasionally attitude, but rarely influence drinking behaviour.

The controllers of broadcast media should ensure that the consequences of alcohol consumption are clearly portrayed and more emphasis given to 'sensible drinking'. However, intimidating motorists with ever-growing penalties for drink-driving offences, without developing an infrastructure of reliable public transport, is pointless and only deals with half the problem.

HIV/AIDS and sexual health

The general objectives of these targets are:

- to reduce the incidence of HIV infection and other sexually transmitted diseases (STDs)
- to develop further and strengthen monitoring and surveillance
- to provide effective services for diagnosis and treatment of HIV and other STDs
- to reduce the number of unwanted pregnancies
- to ensure the provision of effective family planning services for those who want them (DoH 1992).

Examples of health promotion initiatives identified include:

- health promotion roadshows raising public awareness in shopping centres, at football matches and fêtes
- building healthy alliances between the NHS, local authority and voluntary services to provide drop-in centres for counselling, recreational, legal and educational services and clinic sessions
- making services available out of normal hours for those who need them
- improving awareness of the risks associated with unprotected sex, sharing of needles, caring for patients with HIV/AIDS and first aid where blood and body fluids are involved
- identifying the need for services
- focusing services to disadvantaged groups
- using outreach workers to review the needs of homeless people, those whose first language is not English and those with learning difficulties
- facilitating self-help groups
- providing condoms free of charge
- tracing partners to control infection (DoH 1993).

Occupational health nurses are one group involved in addressing environmental aspects of HIV/AIDS, for instance by identifying the implications for:

- refuse collectors of collecting needles and other waste materials from AIDS patients
- home helps working in the homes of those addicted to drugs and those with AIDS
- council workers in streets and gardens who handle syringes and needles left in parks, etc.

Communication skills. Specific counselling skills which enable health workers to discuss sexual matters with clients can be developed (see Ch. 7), so that concerns may be listened to and sexual issues fully considered in a professional but helpful way.

HEALTH PROMOTION IN LATER LIFE

Over the last century, mortality has fallen steadily and life expectancy has increased, as discussed in Chapter 6. The number of people aged over 75 is expected to double over the next 50 years. At present there are about 5000 people in the UK who are over 100 years old. By 2011 there will be close to 30 000 (Age Concern 1994). Improvements in care have shifted the emphasis from merely prolonging life expectancy to increasing the expectation of active life or life free from disability. Many ageing people do not show symptoms of mental or physical decline; on the contrary, they tend to enjoy a level of health that permits them to lead socially and economically active lives, with many being carers for others. Of those aged between 70 and 80 years, 7 out of 10 need no assistance in caring for themselves (WHO 1993). Health promotion efforts with the over-60s should be multidisciplinary, aimed at tackling social, fiscal and economic limitations to health for older people as well as widening health choices at individual levels. Holistic health promotion includes mental and physical aspects of health, taking people's needs, interests and values into consideration. If older people feel accepted, cared for and loved by those with whom they associate, they are more likely to view themselves in a positive way. They will then feel more confident and empowered, in control of themselves and their situation and able to go on to continued growth and self-actualisation. Older people who are disabled can feel autonomous if they are given choices about their care (Hancock & Hancock 1993). The objective should be to maintain maximum functional capacity throughout the later years of life, balanced with appropriate care when needed (Redfern 1991).

Patient education

Health promotion, including health education, can be provided when older people are hospitalised, taking advantage of the nurse–patient relationship to enhance health. Special care may be needed to communicate with those who are visually impaired, deaf or who have learning difficulties, or whose first language is not English. Ewles & Simnett (1992) outline some of the main principles of patient education, based on the teaching and learning strategies discussed in Chapter 9 (see Box 10.7).

Prevention in later life

When health problems occur in later life, people tend to report more than one condition or symptom. The most common problems are arthritis, reduced vision and hearing, dementia, depression, sleep disturbance, incontinence, unsteadi-ness, social isolation, and institutionalisation. These problems should receive priority in both action and research to promote healthy ageing. They are all amenable to primary, secondary or tertiary prevention to improve the quality of life for older people (McClymont et al 1991). Some examples of health promotion and disability prevention in primary care are listed in Box 10.8.

Emotional and sexual needs

Health workers can help people to get the best out of life in later years, with love and sex playing the part that is normal in adulthood, and recognising the extent of individual differences. Advice and counselling may be required about the way in which the natural processes of ageing can sometimes affect sexuality, and how problems can be overcome. The emotional plight of elderly men and women who are living in various types of institution where sexuality may be considered a major problem, is discussed by Gibson (1992).

Mortality and risk factors

The main causes of mortality in the over-60s are ischaemic heart disease, stroke, respiratory disease (for instance influenza and pneumonia) and malignancy. People of Afro-Caribbean origin have a greater risk of high blood pressure, with a consequent rise in the number of strokes. Asians have been found in general to have a higher risk of developing coronary heart disease and diabetes and a lower risk of developing cancer. Afro-Caribbeans have a higher prevalence of disability than white people, while Asians tend to have a lower prevalence than whites. The search for health needs should include an awareness of possible transcultural health differences so that optimum strategies for promoting health can be planned.

Major risk factors for the diseases mentioned above are:

- smoking
- lack of exercise
- poor diet
- raised blood pressure
- alcohol consumption.

Box 10.7 Some principles of patient education (Ewles & Simnett 1992)

- Say important things first.
- Stress and repeat the key points.
- Give specific, precise advice rather than vague guidance—e.g. 'try to take an hour's rest with your feet up every afternoon', not 'get more rest'.
- Structure information into categories—tell the patient the headings you are going to use, and organise your material under these headings as you present it.
- Avoid jargon, long words and long sentences and explain any medical terms you use.
- Use visual aids, leaflets, handouts and written instructions.
- Avoid saying too much at once—three or four key points are all people are likely to remember from one session.
- Ensure that your advice is relevant and realistic for that particular patient's circumstances.
- Get feedback from patients to ensure that they have understood the information or advice given.

Box 10.8 Health promotion and disability prevention (Pickin & St Leger 1993)

- Domiciliary elderly screening service, particularly to pick up:
  —high blood pressure
  —poor vision
  —hearing loss
  —depression
  —dementia
  —Parkinson's disease
  —incontinence
  —poor oral health and ill-fitting dentures
  —diabetes
  —anaemia
  with a system of treatment, referral as appropriate and follow-up

- Chiropody service—domiciliary and health-centre-based
- Easy access to a community physiotherapist and occupational therapist
- Continence adviser
- Community nursing services and health promotion advisers
- Bereavement and other counselling services— domiciliary and health-centre-based
- Assessment and follow-up of people with dementia
- Support for carers—professional and self-help
- Access to complementary therapists employed through the ancillary staff budget

---

Health education has a major role to play, as, for instance, stopping smoking late in life still reduces the risks of heart disease and bronchitis. Modification of lifestyle is, however, only one aspect of health promotion. As Graham (1993) pointed out in her study of younger women, there is a need to broaden the base of health promotion policies, for example tobacco cessation policies, to include interventions which act directly on the circumstances of people's lives. Poverty is particularly associated with old age and the quality of life of an elderly person has been shown to be affected by the amount of disposable income (Pickin & St Leger 1993). Poverty leads to an inability to heat and maintain the home, a poor diet and less access to appropriate private transport to maintain social networks. All of these can lead to increased ill health, for example hypothermia, which is potentially fatal but preventable. It is estimated that in 1991 between 22% and 33% of pensioners who were entitled to income support, and between 5% and 12% who were entitled to housing benefit, did not claim. Health promotion initiatives are needed, therefore, to empower people to obtain money due to them, as well as to try to improve policy strategies (Age Concern 1994).

Older people and work

Research shows clearly that public opinion in all member states of the European Union is against the exclusion of people from opportunity because of their age (WHO 1993). However, during the 1980s there was a mass exodus of older people from the workplace, so that now in many countries in western Europe only a minority of the 55–65 age group have jobs. Youth became more highly regarded than experience, although this attitude is beginning to change. Personnel and training managers are discovering that older workers can learn new ways as surely as their younger colleagues, and that older workers have many positive qualities to offer.

A mature entrant programme was launched in three large supermarket stores which are part of a large retail chain (James 1994). People over the age of 55 were recruited, and the retirement policy for current employees was changed so that they could continue to work if they wished, retaining all of their benefits. A researcher for the World Health Organization studied the mature entry programme. Her results showed that the majority of managers and supervisors rated the older workers the same as younger ones on:

- productivity
- relations with other staff
- likelihood of having an accident
- ability to learn
- willingness to try something new.

Many commented that although the older workers were sometimes slower, they were equally productive because of their greater reliability and sense of responsibility and higher levels of efficiency.

The health and well-being of the older workers was enhanced and they reported the following benefits of work:

- exercise
- human companionship and friendliness
- challenge and stimulation
- a feeling of belonging
- increased confidence and use of problem-solving skills
- independence
- a sense of purpose in continuing to do a good job
- happiness and laughter.

The majority of the older workers were women who worked part-time, and the suggestions for support services needed in the workplace for them included:

- breast screening
- cholesterol testing
- sick room provision
- retirement planning
- occupational health facilities.

The older workers in this scheme were called 'hot house flowers'—ones that need nurturing, but in the best conditions yield the biggest and best blooms (James 1994). Customer service is rated very highly on the business plan of the company concerned, and as the older workers were particularly skilled in this the policy to retain and recruit older workers will continue.

HIV, AIDS and older people

'In the public perception, AIDS is the territory of the young: its cause rooted in youthful behaviour, and its tragedy the cutting short of young lives' (Kaufmann 1993). However, in the UK some 11% of people with AIDS are aged 50 and over. Those diagnosed as HIV-positive may have parents and grandparents who are in their turn deeply affected by the virus, and who need the kind of support usually only offered to younger people who need information, care and counselling. Sometimes people with AIDS go home from the cities to which they have moved, when they become terminally ill, to be cared for by their parents. Areas which lack awareness and understanding of HIV-related issues and where there are no specialist services need healthy alliances to be set up to fill the gaps.

Ageism

Older people have to suffer the negative attitudes of society in general—ageism—in many aspects of life. Physical prowess, the ability to move fast and a youthful appearance are highly regarded, although in some societies old age is respected and venerated. In promoting the health and well-being of older people it is important for society as a whole to value the attributes of old age. A wealth of experience, skills and knowledge is accumulated throughout life, and can be a valuable resource. We should not encourage old people to try to be like the young, but to enjoy and benefit from their maturity as much as possible.

REFERENCES

Age Concern 1994 Older people in the United Kingdom: some basic facts. Age Concern, London

Allen I 1991 Family planning and pregnancy counselling projects for young people. Policy Studies Institute, London

Anionwu E N 1993 Genetics—a philosophy of perfection? In: Beattie A, Gott M, Jones L, Sidell M (eds) Health and wellbeing: a reader. Macmillan & Open University, Milton Keynes

Burns J, Wright C 1993 A trainer's guide to workshops on young people and sexuality in the context of HIV/AIDS. HMSO, London

Chalmers F 1993 Setting standards in schools. Healthlines 5: 18–19

Davies J 1993 Mothers at risk. Modern Midwife 3(4): 31–33

Department of Health 1992 The health of the nation: a strategy for health in England. Cm 1986. HMSO, London

Department of Health 1993 Targeting practice: the contribution of nurses, midwives and health visitors. Department of Health, London

Department of Health 1994 On the state of the public health 1993. HMSO, London

English National Board for Nursing, Midwifery and Health Visiting (ENB) 1994 Sexual health education and training: guidelines for good practice in the teaching of nurses, midwives and health visitors. ENB, London

Ewles L, Simnett I 1992 Promoting health: a practical guide, 2nd edn. Scutari, London

Gaulton-Berks L 1994 Homeless but not helpless. Nursing Times 90(15): 53–55

Gibson H B 1992 The emotional and sexual lives of older people: a manual for professionals. Chapman & Hall, London

Goldman R, Goldman J 1982 Children's sexual thinking. Routledge & Kegan Paul, London

Graham H 1993 When life's a drag: women, smoking and disadvantage. HMSO, London

Hancock B, Hancock D 1993 Mastery of the environment. Elderly Care 5(6): 22–23

James L 1994 Hot house flowers—a UK retailer's response to older workers. In: Health Education Authority (ed) Investing in older people at work: contributions, case studies and recommendations. HEA, London

Kaufmann T 1993 A crisis of silence: HIV, AIDS and older people. Age Concern, London

McClymont M, Thomas S, Denham M J 1991 Health visiting and elderly people: a health promotion challenge, 2nd edn. Churchill Livingstone, Edinburgh

Murray A 1992 Minimal intervention with problem drinkers. In: Plant M, Ritson B, Robertson R (eds) Alcohol and drugs: the Scottish experience. Edinburgh University Press, Edinburgh

National Curriculum Council 1990 Curriculum guidance No. 3. The whole curriculum. National Curriculum Council, York

Parmar A 1993 Safety and minority ethnic communities: a preliminary report on the home safety information needs of the Asian, Chinese and Vietnamese communities living in the UK in the 1990s. Royal Society for the Prevention of Accidents, Birmingham

Paton D, Brown R 1991 Lifespan health psychology: nursing problems and interventions. Harper Collins, London

Pickin C, St Leger S 1993 Assessing health need using the life cycle framework. Open University Press, Milton Keynes

Prendergast S 1992 This is the time to grow up: girls' experiences of menstruation in school. Health Promotion Research Trust, London

Redfern S J (ed) 1991 Nursing elderly people, 2nd edn. Churchill Livingstone, Edinburgh

Robertson C 1991 Health visiting in practice, 2nd edn. Churchill Livingstone, Edinburgh

Seedhouse D 1986 Health: the foundations for achievement. John Wiley, Chichester

Silverton L 1993 A mother's charter. Modern Midwife 3(4): 23

Simmons S 1994 Quality of life in community mental health care—a review. International Journal of Nursing Studies 31(2): 183–193

Spooner B, Rudge G 1993 Tasteful pictures. Nursing Times 89(33): 34–36

Tones K, Tilford S 1994 Health education: effectiveness, efficiency and equity, 2nd edn. Chapman & Hall, London

Wood M 1987 A coordinated approach to smoking cessation. In: Hobbs P (ed) Public education about cancer. Hans Huber, Toronto

Woodroffe C, Williams J 1994 Accidents. In: Jacobson B (ed) East London and the City: health in the East End. East London & the City Health Authority and City & East London FHSA, London

Woodroffe C, Glickman M, Barber M, Power C 1991 Children, teenagers and health: the key data. Oxford University Press, Oxford

World Health Organization 1993 Health for all targets: the health policy for Europe, updated edn. WHO, Regional Office, Copenhagen

Wright C 1994 Safety equipment loan scheme. Community Nursing Association Newsletter Autumn 1994: 2–3

FURTHER READING

Burns J, Wright C 1993 A trainer's guide to workshops on young people and sexuality in the context of HIV/AIDS. HMSO, London

Department for Education and the Welsh Office 1992 Drug misuse and the young: a guide for the education service. Department for Education, London

Department of Health 1993 Ethnicity and health: a guide for the NHS. Department of Health, London

Health Education Authority 1990 Young adults' health and lifestyles. MORI, London

Royal College of Nursing 1990 Guidelines for assessment of elderly people. Royal College of Nursing, London

Royal College of Nursing 1992 Manual of family health: everyday care in the home. Little Brown, London

Squires A J (ed) Multicultural health care and rehabilitation of older people. Edward Arnold, London

Webb C (ed) 1994 Living sexuality: issues for nursing and health. Scutari, London

Broadening the vision for health promotion

SECTION CONTENTS

11. Settings for health promotion   143

12. Inequalities in health and health promotion   157

13. Health and the environment   171

14. Towards an integrated model of health promotion in nursing practice   185

This section adopts a wide-angle view of health promotion, taking in the varying settings in which it is carried out, and looking at relevant issues such as inequality and the effect of the environment. The final chapter puts forward an integrated model for nursing practice.

CHAPTER CONTENTS

Introduction   143

Health-promoting schools   144
Aspects of health education   144
Health education activities   146
The role of the school nurse   147

The health-promoting workplace   148
Look after your heart (LAYH)   150
Disabled people in employment   150
Job stress   150

Health education and the mass media   151
Changing behaviour   152
The media and mental health   153
'Health of the Nation' strategy   153

References   154

Further reading   155

11

Settings for health promotion

Diana Forster

By the year 2000, all settings of social life and activity, such as the city, school, workplace, neighbourhood and home, should provide greater opportunities for promoting health.

(Target 14: Settings for health promotion, WHO 1993)

INTRODUCTION

Much disease, disability and premature death could be avoided, and positive aspects of health promoted, if settings where people live and work gave greater support for healthy living. Promoting healthy settings for living is the strategy for implementing healthy public policy at the local level. Schools and recreation areas can encourage social experiences that help children to choose healthy lifestyles and develop all aspects of their lives. Workplaces can be safe and offer opportunities for self-development and productivity in an environment that encourages health and well-being. Health centres and hospitals can be designed and organised to encourage and motivate people, raising their expectations for health and fitness. Activities to strengthen personal skills and competence and provide relevant knowledge can be incorporated into all the settings of daily life. Vulnerable and disadvantaged groups, however, often have limited access to services, recreation and education facilities outside the normal settings of their lives. Health promotion and health education therefore need to operate on an outreach basis if such groups are to be successfully targeted (WHO 1993).

Activity 11.1

Reflect upon your own setting—where you live, learn or work. Identify one aspect which you would like to change in order to improve your own health and well-being, and which might be influenced by negotiation with others.

The active involvement of people is vital in a settings approach to health promotion. The people who live, learn and work where health is being promoted should help to decide what their settings will be like, negotiating with those in positions of responsibility to choose their own definition of what is important for their health and well-being. This is particularly relevant in a transcultural society where a rich variety of lifestyles and values needs to be recognised. Plans should then be made to carry out strategies to promote health for the whole community.

Many people, including:

- city planners
- social and health workers
- housing and traffic administrators
- teachers
- environmental officers
- business employers
- community activists

have a part to play in promoting health in a settings perspective. Alliances need to be formed to bring community groups, organisations and professional disciplines together (see Chs 3 and 13).

The main advantage of the settings approach to health promotion is that it encourages the active involvement of the people most concerned, and interventions can be tailored to their specific requirements and local circumstances (WHO 1993).

The mass media may be regarded as a wide-ranging setting for health promotion, with their many facets having great potential for helping people to learn about, and choose to work towards, the levels of health and lifestyle they want for themselves and their community. This, with two other examples of settings for health promotion, will be considered in this chapter.

HEALTH-PROMOTING SCHOOLS

Aspects of health education

Health education in schools is concerned with quality of life and with the promotion of physical, social and mental well-being of pupils. It includes not only the imparting of knowledge about what is beneficial and what is harmful, but also includes the development of skills which will help children and young people to use their knowledge effectively. Pupils also need the opportunity to develop attitudes and values which will enable them to make choices now in their present lives and also in the future. The 'hidden curriculum' is also important. In the health-promoting school this is reflected in its care for pupils and staff, the food which is served at mealtimes, and in the provision of a stimulating, safe environment. It is also reflected in the health and caring services' provision of health screening, immunisation, first aid and psychological services (Young & Williams 1989).

There has been a widespread tendency in the past to organise health education in schools around health topics, such as the effects upon health of smoking and the misuse of drugs. A different approach is to identify the competences and attributes people need to develop in order to achieve the level of health they desire. Emphasis might be focused upon developing:

- self-esteem
- self-efficacy
- locus of control
- empowerment
- decision-making
- assertiveness
- advocacy

and other related skills (Tones & Tilford 1994). This fits in with the 'education as freeing' approach discussed in Chapter 9 (Greenberg 1992).

The idea of empowerment applied to children suggests a fundamental change in the manner in which children are perceived. A shift in attitude is required, from thinking about children as recipients of health promotion efforts on their behalf, to children as partners in health promo-

---

Box 11.1 The school health fax (McAleer & Jackson 1994)

The health fax was piloted in 21 schools in inner London for pupils in year seven (11-plus). It was developed as a focus for health interviews and as a tool to empower young people to share responsibility for their own health. In some pilot schools many pupils used English as a second language, and travelled regularly between England and other countries. A readily accessible, up-to-date health record was expected to be advantageous. Evaluation showed that most pupils liked the fax and appreciated having a comprehensive record of their own health status.

Box 11.2 School health profiles (Bagnall 1994)

These will provide an overall picture of the health of children in each school and identify areas of concern. These profiles can then be amalgamated into a neighbourhood or locality profile. Information can then be used to direct resources towards specific areas of need and to inform purchasers of the health needs of the school-age population.

---

tion. Their views and concerns about health should be accepted as valid in their own right, and children's competence to make and implement decisions should be recognised (Kalnins et al 1992). An NHS trust in London has recently introduced pupil-held records, known as the 'health fax' (McAleer & Jackson 1994) and described in Box 11.1 (also see Box 5.5, p 52).

Children with special educational needs

The health-promoting school, either mainstream or special, has great potential for enhancing the physical, social and emotional well-being of children with special needs. Modifications to health education materials may sometimes be required, for example making worksheets clearer and easy to read, making tasks shorter and classes smaller. Most schools give extra help to pupils with specific problems on an individual basis.

The curriculum

The school health education curriculum should ideally be developed around the attributes and competences needed for health in both individuals and the community surrounding them. The school can then play a major part in an integrated model of health promotion, linking the school to its community, particularly in multicultural settings. Major community health initiatives such as those related to road safety, smoking, nutrition, drugs and HIV/AIDS should be coordinated as closely as possible with local school programmes.

In this way pupils can experience community support for what they are studying at school. School health profiles combined with neighbourhood/locality profiles help to identify priorities and set targets appropriately (see Box 11.2).

Health education should be an integrated and continuous programme available to all pupils throughout the school years (DoH 1992). Generally it is true to say that, while teachers should take professional responsibility for the teaching of health education, the school health service provides a vital resource for its planning and implementation. Schools should identify professionals other than teachers, who are committed to targeting young people and who may be able to contribute to health education programmes, including for example:

- members of the school health team—including the school nurse (discussed below) and the school doctor who can provide information about disease and medical conditions
- health promotion officers—who can initiate specific campaigns, for example on dental health
- family planning nurses—for specialist information on relationships, family planning and sexually transmitted diseases
- community mental health nurses—for discussions of substance abuse and promoting mental health
- dietitians—for exploring healthy eating policies (Bagnall 1993).

The psychological services also have an important role to play in the promotion of health in schools. In addition to their traditional role, they can contribute to training courses for teachers, run workshops for parents, and develop courses on approaches to learning difficulties and practical guides on meeting the special needs of children with disabilities.

Irish schools

One of the key recommendations made to the Irish government by its advisors is that relationships and sexuality education should begin in Irish primary schools at junior primary level. Coverage would not be made compulsory, however, but sex education is recommended as a required part of the curriculum of each primary and post-primary school. It should be evident on a timetabled social, personal and health education programme and should reflect the core values and ethos of the school (Ray 1994).

Scottish schools

In Scotland recently there have been several influential reports on health education. National guidelines on curriculum and assessment have been published on a consultative basis by the Scottish Office Education Department (1991). Health education in Scottish schools is seen as a cross-curricular component, but receives less prominent and comprehensive coverage than in the national curriculum of England and Wales (see below). It is dealt with specifically only in 'Healthy and Safe Living', part of environmental studies. Since 1989 a special HIV and AIDS team of seconded teachers has been working with pupils in schools in the Lothian region, as Edinburgh has the highest rate of HIV infection in Europe. This is significantly linked to drug misuse, so health education is directed at this problem also (Eales & Watson 1994).

National curriculum

The 1988 Education Reform Act requires schools in England and Wales to provide a broad and balanced curriculum designed:

- to promote the spiritual, moral, cultural, mental and physical development of pupils at the school and of society

- to prepare pupils for the opportunities, responsibilities and experiences of adult life (National Curriculum Council 1990).

Health education is covered by a guidance document which recommends the components for a health education curriculum for children between 5 and 16 years. How far these are incorporated into the main subjects depends on the school's commitment to health education (Bagnall 1993).

The context for HIV/AIDS and sex education in schools in England and Wales has recently changed. In July 1993, the government accepted an amendment to the 1988 Education Act which had the effects outlined in Box 11.3.

Health education activities

Many health education initiatives have been developed in response to the targets identified in 'The Health of the Nation' (DoH 1992). A follow-up document (DoH 1993a) highlights the considerable health promotion activities targeted at

---

Box 11.3 Effects of the 1993 Amendment to the 1988 Education Act (Department for Education 1993)

- Removing the teaching of HIV and other sexually transmitted diseases (STDs), and the 'teaching of aspects of human sexual behaviour, other than biological aspects' from the revised Statutory Orders for Science at key stage 3 (11- to 14-year-olds)
- Requiring the governing bodies of secondary schools to provide sex education, including the study of STDs, as part of the secular curriculum (i.e. not part of the National Curriculum) and to develop policies which reflect the status of sex education from optional to compulsory
- Requiring maintained or grant-maintained secondary schools to provide sex education for all pupils, which includes those aspects of sex education previously referred to in the revised Statutory Orders for Science
- Requiring the governing body of primary schools to decide whether sex education should take place, and if so, in what form
- Establishing a parental right of withdrawal from those aspects of sex education that take place as part of the secular curriculum in both primary and secondary schools

children with the aim of reducing the death rate for accidents among children under 15 by at least 33% by 2005. It states that the health promotion activities relate:

- to improving awareness and knowledge about the risks involved in everyday behaviour
- to encouraging people, especially parents and carers, to adopt a healthy or safer pattern of behaviour
- to encouraging those at risk to change their behaviour to reduce the risk of accidents.

However, although it is important to raise awareness of road safety behaviour in children, it is also vital to do so in the context of making sure that the environment is as safe as possible. A study was carried out in Glasgow to investigate factors which led to children being at risk from accidents. Researchers found that parents had a good understanding of the causes of accidents in general, clear views on hazards and risks in their own environments, and that they were effective most of the time in keeping children safe in unsafe conditions. The study concludes 'Just as the introduction of child resistant containers for medicine has been associated with a steep drop in childhood poisonings, our work indicates a number of areas where preventive efforts based on environmental rather than (though in association with) behavioural change might usefully focus.' (Roberts et al 1993). Children and their parents need, therefore, to be encouraged and enabled to influence the community and government approaches to reducing accidents.

We need to develop educational approaches which do more than just aim to protect children and young people from illness and risks to their health and well-being. While educational responses to problems like drug abuse, tobacco and AIDS are often effective in the short term, these topics need to be explored in the wider context of the health and lifeskills needs of young people. Issues such as sexuality and relationships should be considered not as problems, but as positive aspects of human development. The developmental stages of children and young people are critical in relation to promoting health, as for

example peer group influences tend to override parental and educational guidance at some stages of adolescence.

This factor can be exploited in health education by developing peer teaching programmes. Phelps et al (1994) describe a programme using 66 selected, trained peer leaders aged 16–17 years who worked with 38 secondary school classes (aged 13–14 years) in the south-west of England. Evaluation showed that the programme positively affected the pupils' knowledge, skills and beliefs relating to social norms; peer leaders gained knowledge, skills and self-confidence.

Child abuse

Every child and young person has the right to life free from abuse. Article 19 of the United Nations Convention on the Rights of the Child, to which the United Kingdom is a signatory, is shown in Box 11.4.

Nurses in collaboration with others can educate children and young people about their right to personal safety. Child abuse prevention programmes can be introduced in schools, although preferably these should be combined with other curriculum topics so that the issue of abuse is placed in a context which is understandable but unalarming to children (RCN 1994). Children need to be introduced to such programmes early, at primary school level as well as secondary school, so that they have the knowledge, skills and language to say 'no' and to talk to a trusted adult.

The role of the school nurse

The school health team has traditionally worked in a task-related way, carrying out routine

---

Box 11.4 Article 19 of the United Nations Convention on the Rights of the Child (United Nations 1992)

Parties shall take all appropriate legislative, administrative, social and educational measures to protect the child from all forms of physical and mental violence, injury or abuse, neglect or negligent treatment, maltreatment or exploitation, including sexual abuse, while in the care of the parent(s), legal guardian or any other person who has the care of the child.

surveillance, medical, screening and immunisation programmes. More recently, medical screening has been rationalised and health promotion is carried out by teams of school nurses and other members of the health care team following guidance in the revised Hall report (1991). The school nurse helps to plan health education programmes and initiatives with teaching staff, based on an identification of need, balanced with the school curriculum, and leading to targets being set and evaluated. It is also vital for school nurses to be available when required for advice, counselling and support for pupils. School nurses are developing skills and undertaking greater responsibilities within the school setting (Bagnall 1993). Many health authorities have reviewed their school health services policies, and communication and collaboration between health and education services are developing in an effort to further improve the health-promoting school, so that children acquire not just an academic education, but skills for life.

THE HEALTH-PROMOTING WORKPLACE

Effort is needed to achieve real improvements in the state of employees' health, from the point of view of both quality of life for the employee and the commercial benefits to employers, which also improve health chances for the workforce.

A Health Education Authority survey of health promotion in 1344 workplaces in England found that only 40% of them undertook some kind of health initiatives, with larger employers more likely to promote them than small ones (HEA 1993). Action on smoking was most popular, with 31% of all workplaces tackling this issue. Box 11.5 contains a list of the range of activities undertaken in all the workplaces.

Alcohol policies in the workplace act as a mechanism for detecting alcohol problems, and can also be used for health promotion and problem prevention (see Ch. 10). However, a study by Baggott & Powell (1994) found that most employers chose to concentrate on disciplinary policies rather than health promotion initiatives in relation to alcohol.

Box 11.5   Range of health promotion activities (HEA 1993)

- Smoking
- Alcohol
- Healthy eating
- Catering
- Stress
- HIV/AIDS
- Weight control
- Exercise/fitness
- Heart health
- Breast screening
- Cervical screening
- General screening
- Lifestyle assessment
- Cholesterol testing
- Blood pressure control
- Drug/substance abuse

Participation in health promotion activities at work, by the workforce and managers alike, has been shown to be more successful than 'top-down' programmes. When employee steering committees took part in developing and implementing stop-smoking programmes, which were evaluated in one study, the participation was shown to be very effective (Dugdill & Springett 1994). An action–research approach was most health enhancing, with the programmes being monitored and changes made as the sessions proceeded. However, it is still important for top management to be involved as well as the workforce, as staff morale remains higher with management support.

A healthy workforce is good for business for many reasons, including:

- absences from work are very costly for employers—see Box 11.6.
- fewer 'core' employees now workforces have been cut back, means that companies cannot afford to lose them through ill health
- workers who retire early because of ill health

Activity 11.2

Outline a health promotion intervention which would enhance the health and well-being of you and your colleagues at work or in a community setting.

> **Box 11.6   Costs of ill health**
>
> The direct cost to industry of sickness absences in the United Kingdom (UK) was recently estimated to be £13 billion annually (CBI, BUPA 1993). 8 million days annually are lost through alcohol and drink-related disease and 80 million days are lost through mental illness, at an estimated cost of over £5 billion. An additional 50 million days are lost in the UK because of smoking-related diseases (DoH 1994).

are costly to employers and represent lost skills and experience
● health promotion boosts morale and reduces staff turnover.

There are also increasing external pressures to ensure employees' health and safety:

● new government legislation on workplace health hazards such as the 'Control of Substances Hazardous to Health' (COSHH) (DoH 1989) and the 'Management of Health and Safety at Work Regulations' (Health and Safety Commission 1992) which reflect EC directives
● legal action by workers suffering from work-related stress, illnesses caused by passive smoking and injuries such as repetitive strain injury
● tougher conditions for employers' liability insurance
● the 'Workplace Task Force Report' (DoH 1993b) which recommended better evaluation of workplace health promotional activity, and the setting up of local health alliances to provide information, advice and support for employers who wanted to increase their health promotion activities.

An engineering company in Gwynedd, north Wales is aiming to be a very effective setting for health promotion. The company canteen offers a range of healthy eating options and cash subsidies for eating in the canteen. Food information is circulated throughout the company. A multi-gym has been set up for the workforce and trips to local leisure centres, with discounts, are arranged. Mobile health units provide screening on dental hygiene and general lifestyle issues, and policies regarding the safe and sensible use of alcohol and

the prevention of HIV/AIDS have been established (Hobbs 1994).

Another company in south-west England, a small cider-making company which employs 550 people, has become a pioneer with its employee protection and health care initiatives. The company introduced safety-at-work practices and manual-handling training years before such procedures became a legal requirement. An ear-defence system has been initiated in its bottling hall to reduce risks from noise pollution. A no-smoking policy was introduced in 1993 into all its public areas and meeting places, and a counselling service to help smokers give up was being introduced (Chalmers 1993).

These examples illustrate some of the requirements of the Health and Safety Commission (1992) which places general duties on employers to ensure the health and safety of their employees by providing:

● safe plant and equipment, with maintenance, and safe systems of work
● safety in relation to the use, handling, storage and transport of articles and substances
● information, instruction, training and supervision
● maintenance of a safe working place (this point does not apply to the homes of patients/clients of health workers as these are not under the employer's control, but it does not dilute the employer's duty to keep staff safe wherever they are)
● facilities and arrangements for welfare at work.

In the community setting, midwives are in an ideal position to provide education to clients about health and safety at work, particularly during pregnancy (Goodwin & Aston 1994). Midwives and health care professionals supporting the pregnant woman at work can consult local health and safety officers for information and guidance about latest regulations, such as those limiting the occupational risks of heavy work and postural stress in pregnancy (Health and Safety Executive 1994).

Employers are now obliged to be able to assess risks to the health and safety of their workforce, and personnel managers need to take into account the effects that mental or physical ill health can have on employees' performance at work. Having assessed the risks there is a need to plan, organise, control and monitor the necessary preventive and protective measures. The employers of health care staff need to take seriously the problem of violence, including racial harassment, and demonstrate a commitment to ensure that their staff are as safe as possible. This is particularly important for the range of community nurse employers—GPs, community trusts, local authorities, and voluntary agencies (RCN 1994).

Sexual harassment

Sexual harassment is unwanted and unwelcome behaviour which may be defined as 'unwanted conduct of a sexual nature or other conduct based on sex affecting the dignity of women and men at work' (UNISON 1994). It can include:

- physical contact, ranging from unnecessary touching through to sexual assault or rape
- demands for sexual favours
- sexual propositions
- unwanted comments on dress or appearance
- leering and suggestive gestures
- the display of pornographic pictures or pin-ups.

Management have a responsibility to protect their employees wherever they are working and to deal swiftly and effectively with any complaints. Life-skills and assertiveness training may help people to respond effectively if they are being harassed themselves, or to support others and perhaps to help to negotiate policies and procedures to counter sexual harassment.

Look after your heart (LAYH)

LAYH is the national coronary heart disease (CHD) prevention programme for England. It was launched in 1987 by the Health Education Authority and Department of Health as a campaign, and subsequently extended as a broad-based, comprehensive and systematically planned programme for 1990–1995 (Lincoln 1992). Its main aims include the development of

programmes in settings including the workplace where health education is concentrated upon:

- smoking and tobacco use
- diet and nutrition
- control of blood pressure
- promotion of physical activity.

Many companies have introduced a LAYH Charter and successfully encouraged their workers to take part in health-promoting activities.

In Glasgow, the Good Hearted Glasgow Campaign was launched in 1986, but was not very successful, partly because of lack of publicity, lack of central support, lack of staff and underfunding (Hanlon 1992). The programme is to be relaunched.

Whitehead & Tones (1990) discuss an evaluation of the LAYH initiative which suggests that lack of resources and facilities and low levels of senior management support sometimes meant that programmes were ineffective. There are new initiatives planned to attempt to overcome these obstacles.

Disabled people in employment

If disabled people are to achieve greater independence, it is important for the labour market to be as accessible as possible to them. The quota scheme which is currently in force is increasingly recognised as unworkable. It requires employers with 20 or more employees to employ at least 3% registered disabled people in their workforce. But only one-third of those eligible to register do so, and employers sometimes discriminate unjustly against disabled people and fail to employ them.

At present the policies are being reviewed, and new legislation may be introduced to protect the rights of disabled people.

Job stress

Stress at work has been associated with:

- high staff turnover
- sickness absence
- increased accident rates
- decreased quality of work

- increased health care costs
- reduced job satisfaction.

In looking at the nursing profession, it can be seen that job-related stress affects all groups. Wheeler & Riding (1994) cite studies which have demonstrated stress in:

- student nurses
- operating theatre nurses
- coronary care unit nurses
- intensive care unit staff
- renal unit nurses
- geriatric ward staff
- hospice nurses.

Their own study of stress in general nurses and midwives found four underlying factors:

- work overload and time pressure
- organisational and management issues
- poor interpersonal relationships
- poor working conditions and facilities.

The key points which emerged from their comprehensive research are shown in Box 11.7.

The nurse's working environment

It is as impossible for nurses as it is for other workers to maintain a healthy lifestyle in an unhealthy working environment. A comprehensive occupational health service should promote health by:

- monitoring, controlling or abolishing hazards in the workplace
- providing health-screening facilities for nurses
- supervising employee nurses' health
- providing health education
- advising on occupational safety and environmental monitoring
- providing and maintaining a confidential counselling service
- advising on rehabilitation and resettlement where this is appropriate, for example for nurses who have experienced illness or disablement (Rogers & Salvage 1988).

Health care workers need to develop their own sense of self-empowerment so that they can feel responsible for their own health and well-being and encourage others to make health enhancing decisions.

HEALTH EDUCATION AND THE MASS MEDIA

An important part of UK government policy towards disease prevention and health promotion in the late 1980s was directed towards high-profile mass media approaches to educate the public. These focused particularly on drug abuse, drinking and driving, heart disease and AIDS. Whitehead (1989) examines government-supported campaigns in England based upon heroin addiction and HIV / AIDS. These campaigns were hard hitting and sensational, intended to shock young people in particular into changing their attitudes and behaviour in relation to such hazards to health. The campaign against heroin use was concentrated around a display of images designed to shock people, placed on public hoardings. The prevention of AIDS campaign contained a series of powerful images on television, also designed to be shocking in their effect. The campaigns raised many anxieties, and their effectiveness was in doubt because of unintended and inappropriate effects. For example, the cam-

---

Box 11.7 Key points—occupational stress in general nurses and midwives (Wheeler & Riding 1994)

- The most common source of nurse stress is pressure of workload/time.
- The general level of stress as perceived by nurses is moderate or mild rather than very or extremely stressful.
- There is little difference in stress level between general nurses and midwives, although general nurses rated the factors of management, relationships and facilities more highly as stressors.
- Most nurses find their jobs satisfying.
- In terms of career commitment, older nurses thought it likely that they would choose nursing again, while younger ones were evenly divided, although they were less likely than the older nurses to choose nursing again.
- Nurses tend to have a high opinion of their professional effectiveness.

paign to raise awareness of AIDS confused the 'worried well', raising high levels of anxiety in people who were unlikely to be at risk. The campaign against heroin unintentionally glamorised victims, and probably perpetuated inappropriate stereotypes. Tones & Tilford (1994) suggest that while the mass media may be very effective in getting simple information across to people, and in raising awareness and starting debates, their ability to change attitudes is limited, and there may be unpredictable and unwanted after-effects. There is usually no personal contact between educator and target audience when mass media techniques are used, and so the influence is likely to be limited. Scare tactics are ineffective because the audience tends to shut out the message if it is too frightening, and so threatening messages can be counterproductive. People may also distort, deny or selectively ignore the media output, supporting their own prejudices, desires and fantasies (Whitehead & Tones 1990).

However, although there are drawbacks, mass media publicity has achieved useful results in the past and, as has been mentioned above, may be expected to have advantages in raising awareness and providing straightforward information. It can also prove useful in disseminating to a wide audience a new recommendation, such as advising older and vulnerable people of the availability of a current flu vaccine. Almost 9 million viewers tuned in to one BBC Health Show to find out how to live a healthier life, and over 1 million people contacted the Health Education Authority for follow-up advice afterwards (Hegarty 1993).

Changing behaviour

The mass media, while not sufficient alone to bring about widespread behavioural change, can provide an entry point to campaigns, such as those related to HIV. A sophisticated campaign should do more than simply provide information related to risk and risk reduction. Information needs to be phased and interrelated to other aspects, such as community support, and opportunities should be used to model appropriate behaviours as well as to teach skills necessary to promote safer sex, including safe condom use.

Critical to the first stage of any campaign is the provision of accurate and relevant information to those at risk. People need to be aware of their own individual risk of HIV infection, the severity of the implications and what they need to do to reduce or eliminate their personal risk. The AIDS 'Iceberg' campaign in the UK and the 'Grim Reaper' campaign in Australia, raised anxieties but provided no means of reducing that anxiety and thus influencing behaviour (Bennett & Hodgson 1992).

Some information on AIDS/HIV and preventive behaviours, such as condom use, may be needed by the community as a whole, but other information concerning sexual practices and details of needle exchange schemes are not necessary for many people. Information should be targeted on relevant groups, perhaps through local or specialist radio, street workers, specialist press (e.g. for gay people) and through the distribution of explicit leaflets to specific groups.

One of the greatest successes of the mass media in recent years has been the alteration of the climate of opinion on cigarette smoking (Whitehead & Tones 1990). This has taken three decades, and has involved many different people, organisations and media campaigns, acting in alliance and reinforcing one another's work. An initiative in 1985 is cited by Whitehead & Tones (1990) as an illustration of how the media have been used editorially to raise awareness of anti-smoking campaigns among national and local policy makers. The Health Education Council (now the Health Education Authority) and the British Medical Association (BMA) launched 'The Big Kill', in which figures for smoking-related deaths and associated NHS costs were detailed for each locality in England, Wales and Northern Ireland. Every local authority, health authority and MP received a copy, as also did a wide variety of the mass media. Within 48 hours of publication, it was quoted in many national and local daily papers, resulting in calls for action on smoking sponsorship and a clamp-down on sales of cigarettes to children. Many health promotion organisations achieve a consistent editorial coverage at little cost by drawing newspaper and radio journalists' attention to newsworthy items. This

Box 11.8 Useful tips on how to keep the local press interested (Street 1993)

- Study each newspaper carefully, noting style, use of features and regular columns.
- Identify relevant journalists—e.g. health correspondents—ring them and ask what kind of stories and features they are interested in.
- A press release should be written in the style of the paper. It should be clear and concise with no 'waffle'. Answer the questions: who, why, what, where, when, and how. It should be accurate with people's names and titles correct.
- Include venue, date and time, and a contact name and telephone number.
- Local radio stations always need good interview subjects—introduce experts known to you.
- Keep stories and features topical and local and be ready to respond quickly.

is particularly so when special campaigns such as 'No Smoking Day' are planned. Local news-papers and radios are prime targets for the health educator (see Box 11.8).

A week-long BBC and ITV scheduling of AIDS educational material provided a good model of how information relating to risk and behavioural change may be carried out. The programmes showed people how to perform certain skills, for example by giving an explicit demonstration of how to put a condom on for safe usage. Programmes were presented by role models who would be liked and respected by the target audience, including youth television and radio presenters. Humour was used, and safer sex was promoted as fun rather than mechanically. Studio discussions aimed to dispel myths and ignorance surrounding sexual practice and HIV infection (Bennett & Hodgson 1992).

The media and mental health

The media have a positive part to play in encour-aging attitudes which are conducive to good health. Where mental health is concerned, how-ever, fears that media coverage contributes to stigmatisation are widespread. To examine this concern, researchers at the Glasgow Media Group undertook a study which involved a content analysis of programmes and a qualitative audi-

ence reception study (Philo et al 1994). The purpose of the content analysis was to find out the dominant messages about mental health issues which were presented in the media. The most common category was found to be coverage linking mental illness with violence to others. Most consisted of news reports of violent crimes in which the perpetrators were labelled as mentally ill through terms like 'mad', 'maniac' and 'psycho'. Similar themes emerged from the fictional accounts in this category. The audience study revealed that almost two-thirds of people in the general sample also believed that violence was linked to mental illness. Most of the people who disagreed with these views did so on the basis of personal experience. The findings suggest that the media can play a significant role not only in informing the public, but also in fuelling beliefs which contribute to the stigmatisation of mental illness. From a health promotion perspective these findings are of considerable concern. As many as one in four people are at statistical risk of having mental health problems in the course of 1 year, and many are embarrassed to seek help because of the stigma surrounding mental illness. Philo et al (1994) suggest that if we are to work towards the lessening of stigma associated with mental illness and the provision of positive, accurate images, then health educators will need to work more closely with the media. Two volun-tary organisations, the National Association for Mental Health (MIND) and Mental Health Media, have recently introduced awards recognising good practice in press reporting and broadcast-ing. The Scottish Mental Health Working Group is producing an information resource for journal-ists and broadcasters which includes guidelines for good practice. Collaboration at a personal, local level is also recommended (Philo et al 1994) and health promotion departments have an im-portant part to play in working with local media on the representation of mental health issues.

'Health of the Nation' strategy

Seven 'healthy settings'—cities, schools, hos-pitals, the workplace, homes, the environment and prisons—were identified in the strategy for health (DoH 1992). People spend at least part of their time in one or other of these settings, all of which can be a focus for local action. At a national level, further initiatives have been developed. The Prison Health Service is evaluating the impact of draft guidance on a wide variety of health promotion programmes issued to five establishments:

- a study of the mental health of unsentenced prisoners was started
- fieldwork for a pilot study of anonymised

HIV surveys in three prisons was completed
- a study of knowledge, attitudes and behaviour related to HIV infection and AIDS was started
- a survey of the physical health of male prisoners is planned (DoH 1994).

The aims of the second year of the strategy are to build upon the momentum generated in the first year, and to focus on the development and provision of help for all those working in health promotion.

REFERENCES

Baggott R, Powell M 1994 Implementation and development of alcohol policies in the workplace: a study in Leeds and Leicestershire. Health Education Journal 53(1): 3–14

Bagnall P 1993 Health promotion, school nursing and the school age child. In: Dines A, Cribb A (eds) Health promotion concepts and practice. Blackwell Scientific Publications, Oxford

Bagnall P 1994 Investing in school-age children's health. Nursing Times 90(31): 27–29

Bennett P, Hodgson R 1992 Psychology and health promotion. In: Bunton R, Macdonald G (eds) Health promotion: disciplines and diversity. Routledge, London

Chalmers F 1993 Building on tradition. Healthlines 5: 9

Confederation of British Industry, BUPA 1993 Working for your health: practical steps to improve the health of your business. Confederation of British Industry, London

Department for Education 1993 Education Act 1993: Elizabeth II. Chapter 35. HMSO, London

Department of Health 1989 The control of substances hazardous to health: guidance for the initial assessment in hospitals. Department of Health, London

Department of Health 1992 The health of the nation: a strategy for health in England. Cm 1986. HMSO, London

Department of Health 1993a One year on: a report on the progress of the health of the nation. Department of Health, London

Department of Health 1993b Health of the nation: workplace task force report. Department of Health, London

Department of Health 1994 On the state of the public health 1993. HMSO, London

Dugdill L, Springett J 1994 Evaluation of workplace health promotion: a review. Health Education Journal 53(3): 337–347

Eales J, Watson J 1994 Health education and special educational needs: Scottish concerns and curriculum framework. Health Education Journal 53(1): 81–91

Goodwin E, Aston G 1994 Pregnant clauses. Nursing Times 90(43): 54–58

Greenberg J S 1992 Health education: learner-centered instructional strategies, 2nd edn. Brown, Iowa

Hall D 1991 Health for all children. Oxford Medical, Oxford

Hanlon P 1992 The good hearted Glasgow campaign. In: Williams K (ed) The community prevention of coronary heart disease. HMSO, London

Health and Safety Commission 1992 Management of health and safety at work: management of health and safety at work regulations 1992: approved code of practice. HMSO, London

Health and Safety Executive 1994 Draft management of health and safety at work (amendment) regulations No. 199: proposals to implement the health and safety provisions of the EC directives on pregnant workers. HMSO, London

Health Education Authority 1993 Health promotion in the workplace: a summary. Health Education Authority, London

Hegarty S 1993 Making the most of the media. Healthlines 3: 15–17

Hobbs A 1994 Healthy profits from a sound business proposition. Healthlines 10: 14–16

Kalnins I, McQueen D V, Backett K C, Curtice L, Currie C E 1992 Children, empowerment and health promotion: some new directions in research and practice. Health Promotion International 7(1): 53–59

Lincoln P 1992 Look after your heart. In: Williams K (ed) The community prevention of coronary heart disease. HMSO, London

McAleer M, Jackson P 1994 The school health fax. Nursing Times 90(31): 29–30

National Curriculum Council 1990 Curriculum guidance No. 3. The whole curriculum. National Curriculum Council, York

Phelps F A, Mellanby A R, Crichton N J, Tripp J H 1994 Sex education: the effect of a peer programme on pupils (aged 13–14 years) and their peer leaders. Health Education Journal 53(2): 127–139

Philo G, Secker J, Platt S, Henderson L, McLaughlin G, Burnside J 1994 The impact of the mass media on public images of mental illness: media content and audience belief. Health Education Journal 53(3): 271–281

Ray C 1994 Sex education for Irish primary schools? Sex Education Matters 3: 1

Roberts H, Smith S, Bryce C 1993 Prevention is better. Sociology of Health and Illness 15(4): 447–463

Rogers R, Salvage J 1988 Nurses at risk: a guide to health and safety at work. Heinemann, London

Royal College of Nursing 1994 Violence and community nursing staff: advice for managers. RCN, London

Scottish Office Education Department 1991 Curriculum and assessment in Scotland: a policy for the 90s. Working paper 13: environmental studies 5–14. HMSO, Edinburgh

Street J 1993 Useful tips on how to keep the local press interested. Healthlines 3: 17

Tones K, Tilford S 1994 Health education: effectiveness, efficiency and equity, 2nd edn. Chapman & Hall, London

UNISON 1994 Sexual harassment: some guidelines for UNISON branches. UNISON, London

United Nations Convention 1992 The United Nations convention on the rights of a child. HMSO, London

Wheeler H, Riding R 1994 Occupational stress in general nurses and midwives. British Journal of Nursing 3(10): 527–534

Whitehead M 1989 Swimming upstream: trends and prospects in education for health. King's Fund, London

Whitehead M, Tones K 1990 Avoiding the pitfalls. Health Education Authority, London

World Health Organization 1993 Health for all targets: the health policy for Europe, updated edn. WHO, Regional Office for Europe, Copenhagen

Young I, Williams T (eds) 1989 The healthy school. Scottish Health Education Group, Edinburgh

FURTHER READING

Evans D, Head M J, Speller V 1994 Assuring quality in health promotion: how to develop standards of good practice. Health Education Authority, London

Ewles L, Simnett I 1992 Promoting health: a practical guide, 2nd edn. Scutari, London

Health Visitors' Association 1991 Project health: health promotion and the role of the school nurse in the community. HVA, London

Whitehead M, Tones K 1990 Avoiding the pitfalls. Health Education Authority, London

CHAPTER CONTENTS

Introduction   157

The health of our population   158
  Mortality   158
  Morbidity   160

Health and lifestyle in contemporary Britain   161

Access to health care   161

Social stratification in modern Britain   162

Gender differences in health status   163
  Explaining gender differences in health   163

Ethnicity and health   164
  The health of ethnic minorities   164

Social class and inequalities in health   165
  Class inequalities in health   166
  Health behaviour and social class   167
  Social class and access to health care   168

Inequalities in health in later life   168

Geographical variations in health   168

**Conclusion: the challenge for health
  promotion   169**

References   170

12

Inequalities in health and health promotion

Christina Victor

By the year 2000, people should have the opportunity to develop and use their own health potential in order to lead socially, economically and mentally fulfilling lives.

(Target 2: Health and quality of life, WHO 1993)

INTRODUCTION

One of the aims underlying the creation of the National Health Service (NHS) was to provide a universal system of health care which would be available to all citizens regardless of their social position. The availability of this system would, it was hoped, eradicate the significant differences in both health status and access to health care which had characterised Britain before 1939. Although the NHS has now been in existence for almost 50 years, Britain is still characterised by profound differences within the population in both their experience of health and access to health care. In this chapter we discuss the current pattern of inequalities in health within the United Kingdom and how health promotion activities at the individual, practice/community and population level can contribute to their reduction. We examine inequalities in health status and access to health care within the population. Before considering the major patterns of health inequalities observed in contemporary Britain, there is a brief overview of the health status of our population. This provides the context for examining the pattern of inequalities in health status. It also states the nature of the health promotion challenge.

THE HEALTH OF OUR POPULATION

Before considering the current pattern of inequalities in health within the United Kingdom it is first necessary to consider the contemporary patterns of health and disease. As we saw in Chapter 6 there are only a limited number of readily available national indicators which describe the health status of our population.

Mortality

As we saw in Chapter 6, our most accessible and complete source of data about the health of our population is concerned with deaths. As we discussed in Chapter 6, it is something of a paradox that we have to use information about deaths to provide a description of the health of our population.

Patterns of mortality

In England and Wales in 1991 there were 570 044 registered deaths and 82% (465 534) were of people aged 65 and over (OPCS 1993). As we saw in Chapter 6, it is usual to describe patterns of mortality (and indeed morbidity) in terms of rates

Table 12.1   Death rates: England and Wales 1991 (OPCS 1993 Table B)

Age (years)	Rate per 1000 Males	Females	Percentage difference (100M/F – 100)
Under 1	8.3	6.4	+29%
1–4	0.4	0.3	+33%
5–14	0.2	0.2	0
15–24	0.8	0.3	+166%
25–34	0.9	0.4	+125%
35–44	1.8	1.1	+63%
45–54	4.6	2.9	+58%
55–64	13.8	8.1	+70%
65–74	38.0	21.8	+74%
75–84	93.0	58.8	+58%
85+	187.1	159.2	+17%
All ages	11.2	11.2	—

> Activity 12.1
>
> Examine the pattern of male and female mortality contained in Table 12.1. From these data which age groups would appear to be likely to benefit most from health promotion? Should health promotion concentrate upon men?

rather than absolute numbers. In 1991 the overall death rate was 11 per 1000 population (see Ch. 6 for a description of how to calculate death rates). Mortality rates are high in the first year of life (8.3 per 1000 for males and 6.4 per 1000 for females), decrease in childhood, and then increase steadily with age (see Table 12.1). For men, death rates increase from 1.8 per 1000 for those aged 35–44 to 187.1 per 1000 males aged 85+. A similar pattern is evident for women.

Recent changes in mortality

How has the pattern of mortality changed in recent decades? We can examine changes in health status over time using three indicators: overall mortality rates, standard mortality ratios and life expectancy.

Overall mortality rates.   Health status in the United Kingdom, as measured by overall mortality rates (also known as crude mortality rates) has improved steadily during this century (see Ch. 2). In 1900–1902 the overall mortality rate was 18.4 per 1000 for men and 16.3 per 1000 for women (CSO 1993) compared with 11 per 1000 in 1991 (OPCS 1993). Age-specific rates have also decreased. In 1948 the rate per 1000 for males aged 45–54 was 8.2 compared with 4.6 in 1991—a decrease of 44% (Ham 1993). Similar improvements have been observed for women. Deaths of children in the first year of life are indicative of the general levels of health within any population (i.e. local, regional, national or international). In England and Wales in 1948 the infant mortality rate was 34 per 1000 live births; this had decreased by 75% in 1988 when the rate was 8.4 per 1000 live births (Ham 1993).

Standard mortality ratios.   In order to make valid comparisons over time in overall mortality rates, we must exclude the influence of changes in population structure. For example, the decrease in death rates may simply reflect an increased number of younger people in the population. An increase in mortality rates over time may simply reflect the 'ageing' of the population. One way of taking out the influence of population change upon mortality rates is by making comparisons of standardised mortality ratios (SMR; see Ch. 6 for a description of the SMR). The SMR for 1971 was 88 and by 1991 this had decreased to 62; this represents a 20% decrease in death rates over the last 40 years (OPCS 1993). From this we may conclude that there has been a significant improvement in the health of our population.

Life expectancy.   Life expectancy is the age to which an average person can expect to live. This is usually calculated at birth but may be computed from any age. For example, we may compute expectation of life for those who are aged 65 or 85. When attempting to summarise the health of the population, it is traditional to use expectation of life at birth. Expectation of life at birth in 1841 was 40.2 years for males and 42.2 for females. In 1950–52 it was 67.7 and 72.4 years respectively and in 1989–91 it was 73.2 and 78.7 years (OPCS 1993). This represents an 8.1% increase in life expectancy for males and 8.7% for females in the last 40 years.

Factors influencing changes in mortality

Several factors explain the decrease in death rates and increase in life expectancy which we have seen in the last 40 years. Viewed in the broadest sense, health promotion has been of considerable significance. Healthier environments, as illustrated by improved housing and standards of living, have been vital in improving the health of the population (see Ch. 2). The creation of specific immunisation and screening programmes has been a contributory factor but is not the only factor involved. Access to both primary and secondary health care services has been of lesser importance in contributing to the improved health of the population. This illustrates that improvements in the health of the population have resulted from widespread social change and not simply the development of modern medicine.

The importance of improved housing and

Activity 12.2

What factors have brought about the decrease in death rates and increase in life expectancy?

---

material circumstances in accounting for the improved health of the population emphasises that health promotion is a much broader activity than simply helping people to give up smoking or participate in screening or immunisation programmes. In seeking to improve the health of the population, health professionals will find themselves working in a variety of different settings. Indeed, the majority of health promotion work may take place outside of traditional health-care settings, especially when working with 'hard to reach' groups such as homeless people, or when involved in environmental issues such as housing or measures to improve the safety of pedestrians.

What are the main causes of death?

Overall patterns of mortality can provide a broad overview but tell us little about the major causes of death. We need to determine the most important causes of death so that we may identify the main sources of ill health within society. Identification of the main causes of death in the major age groups is a prerequisite for defining health promotion strategies and setting targets for health promotion activity at practice, locality and national level.

In 1991, the four main causes of death for both men and women were heart disease (31%), neoplasms (25%), cerebrovascular disease (12%) and respiratory diseases (11%) (OPCS 1993). This broad pattern was not consistent across the age groups. For children under 14, 14% of deaths were caused by accidents; for those aged 15–44, 19% of deaths were the result of accidents compared with 4% of deaths for those aged 45–54 (OPCS 1993).

Each of the main causes of death noted above is, in theory at least, reducible by effective health promotion. For example, smoking is an important contributory factor in deaths from stroke, heart disease, a variety of cancers and most respiratory diseases (see Royal College of Physicians 1977). It is estimated that at least one-third of all cancer deaths are preventable. Deaths from accidents and suicide also have a preventable element.

The importance of different causes of death at different ages means that health promoters must adopt strategies, styles of working and targets which are sensitive to the group or individuals with whom they are working (see Chs 8 and 10).

Morbidity

As we discussed in Chapter 6, data about deaths are used as a proxy or indirect measure of the health status of populations. Nationally collected measures of morbidity are less readily available. The main source of population-based morbidity data is the General Household Survey (GHS) (see Ch. 6). The GHS collects information about the prevalence of both acute and chronic health problems within the population (see Ch. 6 for details of how these measures are defined), whilst the 1991 census was concerned with the prevalence of long-standing limiting illness (a measure of chronic health problems).

In 1992, the GHS reported that 12% of the population stated that they had had an acute health problem in the 14 days before interview; 32% had a chronic or long-term health problem and 19% had a long-standing limiting health problem (OPCS 1994) (see Table 12.2).

The GHS data are a useful way to describe the broad pattern of health status of our population. However, it is doubtful if health promotion could have much of an impact upon the level of acute health problems within the population. The lack of information about the causes of chronic physical long-term health problems within the population limits the scope for health promotion activity.

Table 12.2 Great Britain 1992: health status by age and sex (OPCS 1994)

Age (years)	Long-standing illness		Long-standing limiting illness		Acute illness	
	Male (%)	Female (%)	Male (%)	Female (%)	Male (%)	Female (%)
0–4	15	10	5	2	12	9
5–15	19	18	8	7	9	10
16–44	23	24	10	13	8	12
45–64	42	43	26	26	12	16
65–74	60	58	40	38	15	18
75+	64	67	49	52	17	23
All ages	31	33	18	20	11	14

We must therefore assume that it is problems such as heart disease, stroke and cancers which are the main causes of disability. This assumption is problematic because diseases such as arthritis are important causes of disability but not mortality. For example, Martin et al (1988) report that 46% of all disabled adults are disabled by musculoskeletal disorders.

It is doubtful if the activities of the health promoter can have much of an impact upon the progression of many chronic diseases such as arthritis. However, they may be very effective in reducing the degree of handicap—the 'socially' constructed disadvantage resulting from disability and disease. For example, health promotion activities which focus upon improving public access for people with disabilities may be very effective in improving the quality of life of these groups and individuals. This serves to emphasise that health promotion activities operate on a variety of different levels which may have a variety of different outcomes (e.g. decrease in mortality or increase in quality of life).

The objectives of health promotion may vary according to whether the health promoter is working with individuals, groups, communities or entire populations. Health promotion activity concerned with reducing the ill health associated with tobacco smoking might focus upon getting individuals to quit, preventing groups such as children taking up smoking (group activity), creating smoke-free environments (community or locality based activity) or banning advertising of tobacco products (population level approach).

As was stressed in Chapter 6, it is important to review carefully the sources upon which we are basing our health promotion activity. It is important to note any major groups which the source may not include. For example, the GHS only collects information about a sample of the general population resident in the community and therefore excludes those who are resident in institutions such as prisons, hospitals or nursing homes.

Such groups are often excluded from mainstream health promotion even though their needs may be significant. For example, women in prisons or long-stay institutions may not receive breast or cervical cancer screening because it is assumed that it is inappropriate or that they will be screened by virtue of their residence in a 'caring' institution.

HEALTH AND LIFESTYLE IN CONTEMPORARY BRITAIN

It is widely accepted that certain aspects of modern lifestyles are associated with poor health. Cigarette smoking, high alcohol consumption, poor diet and lack of exercise all contribute to deaths from cancers, respiratory disease and heart disease/stroke. It is estimated that cigarette

smoking is responsible for 100 000 deaths annually in England and Wales. Less tangible social support factors may be associated with mental illness and suicide. These factors are much less easy to quantify and consequently are often 'forgotten' or left off mainstream health promotion activities.

Attempting to change behaviour has been perceived as the main province of health promotion (see Lambert & McPherson 1993). However, such an emphasis concentrates upon individuals and often fails to identify the importance of the effects that social and environmental factors have upon the behaviour of individuals (Breslow 1990). Poverty and poor housing remain important correlates of disease and poor health in contemporary Britain. For example, the health promoter's attempts to reduce respiratory disease, such as wheeze in children, may concentrate upon getting the parent(s) to stop or reduce smoking, rather than looking at the influence that bad housing conditions may be having on the family's health. Wherever they work, health promoters must acknowledge and work within the social and environmental context of their clients' lives.

It is against this rather complex background that the data about the prevalence of aspects of health-related behaviour should be interpreted. These data are available from a variety of sources. The General Household Survey reports that 28% of adult females and 29% of males were currently smokers in 1992 and 27% of males and 11% of females were 'heavy' drinkers (OPCS 1994). Measuring diet in a general health survey is problematic. However, it is accepted that the modern British diet is too high in fats and sugars and too low in fibre. The 'Health and Lifestyles' survey (Blaxter 1990) demonstrated the complex interrelationships between different types of health behaviour and how behaviour was rooted in the social context within which individuals function.

ACCESS TO HEALTH CARE

The National Health Service (NHS) was founded in 1948 and provides both primary and secondary

---

Activity 12.5

Consider the possible contribution and areas of activity which you as a health promoter could undertake with women residents of prisons.

health care services. The system is largely funded out of general taxation. The founding principle of the NHS was to provide a comprehensive system of health care to those in need irrespective of their social circumstances. The system was therefore committed to social and geographical equity and the implicit aim was to bring about equality of health in the population by providing a free service. It is against this objective that the data about social inequality presented later in this chapter should be judged. As created, the NHS was concerned with providing curative services and it was only later in the development of the NHS that attention was paid to prevention rather than cure. However, the system is still dominated by the secondary care sector. There has been little debate about how expenditure should be balanced amongst promotion, prevention and cure. The creation of the internal market following the 1991 reforms has done little to upgrade the importance of health promotion.

Expenditure on the NHS in the UK in 1988 was almost £24 billion and this represented 5.9% of gross domestic product (Ham 1993). It is difficult to calculate how much is spent on disease prevention and health promotion. Lambert & McPherson (1993) suggest that this amounts to only 5% of the amount spent on curative services. Health promotion certainly only accounts for a small part of NHS expenditure.

For the purposes of this chapter we will confine our analysis to the pattern of health service use within the population. The General Household Survey again provides an important source of information about use of NHS services by the general population. The 1992 GHS reports that 15% of the population had consulted a GP in the 14 days before the interview; 14% had been to a casualty or outpatient clinician during the previous 3 months; 4% had been treated in hospital as a day patient in the previous year; and 10% had been a hospital inpatient in the previous year (OPCS 1994). These broad levels of utilisation provide the context within which to examine social and geographic patterns of access to health care. This emphasises that, in any one year, most of the population do not see a health care professional. Consequently, health promo-

> **Activity 12.6**
>
> Why is spending by the NHS on health promotion so low? Would greater expenditure on health promotion improve health?

tion that confines itself to the surgery or hospital will reach only a minority of the population. This reinforces the need for health promotion in the community and the need for all government departments to concern themselves with the health effects of their interventions.

SOCIAL STRATIFICATION IN MODERN BRITAIN

The study of patterns of health and disease from a population perspective involves identifying and describing those segments of the population that experience ill health and those that do not. Identification of the groups that experience poorer levels of health enables the health promoter to target those groups that would appear to be in greatest need. The earlier parts of this chapter have provided an overview of the health of the British population and levels of health service utilisation. However, not all parts of the population experience health in the same way. There remain important and significant differences in both the experience of health and access to health care within our population. The rest of this chapter presents an overview of the main differences in health and access to health care with particular reference to age, gender, class, ethnicity and geography. Whilst the focus of our discussion is upon health and access to health, it must be remembered that health is simply one aspect of a broad group of inequalities linked with these social divisions. In particular, class, gender, race and age all profoundly influence a wide range of social opportunities. For some social groups, illness and poor health is simply one component of a pattern of multiple deprivation which includes poor housing, low income and very limited access to leisure and other recreational activities.

GENDER DIFFERENCES IN HEALTH STATUS

As was indicated in Chapter 2, men and women experience considerable differences in health status. However, the pattern observed varies depending upon whether we are considering mortality or morbidity. As measured by mortality, women have a clear health advantage over men. Expectation of life at birth in 1993 in the UK was 73 years for males and 77 years for females (CSO 1993). Scrutiny of Table 12.1 reveals that at each age women experience considerably lower mortality rates as compared with men. For example, at age 15–24 male death rates are two and a half times as high as female rates—even at age 85 and over, men experience death rates 17% higher than women.

Does the pattern of morbidity reflect the mortality differences described above? Table 12.2 illustrates that for morbidity the reverse pattern is observed; men have better health status than women overall. Women have rates of acute illness 27% higher than men, and 11% for long-standing limiting illness. Hence we have a paradox that men are more likely to die than women but those who survive have better health than their female contemporaries.

How is this gender difference in health status reflected in levels of service use?

Females have overall higher crude levels of service use than males, especially for inpatient hospitals spells and GP consultations (see Table 12.3). However, the pattern of service use is not consistent for each age group. It is only for the 16–44 age group that there are very large differences in inpatient hospital spells and GP consultations between the sexes (inpatient stays—6% for men vs 13% for women; GP consultations—9% for men vs 18% for women), and this largely reflects the use of services by women for

Table 12.3   Great Britain 1992: utilisation of health care by sex (OPCS 1994)

	Male (%)	Female (%)
GP in last 14 days	12	18
Average number of GP consultations per year	4	6
Outpatient or casualty in previous 3 months	13	14
Day patient in previous year	4	4
Inpatient in previous year	8	11

childbirth and gynaecological problems. It is this major difference which largely accounts for the crude male–female difference in overall rates—in all other age groups, males have slightly higher levels of health service use.

Explaining gender differences in health

Little attention has been given to trying to explain gender-based differences in health status. Work in the United States by Waldron (1976) concluded that over half of the observed mortality difference between the sexes resulted from differences in behaviour (e.g. cigarette smoking). The observed differences in morbidity may result from a reluctance by men to report illness or from a greater propensity towards illness by women (or indeed some combination of the two). Whilst the causes of gender-based health differences remain unclear, most studies demonstrate the importance of social and environmental factors in determining the health of both men and women. The activities of health promotion can improve the health of both sexes by improving the built environment, strengthening the social environment, and promoting a healthier lifestyle.

Activity 12.7

Given the patterns of morbidity that have been described, should health promotion concentrate upon men or women?

Activity 12.8

What factors might underlie the differences in mortality and morbidity shown by women and men? What contribution could health promotion make to reducing these differences?

ETHNICITY AND HEALTH

Ethnicity is a major axis of social differentiation within British society. The 1991 census asked detailed questions about the ethnic status of the population. According to this source, 5% of the population of Great Britain were from ethnic minorities. However, the ethnic minority population is not equally distributed throughout the country. In inner London 25% of the population are from minority communities compared with 2% in East Anglia (OPCS 1992).

The 1991 census asked people to record whether they belonged to one of the following minority groups: Black (subdivided into African, Afro-Caribbean and other), Asian (subdivided into Indian, Pakistani and Bangladeshi), Chinese, Arab, and other.

In Great Britain 5% of the population belonged to minority groups. The largest groups were Asian (2.6%) and Black (1.6%). A large but usually neglected segment of the minority community is the 2% of the population (2.25 million people) of Irish descent (Jewson 1993). Those working in health promotion must clearly understand the different cultural backgrounds of these groups and aim to provide appropriate and acceptable services to minority community members.

Minority communities in Britain have their roots in the mass migration of groups from Ireland, the Caribbean and Asia to the UK in order to find employment. Initially, therefore, minority group members were identified by collecting data about place of birth. However, it is now incorrect to think of our ethnic minority population as being predominantly an immigrant population as it is estimated that 50% have been born in the UK (Jewson 1993). From a health and health promotion perspective, it may be necessary to distinguish between the migrant and native-born components of our minority communities. For example, information about cervical and breast cancer screening for women from minority communities may need to be in their own language for migrants but not necessarily for those born here.

When examining the overall pattern of health in contemporary Britain, it was noted that health status, as measured by mortality and morbidity, decreased with age. The age composition of a population is, therefore, an important indicator of its health status. The age profile of the minority community is younger than the rest of the British population. It is estimated that 20% of the white population are aged 60+ compared with 5% of those from minority communities (Victor 1991a). This is an important fact when making comparisons of health status and in determining the need for, and style of, health promotion required by minority communities.

The health of ethnic minorities

There are fewer routine data available about the health status of our ethnic minority communities. Death rates are not routinely published by ethnic origin, partly because of problems in determining ethnic status from the data provided on a death certificate (i.e. name only or place of birth). Many national surveys such as the GHS do not include sufficient ethnic minority members within their samples to produce analyses of data for these groups.

The Immigration Mortality Study (Marmot et al 1984) focused upon those aged 20+ who had been born outside England and Wales. This therefore excluded British-born ethnic residents and included British subjects born abroad. With the exception of Irish migrants, death rates for migrants were lower than for their countries of birth. This reflects the fact that 'healthier' people opted to move between countries to find employment.

Although minority communities have patterns of mortality broadly similar to the rest of the population they do experience elevated rates of certain diseases. Amongst the Afro-Caribbean community death rates from TB, hypertension, cerebrovascular disease, diabetes, accidents and

---

Activity 12.9

What special factors would need to be incorporated if you were setting up an AIDS education programme for minority communities?

liver cancer are elevated. Asians have elevated rates of liver cancer and ischaemic heart disease (Britton 1990). Sickle cell disease is a particular problem amongst Afro-Caribbean populations.

The elevated rates of diseases such as diabetes, stroke, hypertension and heart disease which, in theory at least, have a substantial 'avoidable' component, emphasise the potential role for health promotion amongst minority communities. However, such programmes clearly must be both appropriate and acceptable to the target populations. Concentrating upon diseases such as sickle cell, despite their importance, diverts attention away from the major sources of ill health within minority communities and will have little overall effect upon the health of the population.

As was noted earlier in this chapter mortality rates have been declining over the past decades. Minority groups have not shared equally in this decline. For example, mortality from stroke declined by 28% between 1970 and 1980 but by only 3% in men born in the Indian subcontinent (Balarajan 1991). Infant mortality rates are also elevated amongst mothers born in Pakistan and the Caribbean.

Rates of morbidity amongst minority communities appear to be lower than those for the rest of the population. However, it is misleading to make such comparisons, because of the differences in the age structure of the populations. To overcome this we need to standardise the rates and this may be done for either local or national populations. For example, in Kensington, Chelsea and Westminster Commissioning Agency 11% of the white population reported the presence of long-standing limiting illness compared with 10% for both the Black and Asian populations. However, when the rates are standardised (KCW = 100) then the rate for the white population is 95 compared with 133 for Blacks and 145 for Asians (KCWCA 1994).

Activity 12.10

Given the worse health experienced by members of our minority communities, should we concentrate health promotion upon this group or should we aim to improve the health of the total population?

From this we may conclude that the health of many parts of the minority population, especially those resident in inner city areas, is worse than that of their white contemporaries. There is also some preliminary evidence that the health of older people from minority communities in the inner city is worse than that of their native-born contemporaries (Victor 1994).

SOCIAL CLASS AND INEQUALITIES IN HEALTH

Social class is concerned with the relationships made by people in the labour market. Typically these relationships are important in determining the income of people and their degree of autonomy at work. Clusters of occupations tend to have similar profiles; for example, those in professional jobs such as lawyers, accountants and senior managers have high autonomy in the workplace, exercise considerable authority and autonomy at work and earn high salaries. In contrast, those in unskilled manual jobs, such as labourers, have little autonomy, little opportunity to exercise authority and low incomes.

There are numerous different occupations which would make data analysis impossible because there would be too many categories. Consequently, occupations are classified into six major social classes using the Registrar General's classification (see Table 12.4). This classification was first developed in the 1920s and may trace its origins back to the groupings of occupations developed by Farr in the late nineteenth century (Jewson 1993).

The six-category classification is not without its problems, especially in the treatment of women.

Table 12.4 Social classification by occupation

Class	Title	Example
I	Professional	Doctor, barrister
II	Intermediate non-manual	Teacher
IIIn	Skilled non-manual	Clerk
IIIm	Skilled manual	Welder
IV	Semi-skilled manual	Postman
V	Unskilled manual	Labourer

Men are allocated a social class on the basis of their own occupation whilst married women are often classified on the basis of their husband's job; this is problematic as married couples may not have jobs with the same classification. Furthermore, although the categories are presented as being distinct and uniform, there is a degree of variation within groups which may weaken the inter-group variations in, for example, health status or access to health care.

Class inequalities in health

Table 12.5 presents the SMR by social class for both men and women of working age. This shows that, for both men and women, death rates amongst those in social class V are double those of people in social class I. Social class differences in mortality are at their most extreme in the first year of life. The infant mortality rate (i.e. deaths in the first year) is twice as high amongst babies born to parents in class V (11.8 per 1000) as compared with those in social class I (6.9 per 1000) (see Table 12.5).

Social class gradients in mortality are also observable for specific causes of death. Between 1979 and 1983 (the latest date for which data are available) the SMR for men aged 20–64 was higher amongst those in classes IV and V as compared with classes I and II for 65 out of 78

Table 12.5 Mortality by social class (Jewson 1993)

| Class | Male | | | Female | Infant mortality rate per 1000 live births |
	15–64	65–74	75+	20–59	
I	66	68	73	69	6.9
II	77	81	84	78	6.7
IIIn	105	86	92	87	7.1
IIIm	96	100	105	100	7.7
IV	69	106	108	110	9.6
V	124	109	116	134	11.8
Ratio: Class V / Class I	1.88	1.60	1.59	1.90	1.71

Table 12.6 Great Britain: prevalence of acute and chronic ill health by class, age and sex (OPCS 1994)

| | Acute illness | | | Long-standing limiting illness | | |
	Manual (%)	Non-manual (%)	Ratio	Manual (%)	Non-manual (%)	Ratio
Age 16–44						
M	9	8	1.12	12	8	1.5
F	11	12	0.91	13	12	1.08
Age 45–64						
M	12	11	1.18	31	19	1.63
F	16	15	1.06	28	23	1.21
Age 65+						
M	16	15	1.06	47	38	1.23
F	20	21	0.95	47	41	1.14

causes of death (Townsend et al 1988). The reverse pattern was illustrated for only one cause of death: malignant melanoma. For women, of the 82 causes of death, 62 demonstrate a classic social class gradient, with the reverse gradient for breast cancer and malignant melanoma.

It is not simply in mortality that we can observe class-based differences in health status. Table 12.6 indicates that for long-standing limiting illness and acute illness there are significant variations in prevalence between the classes. When expressed as a ratio, the advantageous position of men in the non-manual occupation groups is readily apparent. For long-standing limiting illness, male manual workers aged 45–64 experience rates which are 63% higher than those of their non-manual counterparts.

Recent trends in class-based health inequalities

Have differences in health status between the social classes decreased? Whitehead (1992) has reviewed trends in both child and adult health. She concluded that although health status has generally improved over the past decades it would appear that those in non-manual occupations have benefited most from these improvements. For the years 1975–1990 she concluded that there was no decrease in the gap between the social classes for perinatal deaths (stillbirths and deaths in the first week of life). Consistently the perinatal death rate for social classes IV and V has been 50% above that of those in classes I and II (e.g. in 1990 the respective rates were 9.5 and 6.2 per 1000 births).

Several studies have pointed to an increase in occupationally based mortality differentials for adults since the 1970s (Marmot & McDowell 1986). Blane et al (1990) and Wagstaffe et al (1991), using 'years of life lost' rather than deaths, reported that social class differences in adult health had not decreased over the last two decades. General Household Survey data for the years 1972–1988 indicate that the gap between the social classes in the prevalence of long-standing limiting illness increased between 1972 and 1984 and has remained roughly stable since then.

Factors influencing class-based health inequalities

There are a variety of complex and interrelated factors which explain why those in social class V have worse health than their contemporaries in non-manual occupations and why they do not seem to have experienced the same improvements in health as non-manual workers. Differential increases in wealth, the rise of unemployment, differences in housing and other material circumstances, and exposure to occupational hazards at work and 'unhealthy' environments are all clearly implicated in the continuing existence of health inequalities in modern Britain.

What can health promotion do about continued inequalities?

Clearly, action at an individual level is very important for it is the result of many individuals changing their habits (e.g. smoking) that produces widespread social change. Health promoters working at local levels may target those at 'highest' risk of ill health by focusing their activities upon groups (e.g. workers about to be made redundant) or areas (e.g. housing estates where

there are concentrations of low-income families). The onus here is upon health promoters to work with local people and help them to take action over, for example, inadequate play space for children living in high-rise accommodation. In many instances the role of the health promoter is to act as a catalyst of local action.

However, the importance of factors such as income, access to stable employment, good housing and healthy environments in determining the distribution of disease and ill health reinforces the importance of health promotion challenging the structural and environmental factors which clearly influence these continued health inequalities. If the goal of health promotion is to reduce health inequalities, then it becomes a very challenging and somewhat controversial activity. Health promotion is not simply about getting individuals to change but about challenging many of the social facts we take for granted.

Health behaviour and social class

There are important differences in health lifestyle between the social classes. In 1992, 15% of those in social class I smoked compared with 38% in class V (unskilled manual workers). Alcohol consumption shows much less clear gradients with 25% of men in class I consuming above the weekly recommended level of 22 units compared with 28% in class V. The situation concerning exercise is also unclear. Those in non-manual groups like more leisure time exercise but manual workers have more strenuous activity at work. Whilst these differences in lifestyle are important they are not the sole explanation for the class-based health inequalities. It is a very narrow conception of health promotion that confines itself only to changes in individual behaviour. Consequently, reducing differences in lifestyle is only one of the

---

Activity 12.11

What factors may underlie the failure of those in social class V to experience the same improvements in health status as their contemporaries in class I?

many challenges facing those undertaking health promotion.

Social class and access to health care

As was noted in the introduction to this chapter, health care in this country is available to all members of the population. One of the founding principles of the NHS was the notion of equal access to health care for all citizens regardless of social position or geographical location. However, not all social groups have equal access to health care and Tudor Hart (1971) coined the phrase 'the inverse care law' to describe his observation that medical services were generally least available where they were most needed. The greater uptake of preventive and screening services by the non-manual occupations is well documented (see Whitehead 1992). There is a paradox that those who actively seek 'health promotion' are usually those who need it least. It is therefore very important that the health promoter goes out to the population to find those who are most in need and try to encourage such 'hard to reach' to participate. Assuming that those who do not turn up for cervical screening do not need it is very far from correct.

INEQUALITIES IN HEALTH IN LATER LIFE

The debate about inequalities in health has largely concentrated upon identifying social class differences in premature deaths (i.e. deaths before age 65) in men. Rarely have researchers extended their analysis to consider inequalities within older age groups, possibly because they have implicitly adopted a biological/medical framework which considers that old age is characterised by universal and inevitable ill health.

Evidence for class-based variations in mortality is provided by Fox & Goldblatt (1982). Using data from the OPCS longitudinal study, they showed that for males class-based inequalities extended into later life. Thus the SMR for males aged 65–74 from the professional and managerial classes (social classes I and II) was 68 compared with 109

for those from unskilled or semi-skilled occupational groups. A similar difference was observed for those aged over 75 years (see Table 12.5).

The prevalence of chronic ill health in later life shows statistically significant differences between social classes (Victor 1991b). Consistently, elderly people from the professional and managerial classes experience better health than their contemporaries from the manual occupational groups. For example, rates of long-standing limiting illness were 27% higher amongst those in classes IV and V compared with those in classes I and II; for acute problems the difference was 29% (Victor 1991b).

The continuation of health inequalities into the later phases of the life cycle illustrates their entrenched nature. It also serves to illustrate that there is always scope for health promotion whatever the age of the target population. Too little attention has been paid by health promotion to the older age groups. However, there are significant benefits which could be achieved by working with these groups. Unmet need in this group is high. Decreased mortality and improved quality of life have been demonstrated to result from annual visits by health visitors. Greater attention by health promotion to the older age groups would certainly reap significant benefits in terms of improved quality of life.

GEOGRAPHICAL VARIATIONS IN HEALTH

As well as socially based variations in health there are also spatial variations in both health status of populations and access to health care. Within Great Britain there are distinct variations between both counties and regions in terms of both child and adult health. Mortality rates are higher in Scotland and three regions—Yorkshire and Humberside, North Midlands and West Midlands. A general north to south-east gradient is observed.

Data on variations in death rates are now added to by information on morbidity and fitness. Consistently, morbidity and fitness data confirm the north–south health divide. However, this is a very broad-brush view of what is a very complex pattern of the spatial distribution of (ill) health. For example, Townsend et al (1988) report that areas within the northern regions demonstrate mortality rates which compare with the best in the country but that at the regional level there are many areas of exceptionally high rates. Inner city districts, irrespective of location, generally experience worse health than suburban areas. However, even within apparently 'healthy' districts, there may exist localities which experience very poor health. Kensington, Chelsea and Westminster Commissioning Agency (KCWCA) in inner London has an SMR of 93 and a standardised long-standing limiting illness ratio of 89. However, within KCW one ward in North Kensington has an SMR of 153 and a standardised limiting illness ratio of 146. Even within one single health district, therefore, there may exist profound differences in the health status of the population, which health professionals must be both aware of and work towards reducing in their daily activities. Locally based health data can be extremely useful in identifying those localities that appear to pose the biggest challenges for health promotion. Given the finite resources which exist, health promotion activity will probably have increasingly to choose between universal and targeted approaches.

CONCLUSION : THE CHALLENGE FOR HEALTH PROMOTION

This chapter has demonstrated that the distribution of health (or ill health) within the population is neither equal nor haphazard. Consistently, particular groups such as women, minority group members or those with unskilled jobs (or indeed no jobs) experience the highest rates of mortality and morbidity. It is also highly likely that they experience the highest rates of mental health problems (Victor & Lamping 1994). What brings about these inequalities in health and what can health promotion do about them?

Four main explanations for the continued existence of class-based health inequalities have been proposed (Whitehead 1992; see Box 12.1). It is unlikely that all the differences we have seen in this chapter are a result of statistical errors (the

---

Box 12.1   The main explanations for class-based inequalities (Whitehead 1992)

- Artefact—the method of measuring social class is unreliable and inaccurate and therefore inflates class differences
- Natural and social selection—people in poor health are downwardly socially mobile
- Cultural/behavioural—people in the lower social class have 'bad' habits (e.g. smoking) and are therefore less well
- Materialist/structuralist—emphasises the role of external conditions under which people live

---

'artefact' explanation) or that they are because of 'social selection' and the downward drift of 'sick individuals'.

The other two main explanations for class differences in health both agree that social circumstances affect health but differ in where the emphasis is placed. The cultural/behavioural theory stresses differences in lifestyle and behaviour between groups and concludes that certain social groups experience 'worse' health because they have chosen less healthy lifestyles such as smoking, heavy drinking or drug use. Based on a detailed review of all the evidence, Whitehead (1992) concludes that differences in lifestyle account for only part of the observed differences in health status between social classes and probably between women and men in health. Such individualistic 'victim-blaming' approaches fail to appreciate how the social context influences the ability of individuals to undertake 'healthy' lifestyles. Exhorting individuals to take more exercise or eat a more healthy diet is not going to be very effective if these individuals are living on low incomes and cannot afford to change their way of life. Health promotion must always be very sensitive to the limitations of an individual-focused approach.

The cultural/materialist perspective stresses the role of the conditions under which people live—their material circumstances and environment—in determining inequalities in health. A vast body of evidence links health with material circumstances such as housing, income and working environment. As well as often being linked directly with specific health problems (e.g. damp housing with respiratory disease in children) material circumstances form the social context which can either limit or enhance opportunities for people to engage in 'healthy' lifestyles. Policies which seek to reduce inequalities in health must therefore tackle these issues if they are to succeed in changing individual behaviour. However, this makes health promotion a very radical activity as it is asking very fundamental questions about the way that society is organised and how this influences the health of the population.

Despite the availability of a universal system of health care funded out of general taxation and free at the point of use, modern Britain is characterised by profound inequalities in health. Their continued existence, despite 40 years of the NHS, suggests that health inequalities are not created by lack of access to health care but are a manifestation of wider variations in material circumstances within society. Health promotion may operate on a variety of different levels ranging from the individual to the population. However, the entrenched nature of the health inequalities identified suggests that only effective health promotion at a structural level which challenges the existence of poverty and bad housing will have any long-term impact. This makes health promotion a radical activity and potentially an important agent of social change.

REFERENCES

Balarajan R 1991 Ethnic differences in mortality from IHD and CVD in England and Wales. British Medical Journal 289: 560–564

Blane D, Davey-Smith G, Bartley M 1990 Social class differences in years of potential life lost. British Medical Journal 301: 429–432

Blaxter M 1990 Health and lifestyles. Tavistock/Routledge, London

Breslow L 1990 A health promotion primer for the 1990s. Health Affairs (Summer): 6–21

Britton M 1990 Mortality and geography. OPCS series D S. HMSO, London

Central Statistical Office (CSO) 1993 Annual abstract of statistics. HMSO, London

Fox J, Goldblatt P 1982 Socio-demographic mortality differentials: longitudinal study, 1971–1975. Series LS, No. 1. HMSO, London

Ham C 1993 Health policy in Britain, 3rd edn. Macmillan, Basingstoke

Jewson N 1993 Inequalities and differences in health. In: Taylor J, Field D (eds) Sociology of health and health care. Blackwell, Oxford

Kensington, Chelsea and Westminster Commissioning Agency (KCWCA) 1994 Health in KCW. Annual Report of the Director of Public Health. KCW, London

Lambert H, McPherson K 1993 Disease prevention and health promotion. In: Davet B, Popay J (eds) Dilemmas in health care. Open University Press, Milton Keynes

McKeown T 1979 The role of medicine: dream mirage or nemesis, 2nd edn. Basil Blackwell, Oxford

Marmot M, McDowell M E 1986 Mortality decline and widening social inequalities. Lancet ii: 274–276

Marmot M G, Adelstein A M, Bulusu L 1984 Immigrant mortality in England and Wales 1970–78. OPCS Studies on Medical and Population Subjects Number 42. HMSO, London

Martin J, Meltzer H, Elliot D 1988 The prevalence of disability amongst adults. HMSO, London

Office of Population Censuses and Surveys (OPCS) 1992 1991 census: Great Britain. National Monitor Cen 91 Cm56. OPCS, London

Office of Population Censuses and Surveys (OPCS) 1993 Mortality statistics: cause 1991. HMSO, London

Office of Population Censuses and Surveys (OPCS) 1994 General household survey: 1992. HMSO, London

Royal College of Physicians 1977 Smoking and health. RCP, London

Townsend P, Phillimore P, Beattie A 1988 Health and deprivation: inequality in the north. Croom Helm, London

Tudor Hart J 1971 The inverse care law. Lancet 1: 405–412

Victor C R 1991a Health and health care in later life. Open University Press, Milton Keynes

Victor C R 1991b Inequality in health in later life. Ageing and Society 11: 23–39

Victor C R 1994 Broken down by age and sex: gender and ethnic variations in the health of older people in the inner city. Paper presented at the University of Surrey conference on Gender and Ageing

Victor C R, Lamping D 1994 Is mortality a good proxy measure for morbidity? Paper presented at the Faculty of Public Health Medicine Summer Conference

Wagstaffe A, Paci P, Doorslaer G 1991 On the measurement of inequalities in health. Social Science and Medicine 33: 545–547

Waldron I 1976 Why do women live longer than men? Social Science and Medicine 10: 349–362

Whitehead M 1992 The health divide. In: Townsend P, Davidson N, Whitehead M (eds) Inequalities in health. Penguin, London

World Health Organization 1993 Health for all targets: the health policy for Europe, updated edn. WHO, Regional Office for Europe, Copenhagen

CHAPTER CONTENTS

The environment affects your health   171
   Air pollution   172
   Water pollution   174
   Noise pollution   174
   Accidents   175
   Health and safety at work   176
   Smoking   177
   The home environment   177

Community safety   177

Environmental inequalities   178

Health and the green agenda   178

Transport and health   179

The environmental professions   180
   Environmental health officers   181
   Engineers   181
   District surveyors   181
   Town planners   182
   Architects   182
   Working across the professional boundaries   182

References   183

13

Health and the environment

David Pike

By the year 2000, all Member States should have developed, and be implementing, policies on the environment and health that ensure ecologically sustainable development, effective prevention and control of environmental health risks and equitable access to healthy environments.

(Target 18: Policy on environment and health, WHO 1993)

THE ENVIRONMENT AFFECTS YOUR HEALTH

It seems almost self-evident to suggest that the environment in which people spend their lives will have a direct impact upon their state of health and well-being. Yet this apparently simple truth is far from being universally adopted by policy makers and practitioners in either the health or environmental professions. There is a strong tradition amongst researchers which says that causal links between environment and health should be established with 100% certainty before policies based upon such links are taken forward. The major exception is the WHO 'Healthy Cities' movement already referred to in Chapter 2 and this will be used as a reference point in this chapter. Without in any sense undervaluing the contribution of careful research (indeed it encourages it) the 'Healthy Cities' project emphasises a quality of life perspective. This recognises, for example, that reducing pollution is desirable even though certain health consequences cannot be guaranteed beyond all doubt.

First we will spell out in as simple terms as possible the actual health impacts of various forms of environmental pollution on individuals. A report by Hardie & Walker (1992) designed to assist collaboration between local authority and health professionals in the London Borough of Camden succinctly summarises these impacts.

Air pollution

Modern industrial processes, and the motor vehicle in particular, produce a cocktail of air pollutants (see Table 13.1) which have a damaging effect on health. Pollution from motor vehicles is of greatest concern because of the seemingly inexorable rise in the numbers of vehicles on our roads. Latest forecasts suggest a doubling of road traffic by the year 2025.

Different groups of people are affected by air pollution in different ways. Young people absorb toxins into their bodies more quickly than older people. However, older people are more prone to respiratory disease which can be caused or exacerbated by air pollutants. Of particular significance is the recent dramatic rise in asthma cases; a recent report of the Parliamentary Office of Science and Technology (1994) provides evidence of a doubling of asthma cases in the last 10 years. On Friday 13 December 1991, London experienced its worst pollution event in recent years when high atmospheric pressure produced cold, still air; ideal conditions for the accumula-

tion of nitrogen dioxide. Research for a BBC 'Panorama' programme showed that admissions of young asthma sufferers to hospitals doubled during the week of 13 December compared with the corresponding week in January. So what are the major air pollutants that affect health and what impacts do they have on individuals?

Sulphur dioxide (SO_2) is generated by fossil-fuelled power stations and diesel exhaust. At high concentrations, it irritates the eyes and mucous membranes and may cause a narrowing of the airways and induce coughing. In healthy people these effects are normally short-lived.

Ozone is generated in a photochemical reaction between nitrous oxides and hydrocarbons from either industrial processes or more commonly from vehicle emissions. A number of major world cities regularly experience photochemical smogs which include high concentrations of ozone. City authorities, Los Angeles for example, are beginning to take active steps to reduce the incidence and intensity of photochemical smogs. These steps include restrictions on some kinds of petrol-engined vehicles and on the use of barbecue lighter fuel. At relatively low concentrations, ozone can cause runny eyes, throat irritation and breathing difficulties in some people. There is also evidence that, at least temporarily, it can reduce the resistance of the lungs to disease. During periods when ozone levels are high, vigorous outdoor exercise should be avoided.

The motor vehicle is overwhelmingly respon-

Table 13.1 Sources of air pollution in UK (1990) (London Research Centre 1993)

	Percentage of total emissions					
	Sulphur dioxide	Carbon monoxide	Nitrogen oxide	Smoke	Volatile organic compounds	Carbon dioxide
Transport	4	90	58	47	42	20
Electricity supply	72	1	28	6	1	34
Other industry	19	4	9	13	52	26
Domestic	3	4	2	33	2	14
Other	2	1	3	1	3	6
Total	100	100	100	100	100	100

sible for the increasing levels of carbon monoxide in the air. The effect of this gas on people relates to its ability to interact with haemoglobin, the substance in the blood which performs the vital role of carrying oxygen around the body. This interaction causes the formation of carboxyhaemoglobin, which thereby reduces the oxygen-carrying capacity of the blood. The poisoning effect on the human body is proportional to the length of exposure. Brief exposures are reversible, but as the exposure increases, people experience headache, vomiting, collapse and eventually death.

Nitrogen oxides are again produced by vehicle emissions and form a component of photochemical smogs. Although highly toxic in high concentrations, they are rarely present in sufficient quantities to seriously affect people. They can, however, cause irritation to the throat and eyes. Particulate matter comprises the substances (dust, smoke and fine ash) generated by industrial processes and by diesel engines. Finer particles can form a health hazard as they are more likely to become embedded in the tissue of the lungs.

Until 1986, when the permitted levels of lead in petrol were substantially reduced and lead free petrol came into widespread use, the high concentrations of lead in dust found in many urban areas were giving cause for serious concern. Lead is a cumulative poison, which once ingested remains in the body for long periods. High accumulations cause damage to the central nervous system. There is also evidence to suggest that even relatively low amounts can cause learning difficulties in young children.

The adverse health effects of benzene and other volatile organic compounds have perhaps been underestimated to date. Benzene is present in petrol (particularly in super unleaded petrol) and evaporates easily. High atmospheric concentrations occur in petrol filling stations. When fuel tanks are near empty they contain high concentrations of evaporated benzene which is dispelled from the tank by the new fuel flowing in. The person filling the tank could therefore be exposed to high levels for a short period. The nozzles on petrol pumps are now almost universally fitted with a flexible protective collar in an attempt to ameliorate any health risk. High or persistent levels of exposure to benzene may cause anaemia. It is also a carcinogen and has been linked to cases of leukaemia.

Table 13.2 summarises information about the major air pollutants and their effects on health.

Table 13.2 Air pollution and health

Pollutant	Source	Health impact
Sulphur dioxide (SO_2)	Coal-fired power stations Diesel exhaust	Exacerbates asthma, chronic bronchitis
Ozone (O_3)	Photochemical reaction between nitrogen oxides and hydrocarbons (photochemical smogs)	Irritates eyes and throat. Triggers asthma attacks. May increase risk of infection
Carbon monoxide (CO)	Petrol car exhausts	Reduces oxygen-carrying capacity of blood. Lethal in high doses
Nitrogen dioxide (NO_2)	Vehicle exhaust	Irritates eyes and throat. May exacerbate asthma
Particulates (smoke)	Particularly diesel exhausts. Wide range of solid and liquid particles in air	Can carry carcinogenic material to lungs. Wide range of respiratory difficulties
Lead	Dust and vehicle exhausts	Impairs intellectual development of children
Benzene and other volatile organic compounds (VOCS)	Emitted from evaporation of solvents and petrol. Present in vehicle exhaust	Benzene is carcinogenic. Can cause leukaemia in high doses

Water pollution

Drinking water can become a health hazard through the presence of either microorganisms or chemicals that find their way into the water supply at various points in the water cycle. Microorganisms are removed from drinking water through the process of chlorination but the presence of chemicals is less easily dealt with and demands constant monitoring by the water suppliers. We shall deal briefly with those chemicals most likely to pollute the water supply.

Some researchers have claimed to have established a link between Alzheimer's disease and the presence of aluminium in water. This is supported by other evidence relating to patients undergoing renal dialysis. A form of dementia accompanied by muscle weakness and bone fractures has been noted when the aluminium levels in the water used for dialysis rise above a certain very low threshold, a threshold which is one-quarter of that considered acceptable for drinking water. However, to put this evidence into perspective, water is responsible for less than 4% of the body's average daily intake of aluminium.

Relatively high levels of lead in the water supply have been measured in areas of older housing where lead pipework is still present. As with airborne lead, there is evidence which associates learning impairment in children with low-level exposure to lead in water over a long period.

In rural areas, nitrates used in fertilisers and generated by decaying animal and vegetable matter can contaminate the water supply. Ammonia, a common disinfectant, also generates nitrates as it breaks down in the sewerage and water distribution systems.

Nitrates are converted into nitrites in the stomach. A link between nitrates/nitrites and gastric cancer has been demonstrated in animals, but epidemiological research in the UK has failed to establish a link in human beings.

Perhaps one of the most contentious issues in environmental health is the extent to which pesticides that enter the water supply pose a hazard to health. 'Pesticides' is a generic term for a number of substances which can enter the water supply system as runoff from soil or the hard surfaces of cities. They include insecticides, herbicides, fungicides and algicides. The use of two herbicides commonly used by local authorities to control weeds, atrazine and simazine, has recently been banned by the Government. The health effects of long-term exposure to pesticides is simply not known with any confidence. Until there is reliable evidence one way or the other, a precautionary approach is being adopted by the authorities.

Noise pollution

The noise generated by so many of the activities of modern life and experienced in the street, home or working environment can affect people's health in two fundamental ways. First, regular exposure to high levels of noise, particularly in the workplace, can permanently damage hearing. Through the enactment of health and safety at work legislation, it is now common practice for employees working in noisy environments to be required to wear ear protectors, although one suspects that enforcement is not always rigorous. It is estimated that approximately 2 million people suffer some permanent hearing loss due to occupational noise.

Secondly, there are the psychological effects on people who are exposed to lower levels of noise during their everyday lives. Living with the constant noise of aircraft or road traffic, for example, can cause stress and hence stress-related illness. Way back in 1963, the then Minister of Science set up the Committee on the Problem of Noise (the Wilson Committee). In its report (1963), this committee proposed some tentative standards for acceptable noise levels inside dwellings in urban areas. The conventional unit of noise measurement is the decibel A (dBA) which takes into account the varying sensitivity of the human ear to different sound frequencies. The Wilson Committee suggested that for living rooms and bedrooms in dwellings in busy urban areas, a daytime level of 50 dBA and a night-time level of 35 dBA should not be exceeded for more than 10% of the time. Typical noise levels in a busy street are 75–80 dBA during the day and 50–55 dBA at night. If a closed window attenuates noise levels by 20 dBA, it can be seen that even with windows closed the Wilson 'standards' are rarely met; and people like to open their windows occasionally!

The Committee also concluded that 'in London (and no doubt this applies to other large towns as well) road traffic is, at the present time, the predominant source of annoyance, and no other single noise is of comparable importance'. There is little to suggest that this statement is not equally true 30 years later.

Noise from commercial activities can also give rise to considerable annoyance to members of the public. The central London Borough of Camden's Environment Department is experiencing a growing number of complaints relating to commercial noise. Numbers of complaints have risen from 547 in 1989/90 to 756 in 1991/92, an increase of 38% in 3 years. Noise from construction sites accounted for 44% of these complaints in 1991/92, with 17% from music and entertainment, and 12% from mechanical plant and machinery. To control noise nuisance from construction sites, local authorities are increasingly resorting to 'Considerate Contractor' schemes and codes of practice for construction works linked to the granting of planning permission. Recently, Camden successfully prosecuted a major national building contractor for failing to adhere to guidelines and causing a severe nuisance to the residents of adjoining properties.

Accidents

Accidents, whether they occur in the public domain, in the home or at work, can have a variety of causes including the human factor. However, the physical environment is frequently one of their most important causes. Road traffic accidents, for example, can be caused by poor road layout or inadequate street lighting. In 1993, road accidents killed 3820 people, caused 44 890 serious injuries and involved over a quarter of a million other casualties in the UK. However,

Table 13.3 Road deaths in some European countries (1991) (DoT 1993)

Country	Death per 100 000 vehicles
UK	21
Belgium	43
Denmark	35
Eire	52
France	39
Greece	75
Netherlands	21
Spain	66

deaths in road accidents have halved in the past 30 years and injuries have reduced by a third in spite of the very large increase in traffic. Also, as Table 13.3 shows, the rate of road deaths in the UK compares favourably with a number of other European countries. The Government has set a target of reducing reported road accidents by one-third by the year 2000.

As well as causing injury to those directly involved, these accidents cause stress, pain and suffering to friends and relatives with consequential effects on their health. Transport economists have attempted to estimate the full costs to society of road accidents, including the costs to the health service of hospitalisation etc. Latest figures (1993) used by the Department of Transport suggest the cost of a fatality as being £744 000 and a serious casualty £84 000.

The kind of changes to the street environment which have succeeded in reducing accidents are the introduction of pedestrian crossings, guard-rails to encourage people to cross busy roads at relatively safe points, various kinds of traffic-calming measures (including speed-humps) and improved street lighting. Many local authorities have in recent years introduced networks of protected cycle routes and other measures to reduce the alarmingly high number of accidents involving cyclists.

Accidents in the home account for just over one-third of all accidental deaths including one-third of all childhood deaths. They are the most common cause of death amongst children aged less than 1 year. Accidents to children in the home can be caused by disrepair, inadequate lighting, unsafe electricity supply and lack of gates on stairs.

Older people are particularly prone to accidents in the home because of poor sight and mobility, and the fact that they tend to spend more time at home than other people. Environmental causes of such accidents include the presence of poorly maintained equipment, open or portable fires, poor lighting and poorly designed home interiors.

Deaths and injuries from fires in the home account for three-quarters of all fire casualties. Nearly 20% of domestic fires are caused by faulty appliances and wiring. Houses in multiple occupation (HMOs) are vulnerable to fire because of their intensity of use and their frequent lack of adequate means of escape. Local authorities have specific powers to control the use and operation of HMOs.

Health and safety at work

There is a wealth of evidence to suggest that the environment in which people spend their working lives can have serious adverse effects on their health. The Health and Safety at Work Act 1974 places a general duty on the employer 'to ensure, as far as is reasonably practicable, the health, safety and welfare at work of all his employees'. Having said that, a number of well-publicised attempts by victims to extract compensation for damage to their health from employers have demonstrated how difficult it sometimes is to establish cause and effect.

Traditional heavy industries such as coal mining or asbestos manufacture are carried out in dust-laden environments which, unless protective equipment is provided, place workers in severe risk of contracting pneumoconiosis, asbestosis and other forms of lung disease. There have always been financial disincentives, for employers and employees alike, to the wearing of protective clothing and equipment; for employers because of loss of productivity and profitability and for employees because of loss of earnings.

However, it is not only in the traditional heavy industries that the working environment has a direct impact on health. The modern office block has brought with it a whole new set of health and safety problems including the so-called 'sick building syndrome'. In recent years, this phenomenon has seen a flurry of research activity and reports, including the House of Commons Environment Committee's 'Sixth Report on Indoor Pollution' (1991), a review by the Health and Safety Executive (which shares with local authorities responsibility for the monitoring and promotion of health and safety at work) (1992), and a report by the Institution of Environmental Health Officers (1991). All agree that there are problems of defining what is meant by 'sick building syndrome', that there is a need for more research and that guidelines should be prepared to ensure that local authorities adopt a consistent approach to their investigations and data collection.

Sykes (1988) has suggested that

the common feature of sick buildings is that their occupants suffer, or appear to suffer, a measurably higher incidence of illness than expected for no readily identifiable reason. Clinically diagnosed illnesses which can readily be attributed to a particular cause such as humidifier fever, Legionnaires disease or to exposure to a toxic agent in the environment are not usually regarded as 'sick building syndrome'.

The World Health Organization has compiled a common list of symptoms as follows:

- eye, nose and throat irritation
- sensation of dry mucous membrane and skin
- erythema (skin rash)
- mental fatigue
- headaches, high frequency of airway infections and cough
- hoarseness, wheezing, itching and unspecified hypersensitivity
- nausea, dizziness.

Activity 13.1

A patient claims to be suffering from sick building syndrome. What symptoms would you be looking for and what are the likely causes?

A number of interesting patterns have emerged from UK studies. Symptoms are most common in air-conditioned buildings; clerical staff are more likely than managerial staff to suffer; and symptoms tend to be more frequent in the afternoon than the morning.

The most commonly suggested causes of sick building syndrome are:

- airborne pollutants (including chemical pollutants, dust and fibres and microbiological contaminants)
- odours
- lack of negatively charged small air ions
- inadequate ventilation and fresh air supply
- low relative humidity
- high temperatures
- poor lighting.

There is little evidence to suggest that any one of these is the prime cause, although poor ventilation and low relative humidity certainly appear to be responsible for some of the more common symptoms.

Smoking

The effects of smoking on the health of those who smoke has been well documented elsewhere; but smoking also affects the environment in which non-smokers live, work and travel. The well-publicised case of the show-business personality, Roy Castle, who died recently from cancer was a dramatic illustration of this. A non-smoker, he claimed that his lifetime spent performing in smoke-filled night clubs was a contributory cause of the disease.

Although in the medical world the link between passive smoking and lung cancer is disputed by some, there is little doubt that the gases found in cigarette smoke (e.g. aldehydes, ammonia, acetone, hydrogen cyanide) have toxic or irritant properties. The World Health Organization has admitted that more research needs to be done on the health effects of passive smoking but nevertheless advocates more vigorous efforts to curtail smoking in public places. The Independent Scientific Committee on Smoking and Health (the Froggatt Committee) in its fourth report

(1988) concluded that passive smoking presented some hazard to non-smokers and pressed for the separation of smokers from non-smokers at work and in public places. Very considerable strides have been made in recent years towards achieving smoking-free environments on public transport. Smoking is not allowed on the London Underground system or on London's buses. A number of airlines do not allow smoking during flight.

The home environment

We have already seen how environmental factors can affect safety in the home, but the physical condition of housing can have other effects on health. Poor housing conditions were a major driving force behind the public health reforms of the nineteenth century and the establishment of the environmental health profession.

Jacobson et al (1991) refer to studies which have identified a relationship between poor health and factors such as overcrowding, structural deficiencies, lack of privacy and lack of play space. Other studies concerning the impact of housing conditions on the health of children have found that respiratory and bronchial symptoms, headaches and diarrhoea were more common in children living in damp housing once other factors such as smoking in the household and low income had been discounted.

COMMUNITY SAFETY

In many inner-city areas, partnerships between the police, local authorities and local communities are being established under the banner of 'community safety'. The main emphasis is on crime-prevention but one of the underlying concerns is the degrading and dangerous effects that criminal activities such as drug dealing and prostitution can have on the environment in which people live and work. Living in such an environment can have direct effects on health (e.g. the dangers of discarded needles) as well as indirect effects caused by high levels of stress.

The environmental contributions to these partnerships have included devoting more resources to the cleaning of the streets and other public spaces, improving street and housing estate lighting and introducing traffic management schemes to discourage kerb-crawling. Some authorities are seeking to broaden the scope of community safety beyond the narrow confines of crime prevention. In the London Borough of Camden, for example, a partnership initiative has been taken to improve public safety at the Camden Lock markets.

These markets attract hundreds of thousands of shoppers and visitors on most Saturdays and Sundays into a relatively confined area. The police, fire brigade, local authority and the market operators meet regularly to establish agreed codes of practice as to the safe operation of the markets (maintaining adequate aisle widths etc.) and to develop emergency plans.

ENVIRONMENTAL INEQUALITIES

In Chapter 12 we considered the question of inequalities in health and the commitment of the World Health Organization to the reduction of such inequalities. O'Keefe & Newbury (1993) have referred to analysis in London which shows a strong correlation between the health of the population and environmental deprivation when expressed geographically. In other words, areas of inner London with poor levels of health also suffer from high levels of environmental deprivation (as well as socioeconomic deprivation). Thus if one aim of public policy makers is to reduce inequalities in health then an important component of their strategy should be to tackle environmental inequality.

HEALTH AND THE GREEN AGENDA

Earlier in this chapter we have seen quite precisely what impact various forms of pollution have on the health of individual people. In this section we shall set these impacts in the much broader context of the so-called 'green agenda'.

There is a growing realisation that the past levels of economic growth seen in the developed world cannot be sustained without serious (and some believe catastrophic) effects on the earth's environment and life-support systems caused by

dramatic increases in pollution levels. When the claims of the developing world for a fair share in the fruits of economic prosperity are added, then the potential crisis deepens.

Governments throughout the world have responded to this challenge by individually and collectively attempting to pursue strategies for 'sustainable development'. The definition of this term has caused much confusion but basically it means environmentally sustainable economic development. This constrains economic growth to that which can be achieved without irreversibly damaging the earth's environment or using up the earth's supply of finite resources including its atmosphere.

Clearly in the short term this is an impossible target; coal and oil, which are both non-renewable resources and produce damaging atmospheric pollution, will continue to be used to generate electricity. In the medium to long term, however, sustainable development will require a switch to renewable energy sources such as solar power or energy from waste. It will also require huge changes in human behaviour particularly in relation to the motor car, but more of that later.

As a result of the Earth Summit on Environment and Development held in Rio de Janeiro in 1992, individual governments agreed to prepare strategies and action plans to implement the collective agreements reached at that summit. In 1994, the UK Government published its strategy—'Sustainable Development: the UK Strategy', having produced a White Paper 'This Common Inheritance' in 1990 prior to the Rio Summit.

The green agenda has many strands but perhaps of most significance to health is the question of global climate change. There are two key climatic effects of the air pollutants produced by industrial societies. The first is known as 'global warming'. It is caused by the build-up of gases such as carbon dioxide and methane (so-called greenhouse gases) in the earth's atmosphere, which in turn causes the surface of the earth to become warmer with consequent climatic change. The second is the damage to the ozone layer caused by chemicals such as chlorofluorocarbons (CFCs) commonly used as coolants in refrigerators. When released, these chemicals do not break down until they reach the upper atmosphere where ultraviolet radiation turns them into chlorine or bromine which help destroy ozone. The ozone layer acts as a filter to harmful ultraviolet rays, which can cause skin cancer.

Sustainable development strategies need, therefore, to place considerable emphasis on reducing the emissions into the atmosphere of both greenhouse gases and ozone-depleting chemicals. Taking the latter first, over 100 countries have signed the Montreal Protocol on Substances that Deplete the Ozone Layer (UNEP 1987), which controls the production and consumption of the worst offenders. It is sobering to note that, as a result of this and subsequent revisions to it, the quantities of ozone-depleting substances in the atmosphere will only be restored to today's levels in 2012, because some of these substances take up to 15 years to break down.

Similar commitments have been made by world governments to reduce greenhouse gas emissions, particularly of carbon dioxide. The UK Government has set a target to return CO_2 and other greenhouse gas emissions to their 1990 levels by the year 2000. To achieve this target, the government is proposing to concentrate action in the transport and energy sectors which together will account for well over half of all CO_2 emissions in 2000. In the energy sector, government initiatives will be directed towards encouraging greater efficiency of energy production, energy conservation and increases in renewable energy capacity.

The transport sector is a special case which is at the core of the relationship between health and the environment. As we have seen, transport has a very direct impact on the health of individuals, through the pollutants it creates and the large number of accidents that result in personal injury with which it is associated. But it also has a profound effect on the health of the planet as a major generator of greenhouse gas. Because it is so significant, we shall now examine the relationship between transport, the environment and health in more detail.

TRANSPORT AND HEALTH

Transport serves both economic and social purposes and also has considerable effects on the environment. Any successful economy must have efficient means of transporting raw materials, finished goods and people. As an economy grows so will the amount of travel. More goods will be moved and people will choose to spend more of their disposable income on travel.

Transport is also of key importance to social interaction in the modern world. To have access to safe, convenient, relatively cheap transport is a major contribution to a good quality of life. But as we have seen, the price for this increased mobility and accessibility is the damage which the motor vehicle in particular does to the local and global environment and to people's health. Hillman (1991) has succinctly summarised the impacts of transport on health as follows:

- physically, owing to death and injury in road accidents
- psychologically, in distress due to accidents and the fear of accidents
- pathologically, as the pollution and noise from motor vehicles are sources of disease and mental impairment
- ecologically, as exhaust emissions from traffic are a major contributor to global warming.

Transport gives the clearest possible illustration that the new public health and sustainable development agendas are inextricably linked and that a coherent set of transport policies needs to be developed to address both agendas. In the same week in October 1994, two important reports were published both dealing with transport, the environment and health. The first was the eighteenth report of the Royal Commission on Environmental Pollution on 'Transport and the

Environment' (1994) and the second the sixth report of the House of Commons Transport Committee on 'Transport-related Air Pollution in London' (1994). Both these reports are key references for the policy proposals that follow.

So, what transport policies would simultaneously address both the sustainability and health agendas? Firstly, the need for travel should be reduced. Most major cities have experienced a dispersal of activities and development during the greater part of this century. This means that more travel has to take place for both business and pleasure. The classic example of this phenomenon is the growth of out-of-town shopping centres. These have been built on relatively cheap land to capture the high-spending car owners by offering plentiful parking on the congestion-free peripheries of towns. This has had a number of serious adverse effects.

Existing town centres decline as much of their trade is siphoned off to the out-of-town centre. Car owners travel further, use more non-renewable energy, emit more pollution (particularly CO_2) and are involved in more accidents. Those who do not own cars will find it difficult, if not impossible, to reach the new centre by public transport. They will be forced to continue to use the existing centres where, of course, choice has been reduced because of their decline.

Town planners are now beginning to realise that largely market-driven dispersal has to be checked in the interests of environmentally sustainable development. Emphasis is now being placed upon compactness by encouraging the revival and growth of existing town centres or the creation of self-contained new communities. The fast-developing telecommunications revolution may considerably reduce the need for travel.

The second policy strand should be directed at reducing the use (as distinct from the ownership) of motor vehicles. Policy instruments could include making vehicle users pay a charge for the use of road space (road pricing), increasing taxation on fuel, providing incentives to industrial firms to transport their goods by rail, reducing the amount of road space for general traffic use particularly in town centres (e.g. pedestrianisation schemes), improving public transport and encouraging other modes of travel such as cycling and walking.

Thirdly, measures can be taken to improve the environmental performance of vehicles. Since 1992, European Commission standards require that all new cars in the UK have catalytic converters fitted. These substantially reduce emissions of nitrous oxides, hydrocarbons and carbon monoxide. However, a major problem with catalytic converters is that they do not operate when the vehicle engine is relatively cold in the period immediately after starting. This of course is the period when emissions are highest. For the typical short urban journey the catalytic converter may only operate for a small proportion of the journey or even not at all.

The use of alternative fuels is another possibility. Much interest has focused on the development of electric vehicles, in part stimulated by Californian legislation which requires that 2% of cars sold should be 'zero emission vehicles' from 1998 onwards, and 10% from 2003 onwards.

Electric vehicles pose an interesting dilemma for policy makers because the generation of the electricity used to charge vehicle batteries gives rise to the release of more carbon dioxide into the atmosphere than the use of conventional vehicle fuels. In the shorter term the expansion of the use of compressed natural gas (CNG) and liquid petroleum gas (LPG) will reduce emissions of particulates, ozone-forming hydrocarbons and nitrogen oxides. The use of these fuels is particularly beneficial for fleets of medium-sized vehicles operating in urban areas, e.g. buses, minibuses and refuse collection vehicles.

This concludes the part of this chapter concerned with the quite complex issues surrounding health and the environment. We shall now turn our attention to the people who work in the environmental field and discuss how they can contribute to health promotion.

THE ENVIRONMENTAL PROFESSIONS

One of the most important tenets of the 'Healthy Cities' movement is that, in addition to health service professionals, there are many other professional groups whose work has a direct impact upon people's health. It is essential that these groups and health professionals learn to work together effectively. The public is often not concerned with understanding the fine distinctions between professional boundaries; it simply wants a seamless service.

What are the environmental professions and how do they assist in promoting health? It may first be worth noting that many of these professionals would probably not perceive themselves as having a health promotion role. The broader 'Healthy Cities' definition of health needs to be more widely understood within the environmental professions.

Environmental health officers

Environmental health officers (EHOs) are the environmental professionals with whom health service professionals are probably most familiar and where connections are most direct. The Institution of Environmental Health Officers was founded in 1883, its first President being Edwin Chadwick, the great public health reformer. Today's local authority EHOs are responsible for the enforcement of a whole raft of environmental legislation relating to housing condition, the regulation of food premises, the monitoring of air and water pollution, health and safety at work and in places of public entertainment, pest and rodent control and the control of noise nuisance. Resources permitting, EHOs also undertake a health education and promotion role on behalf of local authorities.

Engineers

Public health engineers also helped provide Victorian cities with the clean water supply and sewerage and waste disposal systems necessary for their survival and expansion. Most of today's public health engineers will be employed by the national water regulatory bodies (e.g. the National Rivers Authority), the regional water companies (privatised in 1989), the waste collection and disposal authorities and private engineering consultants. The professional body

which represents and promotes the interests of this group is the Institution of Civil Engineers.

Traffic and highway engineering is a comparatively young professional discipline with the origins of most modern practice being in the USA. The notable exceptions were the great British roads and bridge engineers, Telford and Macadam.

Of primary concern to traffic engineers is the prevention of road accidents through the careful design of road carriageways, road junctions, pedestrian crossings, speed reduction measures (road humps etc.), parking control schemes, and the segregation of traffic, pedestrians and cyclists. The police accurately record the details of traffic accidents involving personal injury, and these data are used by traffic engineers to identify accident black spots and to find measures to reduce traffic and pedestrian conflicts. Most traffic engineers work either in local authorities or as private consultants. In future, more work is likely to be undertaken by consultants as compulsory competitive tendering of local authority services is introduced. Their professional bodies are the Institution of Civil Engineers and the Institute of Highways and Transportation.

Many local authorities also employ specialist road safety officers to promote road safety particularly amongst children and older people.

District surveyors

Related to engineers, but undoubtedly wishing to maintain a strong separate identity, are the district surveyors responsible for the building control function of local authorities. One of the oldest environmental professions (Sir Christopher Wren was the City of London's Surveyor), it is presently responsible for ensuring that all buildings are designed and constructed according to statutory building regulations and codes of practice so as to guarantee public safety. Although most district surveyors currently work for local authorities, this area is being increasingly opened up to private competition. The professional body for this group is the Institute of Building Control.

Activity 13.3

As a locally based community nurse you are keen to develop a health promotion initiative in your locality. What environmental issues would you focus upon, which environmental professionals would you ask to contribute and what outcomes would you hope to achieve?

Town planners

Once again born out of the widespread abhorrence of living conditions in Victorian cities, the town planning profession claims the integrating role necessary to prepare and implement plans to shape the physical development of towns and cities, and indeed rural areas as well.

Local authorities have the statutory responsibility for preparing these plans and for dealing with applications for planning permission. The policies and criteria used to determine planning applications relate to the need to achieve adequate densities of development, to protect daylighting, to minimise the impact of traffic and to promote environmentally sustainable development. The professional body—the Royal Town Planning Institute—encourages people from a wide range of disciplines to become town planners also. These include architects, engineers, transport planners, geographers and economists. Although most town planners work in the public sector, an increasing number are being attracted to private consultancies.

Architects

As the lead profession for building design, architects have a profound influence on the environment in which people spend most of their lives. Architects are most commonly associated with the aesthetics of buildings but they are technicians as well. They have a crucial role in the creation of safe, healthy, environmentally friendly buildings and have to collaborate closely with mechanical, structural, and heating and ventilation engineers.

In the recent past, architects have been heavily criticised for their designs of high rise, public sector housing estates which have sometimes had disastrous consequences for the health of the people living in them. It is unfair to attribute blame entirely to the architects. Political and financial pressures to achieve very ambitious post-war housing programmes were at least as responsible. Over the past 15 years there has been a very pronounced movement of professional architects from the public to the private sector. The professional body which represents their interests is the Royal Institute of British Architects.

Working across the professional boundaries

This chapter has, hopefully, made the case that the environmental professions have an important contribution to make to health promotion. Many local authorities, health authorities and voluntary sector organisations in the UK, Europe and throughout the world are participating in 'Healthy Cities' and 'Health for All' networks. Different professional groups across all sectors come together when appropriate to develop joint plans and policies or to solve particular problems. This kind of networking will become increasingly significant as organisations become more complex and fragmented.

Nurses and other health workers, even those working in local health centres, may not encounter an environmental health officer or a traffic engineer or a town planner very frequently. But occasionally they will prove useful. What is certain is that the physical environment does have an impact on the number and medical condition of people using the health services. The environmental professions have a key role in reducing sickness and promoting health.

REFERENCES

Department of Transport 1993 Transport statistics of Great Britain 1993. HMSO, London

Hardie R, Walker A 1992 Environment and health in Camden. Department of Public Health, Bloomsbury and Islington Health Authority, London

Health and Safety Executive 1992 Contract research report 42/92. Sick building syndrome: a review of the evidence on causes and solutions. Health and Safety Executive, London

Hillman M 1991 Healthy transport policy. In: Draper P (ed) Health through public policy. Green Print, London

House of Commons Environment Committee 1991 Sixth report: indoor pollution, volume I and II. HMSO, London

House of Commons Transport Committee 1994 Sixth report: transport-related air pollution in London, volume I. HMSO, London

Independent Scientific Committee on Smoking and Health 1988 Fourth report. HMSO, London

Institution of Environmental Health Officers 1991 Report on a survey into the incidence of sick building syndrome and other methods of controlling it. Institution of Environmental Health Officers, London

Jacobson B, Smith A, Whitehead M 1991 The nation's health: a strategy for the 1990s, 2nd edn. King's Fund, London

London Research Centre 1993 London energy study. London Research Centre, London

O'Keefe E, Newbury J 1993 Divided London: towards a European public health approach. University of North London Press, London

Parliamentary Office of Science and Technology 1994 Breathing in our cities—urban air pollution and respiratory health. HMSO, London

Report of the Committee on the Problem of Noise 1963 Cm 2056. HMSO, London

Royal Commission on Environmental Pollution 1994 Eighteenth report: transport and the environment. Cm 2674. HMSO, London

Sykes J M 1988 Sick building syndrome: a review. Health and Safety Executive Specialist Inspector Reports Number 10. The Health and Safety Executive, London

UK Government 1994 Sustainable development: the UK strategy 1994. Cm 2426. HMSO, London

United Nations Environment Programme 1987 Montreal protocol on substances that deplete the ozone layer. UNEP

World Health Organization 1993 Health for all targets: the health policy for Europe, updated edn. WHO, Regional Office for Europe, Copenhagen

CHAPTER CONTENTS

Introduction   185

Health promotion in nursing philosophy and
   practice   186
   Philosophical influences on present-day
      nursing   186
   An integrated model of health promotion   187

Models of nursing and health promotion   188
   Nursing process and the integrated approach   189
   How could a nursing model be used within the
      integrated approach to practice?   190

Multisectoral collaboration and equity in health
   promotion   191
   Locality profiling   192
   Collaboration with others   193
   Healthy Islington 2000—a model of multisectoral
      collaboration   193

Conclusion   196

References   196

14

Towards an integrated model of health promotion in nursing practice

Jo Skinner

Nurses and midwives need to develop their own nursing strategy for promoting health.

(ENB 1994 p. 42)

INTRODUCTION

This chapter aims to draw together the central ideas from previous chapters and propose a new strategic approach for health promotion as an integrated part of nursing philosophy and practice. In the past nursing, like medicine, tended to separate health promotion from mainstream care and it became rather like an 'optional extra'. Health promotion is an important and integral part of health care. It must be a central principle of nursing care. The chapter has three main parts:

- health promotion in nursing philosophy and practice
- models of nursing and health promotion
- multisectoral collaboration and health promotion.

Each part explores how nurses can be active in promoting health at micro and macro levels. The section that follows this chapter has activities which relate closely to central concepts explored here; other activities are included within the chapter. Key policy initiatives like the 'Health of the Nation' (DoH 1992) and the World Health Organization 'Health for All' (WHO 1993) strategies provide the background to the discussions in this chapter. In the first part, a new approach to nursing is advocated in the form of an integrated model of health promotion and this concept recurs throughout the chapter. This innovation is partly a response to the radical changes in nurse education through the introduction of Project 2000 (UKCC 1986). Earlier themes are revisited, particularly ideas relating to values in care and individual and collective responsibility and equity. They are important as they have direct relevance for nurses giving care and clients receiving care.

HEALTH PROMOTION IN NURSING PHILOSOPHY AND PRACTICE

This first part of the chapter explores some of the philosophical and emerging ideas which shape present-day nursing. It explores the role of health promotion in relation to nursing practice and suggests that a new approach is required through an integrated model of practice. This relates closely to the discussion in Chapters 1 and 4.

Nurses are primarily concerned with care of patients, clients and families as opposed to seeking cure(s). Nursing care and practice from whatever theoretical base (e.g. model of nursing used) must include health promotion within it. Is it always possible or practicable to do this?

What is proposed here is that health promotion is not something that is 'done to' a patient or client, like giving an injection or even advice, but rather informs and pervades every aspect of nursing care. This *integrated approach* should be equally applicable to any specialisation in nursing, whether acute or community care, mental health, learning disabilities, child or adult health. It is particularly important for new nursing students, as well as qualified practitioners, to adopt this approach because they will work in a variety of settings and deal with all factors affecting health. They will work with individuals, families, groups or whole populations.

Health and well-being are the constant goals of nursing rather than focusing solely on immediate clinical problems. This does not mean that clinical problems are unimportant but that they must be viewed in a broader context. As we saw in Chapter 2, when looking at the successes of the nineteenth century public health initiatives,

health promotion is not new. Indeed when the NHS was set up in 1948 a major aim was to prevent ill health. NHS development has been stunted by its focus on illness and acute care provision (Hart 1988). The growth in new technologies in medicine has ensured that this remains the case (Mays 1993). This is reflected in nursing practice, with the majority of nurses working in hospitals. How has health promotion become so distanced from mainstream nursing philosophy and practice?

Philosophical influences on present-day nursing

Throughout its history, western nursing has always subscribed to certain values and beliefs that are largely founded on Christian ideals. Florence Nightingale's values, beliefs and ideas about what was healthy shaped modern nursing greatly. Much emphasis was given to hygiene and organising and controlling the patient's environment to promote healing and recovery. Nightingale's ideas remain influential in shaping the sort of nursing we have in Britain today (see Ch. 2); in fact, many hospital wards conform to her original design for optimum surveillance.

The development of nursing as an academic discipline from the 1960s onwards has allowed ideas and values to be articulated. American nursing academics, in particular, began to describe nursing and apply theoretical models to practice. Since the 1970s, nursing theory has had a direct influence on nursing education and later practice. The growth or re-emergence of holistic care and now 'new nursing' (Salvage 1992) have become accepted as desirable. These sorts of trends and ideas emerge from time to time and leave a considerable impression on the professional culture.

Influences may also be indirect, reflecting changes and theoretical debates happening 'outside' the profession, like feminism or more recently chaos theory. The result of this is a wealth of writing and research which has increased the professionalisation of nursing and led to greater autonomy for nurses. In many cases these developments were a deliberate attempt to move away from the medical model of health (Aggleton & Chalmers 1986, Salvage 1992). Challenges to orthodox medicine have also been reflected in nursing; for instance complementary therapies, which were frowned upon as 'unscientific' until comparatively recently, have now been brought into mainstream medical and nursing practice (Thompson 1994). In the 1980s, the global resurgence of environmental concerns has also been reflected in nursing. It is contended here that nurse academics have not tackled health promotion as a core aspect of practice and it tends to remain peripheral.

The emergence of patients as consumers with rights and responsibilities, together with new health policies in the 1980s and 1990s, has further shaped nursing ideas. Major steps have been taken to redress the balance of power between nurses and clients by challenging the idea of the nurse as 'all-knowing' expert with an absolute right to intervene in an individual's life for his or her 'own good'. Nurses, or other health professionals for that matter, are not the sole source of knowledge. The concepts of negotiated care and partner relationships with clients have emerged within theoretical nursing developments over the past 30 years.

Such values and principles, including the growth of ethics as a discipline within health care and an emphasis on the social values needed, underpin nursing practice and reflect who we are as professionals (see Ch. 5). The UKCC code of professional conduct specifies core values and characteristics of acceptable practice in order to safeguard the public through the individual accountability of the nurse (UKCC 1992). The sum total of all these directives and theoretical debates contributes towards a collective philosophy of care. In particular, the UKCC code refers to the nurse's responsibility for enhancing well-being by taking into account all relevant circumstances which affect the individual's health and thereby:

act always in such a manner as to promote and safeguard the interests and well-being of patients and clients; ... recognise and respect the uniqueness and dignity of each patient and client, and respond to their need for care, irrespective of their ethnic origin, religious beliefs, personal attributes, the nature of

their health problems or any other factor; ... having regard to the physical, psychological and social effects on patients and clients, [and] any circumstances in the environment of care which could jeopardise standards of practice.

(UKCC 1992)

It is by these standards and values that nurses are judged by their peers, colleagues and public alike; they reflect the idea of partnership and respect between client and professional carer. It is interesting to note that the UKCC code precedes the Citizens' and Patients' Charters (see Ch. 3) and reflects the idea of clear standards that clients and patients should expect and receive. Having said this, many values and practices are not written but still remain. There is always a 'time lag' between what is written and what actually happens in practice or how written codes or philosophies are put into practice; the influence of peers is very great. This is of importance to learners who will observe differences in practices and culture within nursing in different work settings.

An integrated model of health promotion

The relationship between health promotion and nursing practice is crucial to this common nursing philosophy and is illustrated in Figure 14.1. It is

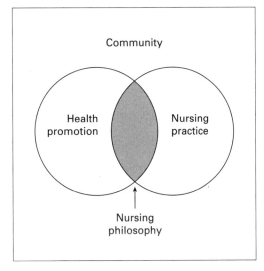

Figure 14.1 An integrated model for nursing practice.

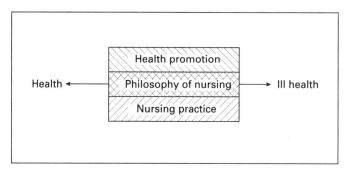

Figure 14.2 Philosophy of nursing.

important to state that all components shown in the figure may be defined and described independently; what is proposed here is to show their relative *interdependence*. Thus health promotion, rather than being a marginalised and 'optional extra', is firmly placed within the sphere of nursing practice. The natural result of this is that it is an essential and integral element of nursing assessment and care planning with patients, clients, carers and others. This approach is applicable to groups and whole populations too.

Chapter 1 examined the importance of thinking about how health is defined, as this will influence both how health promotion is viewed in nursing and the type of care given. Figure 14.2 shows the relative position that health promotion occupies depending on the patient's condition. The continuum shows that nursing may be required to maintain health and improve health or minimise the effects of ill health within the integrated model. In other words, it is not possible to separate health promotion from health needs as both can be seen as a whole. It is essential that health education, although important, is not seen as the only approach within health promotion (see Ch. 4).

Health promotion, like any other aspect of nursing care, must be tailor-made to the individual's circumstances, including the wider community in which the person lives or works. Nursing activities thus take on a much broader approach and become proactive rather than reactive. There must be a relationship between health promotion at an individual level and national and local initiatives. This will be discussed later in this chapter. Thus, health promotion within nursing

practice is an integral part of nursing care and must relate to the whole range of the individual's experience.

MODELS OF NURSING AND HEALTH PROMOTION

The second part of this chapter examines the role of three nursing models, Roper, Logan & Tierney (1990), Orem (1980) and Neuman (1982), in adopting and using the integrated approach in practice. These nursing models are evaluated to consider to what extent they are health-oriented. Models of nursing are most useful in helping students learn about nursing practice by examining key elements of nursing within a safe framework. For further reading on nursing models, see a standard text such as Pearson & Vaughan (1992) or Aggleton & Chalmers (1986). An overview of these three models is provided in Chapter 15.

Named nursing models reflect the individual philosophy of their authors whilst remaining consistent within the collective philosophy of nursing. Each theorist has certain unique in-

---

Activity 14.1

a. Read one of the case studies in Box 15.1 (pp. 201–202) and discuss in small groups how you think the integrated model would work in practice.
b. Identify where you think the patient/client and carers fit along the continuum in Figure 14.2. Keep in mind the distinction between disability and illness.
c. Can you see any difficulties with adopting this integrated approach?

sights which shape nursing practice. Common concepts in nursing theories are explored, such as the individual, health, health systems, nursing and society. How these concepts are constructed will influence all aspects of care including health promotion. As we saw in Chapter 1 with regard to defining health, how we perceive the nursing role will influence greatly the sort of care we give. For example, if our view is from a rather narrow clinical perspective then care may focus solely on symptoms.

Nursing requires a comprehensive framework for assessing, planning and evaluating care. Nursing models are a useful way of doing this. Many models claim to be health-oriented or include health promotion within their philosophy, for example the models of Orem and Neuman. However, nurses need to examine any assumptions inherent within the models themselves. For instance, some models, like those of Roper et al and Orem, focus exclusively on the individual and the individual's ability to make choices but do not acknowledge sufficiently that people do not live in isolation and often cannot make real choices about their health due to outside constraints. This is important in relation to concerns such as disadvantage and inequality.

Nursing process and the integrated approach

The nursing process has been a useful, but not foolproof, way of organising and managing care. Its four stages of assessment, planning, implementation and evaluation provide a dynamic framework within which to assess and deal with change rationally (Yura & Walshe 1986). Many nursing students find that assessment poses the greatest challenge.

Nursing assessment

Nursing assessment is a central part of nursing care and is a key part of both the nursing process and nursing models. Accurate assessment allows nurses to plan and carry out relevant care which is tailor-made for the individuals, their families and carers. It is important that nurses recognise

their powerful position in the assessment process, as they are responsible for identifying health needs including health promotion and deciding how these needs will be met. Health promotion initiatives often fail because health workers do not identify correctly 'where people are at' in the beginning. This may be viewed as a 'top-down' approach. It is not only unsatisfactory to clients and patients but is costly to the health service too. Assessment must allow for a broad perspective including the wider involvement of other workers (this will be discussed more later).

Planning care

By adopting an integrated approach from assessment onwards, health and health-promoting goals can be negotiated and set with clients or groups for short-, medium- and long-term planning. For example, care for a child suffering burns following an accident at home will include planning for prevention of further accidents. This provides nurses with the opportunity to think clearly about what they (and others) expect to be achieved. These nursing outcomes need to be measurable in a meaningful way.

Implementing care

This is often the area that nurses and other health workers find easiest to understand and implement, and clinical aspects of health often predominate. Using an integrated approach, many other factors can become part of care-giving. Clients' motivation and participation in health can be considered. The resources that are required and their availability to deliver appropriate care should be examined. This can include the involvement of other workers and carers. Further education and support may also be required. In the case of the child with burns who is returning home, it will be vital to consider environmental factors and ways of coordinating with other child care services.

Evaluating care

The nurse must have a clear idea of how success

will be gauged. This is not always easy, particularly with health promotion. However, increasing emphasis on health outcomes is recognised as desirable and necessary (Buchan & Ball 1991). What of the child with burns? Measurement of care is not just about the speed of recovery or degree of scarring but also about future recurrence. Therefore, outcomes are linked to broader health promotion policies, for example childhood accident targets (DoH 1992). Evaluation offers the practitioner the opportunity to examine his or her own practice, what went right and why, or the reverse. This may lead to changes including reassessment of clients, staff development, research opportunities and standard setting.

How could a nursing model be used within the integrated approach to practice?

There are no perfect nursing models. When using models, nurse practitioners need to identify how each represents health promotion in relation to nursing practice. Selection of the models of use will also depend on the level of the nurse's knowledge as well as the individual client's situation. For instance, if nurses do not really understand the main principles of the model they will not be able to use it effectively; or if clients are severely depressed they may not be able to participate in their own care. When selecting a model of nursing, in order to ensure that you adopt a more integrated approach, you should ask the questions that are listed in Box 14.1.

Box 14.1   Selection criteria for nursing models in the integrated approach

- Is this model health-oriented?
- Does it focus on health promotion and, if so, how?
- What kind of health promotion—primary, secondary or tertiary?
- To what extent is this integrated into the assessment framework?
- To what extent does the model focus on the individual alone?
- How could the model be adapted to integrate health promotion into nursing practice?
- How could the model be used to evaluate health promotion outcomes?

Limitations of models

Many models of nursing seek to be health-oriented as opposed to being illness-oriented. They relate in the main to hospital and institutional care rather than community or other care settings. Their focus, therefore, is on acute illness or crisis and physical problems rather than chronic illness, disability, psychological or emotional needs. This is relevant given the drive to reorientate health care in the community and changes in 'traditional' nursing roles (DoH 1990, UKCC 1994).

Models tend to encourage nurses to single out patient or client problems so that they are often perceived separately. Problems by their very nature are multifaceted and are often closely related or clustered. For instance, if people have problems with mobility this will have a major effect on other aspects of their lives, like washing, working, shopping or self-perception. It is often more appropriate to tackle these areas as one interrelated 'problem'.

Where models have tried to maximise health, or opportunities for health, they have been limited as they tend to focus almost exclusively on the individual and do not relate to the community as a whole (see Ch. 6). This does not invalidate models of nursing, but nurses need to be aware of such limitations particularly outside of an institutional setting where the environment and context of care is not controlled. Clearly, some models address the needs of groups and have been used successfully by community nurses working in public health (see Ch. 8). As we discussed in earlier chapters, effective health promotion strategies must take into account population and community approaches.

Nursing models tend to emphasise health education activities rather than health promotion strategies. But if nursing models are viewed as aids to be developed and shaped by use in practice, then it is clear that they are open to scrutiny by practitioners and open to adaptation.

How useful are models to an integrated approach?

An overview of the basic concepts and character-

Box 14.2   An integrated approach to health promotion: positive and negative aspects of three nursing models

Roper, Logan & Tierney's model (1990)
- Positive aspects:
  - —incorporates a range of factors that influence health (e.g. environment, sociopolitical, economic, etc.) with activities of living
  - —examines 'normal' patterns of the individual behaviour so that care is more likely to be relevant to the person and start where the client actually is
  - —potential problems are identified, which is very important in preventive work and allows nurses to identify and plan for health risks
  - —encourages nurses to identify the resources required whether staff or equipment
- Negative aspects:
  - —activities of living are often the focal point of assessment and care
  - —assessment can be a negative process as it focuses on what the patient can no longer do for him or herself
  - —medicalised approach as physical aspects tend to dominate
  - —practitioners marginalise factors influencing health
  - —nurses maintain dominant role as professional carers

Orem's model (1980)
- Positive aspects:
  - —health-oriented
  - —responsibilities and choices for health remain with the client
  - —attempts to redress the balance of power between clients and nurses through negotiated care
  - —identifies specific helping activities of the nurse, including education and support; nurses act in a compensatory way

  - —carers are clearly identified as important to care assessment and planning
- Negative aspects:
  - —assumes that individuals are able and capable of self-care, i.e. have material or personal resources to provide for themselves
  - —ignores greater public health issues over which individuals have little control
  - —teamwork is absent

Neuman's model (1982)
- Positive aspects:
  - —a broad approach is taken towards health
  - —the client is central within his or her environment
  - —stress is a central concept which is flexible and counters a biomedical approach
  - —various levels of intervention, primary, secondary and tertiary, relate well to health promotion approaches
  - —useful for assessing the needs of groups
  - —recognises that client and nurse perceptions of a situation may differ
- Negative aspects:
  - —concepts appear vague and difficult to assess
  - —implies that individuals are somehow separate from their environment
  - —individuals respond to events rather than influence or control them
  - —resolution of differing client and nurse perceptions is difficult to address
  - —stress is viewed as only a negative experience to be avoided

---

istics of each of the three models considered here is given in Chapter 15. Positive and negative aspects are summarised in Box 14.2 in the context of an integrated approach to health promotion.

Activity 14.2

Select another case study from Box 15.1, read it carefully and answer the following questions:

a. How could you use a nursing model within the integrated approach to practice?
b. What are the key health promotion opportunities in this study?
c. Using the criteria given earlier, which nursing model would you select for this patient/client's situation?
d. How would the model you have selected allow you to assess and plan nursing intervention to maximise these opportunities?

Each model is flexible enough to accommodate some health promotion activities. It is more appropriate to incorporate the whole model into the integrated framework, as nursing models themselves are often incomplete (see Fig. 14.1) and a broader health promotion strategy is necessary.

MULTISECTORAL COLLABORATION AND EQUITY IN HEALTH PROMOTION

We now go on to examine the relationship of the integrated model and collaborative working within health policies as a means to achieving a healthier population. Implicit within this approach is the need to address inequalities in health both nationally and locally, which is central to the WHO initiatives discussed through this book (WHO 1993, DoH 1992). The challenge to current health care in Britain as elsewhere is to recognise the importance of technological and demographic trends. The move to quicker, cheaper and less invasive forms of acute care, as well as genetic discoveries, will permanently alter the shape of health provision. Rapid growth in the number of elderly people in the population as a whole is important (Victor 1990). Older people often suffer from multiple chronic illness which may be physical and/or mental, and most of their care occurs outside of hospitals. In the face of potential 'infinite demand', it is essential to make the best use of existing expertise and resources. As we discussed earlier in this chapter, health problems are complex and multifaceted. This means they require careful analysis and long-term strategies.

Health promotion is seen by many planners and politicians as the way forward. It offers the possibility to reduce costs, meet health needs and transfer greater responsibility to individuals. Nurses are important agents in carrying out health policies but must also be actively involved in directing attention to health needs and new priorities. Nurses do not practise in isolation. There must be a partnership between practitioners, service users and those taking policy decisions.

In the past, nursing has condoned, sometimes reluctantly, the dominant medical model of health rather than a holistic one. This is not surprising as the majority of nurses were employed in hospitals, and even though community nurses retained more autonomy they were rather marginalised within the system. This medicalised approach to health has been challenged from a number of sources in recent times and successive governments have supported a major policy shift towards primary and community care (see Chs 2 and 3).

New nurse education, and particularly Project 2000, plays a part in the strategy by ensuring that nursing education is more health-oriented (UKCC 1986, UKCC 1993). Newly qualified practitioners are able to work in any setting. Health promotion policies allow nurses to become involved in planning and delivering services to meet current and future health demands at a

variety of levels (see Ch. 4). The integrated approach advocated in this chapter allows nurses to respond to policies at each level through a reorientation of nursing practice. This chapter has, so far, concentrated on the care of individuals, families and carers regarding health promotion. However, within a broader philosophy of health care, nurses must extend their accountability to provide for whole client groups and communities. This will sometimes require specialised care for key groups with particular health needs, for example diabetes in the Asian population, while at other times a broader public health approach is required (UKCC 1994).

The current targets in the 'Health of the Nation' document (DoH 1992) and the WHO European targets (WHO 1993; see Ch. 3) are clear indicators of national priorities. Local priorities are equally important as they can vary considerably. There may be gaps in provision not covered by national targets and, at local level, there may be needs that are not being identified or met, for example the health needs of refugees. Nurses play an important role because of their first-hand knowledge of localities and their direct patient or client contact. This information can be fed into the decision-making process so that new priorities can be set, for example through population and locality profiling. This is vital to ensure both equity of access and provision.

Locality profiling

The integrated model focused earlier on individuals and smaller groups. These principles can be applied to the population as a whole. This population may be local, regional or national. Thus, whatever aspect of practice nurses are involved in or wherever they are located, these wider issues inform their practice. In order to work in an enlightened way and contribute to policy, nurses must make use of all the available information sources so that they can construct detailed profiles of their locality (see Chs 6 and 15). These can then be integral to the assessment and planning process, which should also include effective teamwork (see Ch. 8).

Nurses can build up a picture of the locality

and match it to local policies in a number of ways. The geographical area in which the nurse works is likely to be divided in a number of ways. It may have differing administrative boundaries between health authority, hospital and community trusts, family health service authorities, and local authorities. Physical boundaries and environmental hazards, as discussed in Chapter 13, will also inform this picture, for example main roads, canals, location and nature of industrial units and shopping areas. The local population can also be described by major groups within it, for example groups defined by age, gender, ethnicity, socioeconomic factors (see Ch. 15).

The UKCC Code of Professional Conduct (1992) clearly identifies the reporting responsibilities of the nurse in bringing to the attention of managers and others, unmet need or deficiencies in the environment of care. It is also important that nurses monitor quality to identify and meet appropriate targets, especially long-term health goals.

Collaboration with others

If health promotion policies are to improve the nation's health, inter-agency collaboration is essential. In other words, all factors in our communities which impact upon our health must be coordinated to achieve the health goals identified. These include employment or lack of it, environmental issues such as clean air and water, housing, access to health care and so on (see Ch. 13).

The UKCC code makes it clear that nurses need to: 'work in a collaborative and co-operative manner with patients, clients and their families, ... work in a collaborative and co-operative manner with health care professionals and others in providing care, and recognise and respect their particular contributions within the care team' (UKCC 1992).

As we discussed earlier in this chapter, nursing does not occur in a vacuum—isolated from other health workers. Increasingly, nurses work in skill-mixed teams. Our definition of who is a health worker may be flexible depending on the particular situation, for example social worker or fire fighter. Nurses often work closely with a variety of agencies at individual practitioner level, for example health workers like dietitians, social services, housing and education bodies, voluntary agencies, pharmacists, police, etc. Since the introduction of the NHS and Community Care Act (DoH 1990), changes to health and social care delivery rely on effective collaboration between workers to ensure that clients and patients receive the appropriate care from the right agency at the right time. Figure 14.3 shows interagency collaboration in relation to health promotion as an integral part of this care. Thus nursing practice must articulate well with other services to maintain current provision and develop future services. This is not always easy, and an increasing emphasis on resources requires a clear demonstration of efficiency and effectiveness.

There is a parallel between the roles of the nurse and patient/client in participating in health activities. There is a tension between the potential and scope for involvement on the one hand and, on the other, the natural restraints on them as individuals. For example, a nurse visiting an elderly person with mobility difficulties may have reached a point where the health of the patient cannot be 'progressed' without wider action from the local authority to provide adaptations to the home or replace pavements. The nurse would be expected to contribute to the individual and overall health of people in a locality by bringing health needs and concerns to the attention of the appropriate authority. Supportive management structures and shared health-promoting strategies amongst local providers would facilitate effective teamwork.

Healthy Islington 2000—a model of multisectoral collaboration

The following examples demonstrate the effectiveness of promoting health in collaboration with others. The roles of health workers, including nurses, can be seen and the principles of the integrated approach identified. Healthy Islington 2000 (HI2000) is a multi-agency, multisectoral initiative between health and social services and the voluntary sector. The health services span the range of acute and community services. The

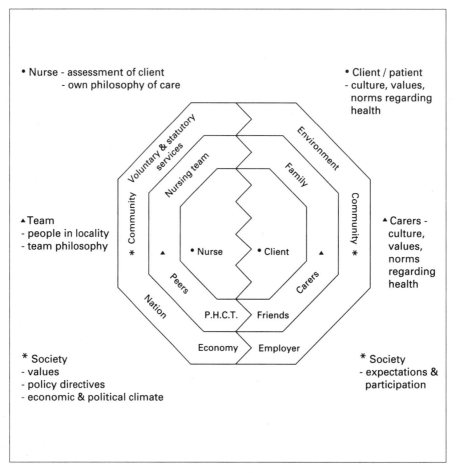

• Nurse - assessment of client
  - own philosophy of care

• Client / patient
  - culture, values,
    norms regarding
    health

▲ Team
  - people in locality
  - team philosophy

▲ Carers -
  culture,
  values,
  norms
  regarding
  health

* Society
  - values
  - policy directives
  - economic & political climate

* Society
  - expectations &
    participation

Voluntary & statutory services · Nursing team · Community · Peers · Nation · P.H.C.T. · Economy · Nurse · Client · Environment · Family · Community · Carers · Friends · Employer

Figure 14.3 The relationship and practice activities of nurses and other health care workers in providing comprehensive care to individuals and the wider society.

community health trust provides community nursing and other health services; family health services authority includes general practices, community pharmacy and dentistry (see Ch. 3). The social service departments include housing, education, environmental services, race and ethnicity unit and personal social services. The voluntary sector includes a wide range of local organisations, for example Age Concern represented through an umbrella organisation called IVAC (Islington Voluntary Action Council). HI2000's remit is to respond to the WHO challenge to make measurable improvements in health. It is based on the three key principles of equity, community participation and multisectoral collaboration. Representatives from the above agen-

cies are members of a steering committee which includes the HI2000 coordinator. This steering group reports directly to the Joint Consultative Committee (JCC). HI2000 has identified four key areas for collaborative work:

● devising a health plan
● equity and access to health services
● health and environment
● accident prevention.

This last area will be explored in greater detail to demonstrate effective joint working.

Accident prevention

The programme was designed to respond to the

WHO targets (initially Targets 11, 17, 24 and 25, and later corresponding 'Health of the Nation' targets) for under-fives, older people and in the workplace. Three joint initiatives addressed these targets. First, the under-fives' scheme which involved lending safety equipment to local families on low incomes, such as stair gates, saucepans and fire guards. The equipment was based at a health centre and advertised locally. Health visiting staff could refer clients directly to the scheme or parents could just 'drop in'. Many mothers and child minders attended for safety talks and exhibitions. The loan service itself was staffed with volunteers and the equipment bought by social services. The pilot service was monitored and found to be effective by service users. As a result the community health trust has agreed to continue this work and provide funding. The service has grown and nearly 200 families participate in the scheme.

Secondly, an initiative to prevent accidents to older people led to the joint development of a resource pack. Representatives from Pensioners' Link, Age Concern, Pensioners' Forum and Islington Council and District Health Authority were involved. The pack includes home safety information, for example on wiring, and useful contact numbers across the services. The pack was distributed widely in the borough with a questionnaire. The questionnaire was intended to determine present safety strategies adopted and indicate training needs for the future. A training strategy is being developed and the pack is being translated into five community languages.

Thirdly, accident prevention in the workplace has presented a considerable challenge, in part due to the great diversity of work environments and workforce profiles within the borough. Currently a multisectoral working group is examining the ways in which joint working can occur. The data collected have highlighted wide discrepancies in practice for reporting accidents. It is recognised that there is a need to standardise these systems and to provide translated information for employees.

These are just a small aspect of the joint working initiatives that have taken place through HI2000. Box 14.3 shows other joint projects that

---

Activity 14.3

Choose any case study from Box 15.1 which could involve at least three different agencies. You can use one that you have used before.

a. What are the opportunities for and obstacles to effective collaboration?
b. Identify a health promotion need in your own locality which can only be solved in collaboration with others, plan out a strategy for this, discuss how you might go about raising this issue.

---

are in progress. It should be noted that, even though these projects are necessary and address both local and national objectives, funding is often problematic and short-term. What is interesting about such projects is the 'spin off' that has come by further collaboration on other health-promoting initiatives. An example of this is shown in the HI2000 annual report:

Joint working through the *(under 5's)* project's steering group has highlighted problems of safety in hostels, bed and breakfast temporary accommodation and the private rented sector. These matters have been taken up by the relevant council departments and have provided a liaison point for health authority staff to work with council and voluntary organisation staff.

(Healthy Islington 2000 1994)

Box 14.3   Other activities and projects in progress as a result of the Healthy Islington 2000 initiative

Equity and access
- Black and ethnic minority health project
- Anti-poverty work–benefits advice service
- Homelessness project
- Women's health subgroup
- Health and fitness subgroup
- Community initiative grant scheme
- Refugees

Health and environment
- Transport and health
- Air quality

Health plan
- Sharing good practice
- Identify problems
- Create framework for outcome measurements for monitoring health promotion activities
- Strategic plan

CONCLUSION

In this chapter it has been stated that nurses need to adopt a much broader philosophy of health to include health promotion through the integrated model. This will enable them to promote health and well-being effectively in the population where they work. The integrated approach underpins nursing care and is a natural part of nursing practice. Health in the broadest sense is the goal of all care. By implication, nurses are not solely responsible for enabling clients and patients to achieve health but need to coordinate their efforts with others. This shift will allow nurses to be more attuned to national and local health needs and policies. They are then better able to initiate and respond flexibly, creatively and effectively to these health needs and policies to improve health for all.

REFERENCES

Aggleton P, Chalmers H 1986 Nursing models and the nursing process. Macmillan, Basingstoke

Buchan J, Ball J 1991 Caring costs, nursing costs and benefits—a review for the Royal College of Nursing. Institute of Manpower Studies, University of Sussex, Brighton

Chapman C 1985 Theory of nursing: practical application. Harper & Row, London

Department of Health 1990 NHS and Community Care Act. HMSO, London

Department of Health 1992 The health of the nation: a strategy for health in England. Cm 1986. HMSO, London

English National Board for Nursing, Midwifery and Health Visiting (ENB) 1994 Project—philosophy of health. RCN, London.

Hart N 1988 The sociology of health and medicine. Causeway Press, London

Healthy Islington 2000 1994 Report of the steering group to JCC. June

Mays N 1993 Innovation in health care. In: Davey B, Popay J (eds) 1993 Dilemmas in health care. Open University Press, Milton Keynes

Neuman B 1982 The Neuman systems model application to nursing education and practice. Appleton-Century-Crofts, New York

Orem D 1980 Nursing: concepts of practice, 2nd edn. McGraw-Hill, New York

Pearson A, Vaughan B 1992 Nursing models for nursing practice. Churchill Livingstone, Edinburgh

Roper N, Logan W, Tierney A J 1990 The elements of nursing: a model for nursing based on a model of living, 3rd edn. Churchill Livingstone, Edinburgh

Salvage J 1992 The new nursing: empowering patients or empowering nurses? In: Robinson J, Gray A, Elkan R (eds) Policy issues in nursing. Open University Press, Milton Keynes

Thompson J 1994 Complementary therapy: increasing patients' options. Community Outlook 4(9): 19–21

United Kingdom Central Council for Nursing, Midwifery and Health Visiting 1983 The nurses, midwives and health visitors rules approval order. UKCC, London

United Kingdom Central Council for Nursing, Midwifery and Health Visiting 1986 Project 2000: a new preparation for practice. UKCC, London

United Kingdom Central Council for Nursing, Midwifery and Health Visiting 1986 Project 2000: the project and the professions. Project paper. UKCC, London

United Kingdom Central Council for Nursing, Midwifery and Health Visiting 1992 Code of professional conduct for nurses, midwives and health visitors, 2nd edn. UKCC, London

United Kingdom Central Council for Nursing, Midwifery and Health Visiting 1994 Post registration preparation and practice. UKCC, London

Victor C 1990 Health and health care in later life. Open University Press, Milton Keynes

World Health Organization 1992 Health for all: 38 European targets. WHO, Geneva

World Health Organization 1993 Health for all targets: the health policy for Europe, updated edn. WHO, Regional Office for Europe, Copenhagen

Yura H, Walshe M B 1986 The nursing process. In: Aggleton P, Chalmers H 1986 Nursing models and the nursing process. Macmillan, Basingstoke

Further activities

SECTION CONTENTS

15. Organising information and exploring ideas   199

This section consists of a single chapter, which, although the last in the book, is key in that it gives students practical advice on building up a portfolio, using the activities completed as they worked through the book and the additional activities included in this section.

CHAPTER CONTENTS

Introduction 199
Notes to teachers and independent students 199
Developing a health promotion portfolio 200

Portfolio formulation 200

Applied activities 200
Using the case studies 200
Overview of nursing models 202

Locality profiling 206
What to include in a locality profile 206
Data sources for profile 207

References 208

15

Organising information and exploring ideas

Jo Skinner

INTRODUCTION

The main aim of this book is to reassert that health promotion is central to health care. Health workers are not just those employed in the NHS but include those employed in other health activities, such as public health. Health care is changing rapidly and requires responsive health workers. Health workers, like nurses, need to develop new approaches to practice in order to achieve health goals. Many concepts explored in the book may be applied to a wide range of health workers. However, the main health workers focused upon here have been nurses.

Notes to teachers and independent students

Activities throughout the book are intended as building blocks to learning. Each chapter is free-standing and has its own related activities. Even though chapters are separate, many important issues and common themes recur. In this chapter, activities involving given case studies and named nursing models have been included to facilitate this learning process. All the activities may be incorporated into a portfolio (see below).

These activities can be used by individuals and/or groups with or without supervision. Multidisciplinary group work, where possible, would be advantageous to enhance learning and increase the potential for change in practice. They also relate to other study areas within course programmes, e.g. research, sociology, social policy and psychology.

Developing a health promotion portfolio

One framework for using the book, suggested here, is based upon the development of a health promotion portfolio. The portfolio provides an opportunity for readers/students:

- to identify and correlate themes and issues within the book
- to collect and collate comprehensive health data in one or more environments
- to understand and apply concepts developed in the book to 'real life' situations
- to use their own experiences and localities to develop health promotion in practice
- to reflect on practice and help identify ways to develop practice
- to foster teamwork in practice
- to develop new areas of knowledge and skills
- to gather all the chapter activities together.

The remainder of this chapter is divided into three linked segments:

- portfolio formulation
- applied activities
- locality profiling.

Both the applied activities and locality profiling can be undertaken separately if wished.

PORTFOLIO FORMULATION

The portfolio should consist of all the material and activities that you have gathered or will gather whilst using this book. How you choose to organise this material is optional, but your method must be flexible and capable of change, e.g. on computer disk or large loose-leaf file. The material should be collated and cross-referenced in a logical sequence. A suggested format is given here:

- personal details and goals for health promotion
- practice opportunities, e.g. observational visits, learning new skills
- record of achievements, i.e. specific chapter activities and *applied activities*
- *locality profile*

- selected health policies
- health promotion initiatives planned and/or delivered
- review of goals and future development
- references.

The portfolio should not be a mass of unconnected and meaningless information, e.g. leaflets. Time should be spent deciding what information should be included and why. Material that has to be omitted may serve a better purpose elsewhere: thus, the portfolio should provide pegs by which self-development can be recorded.

APPLIED ACTIVITIES

Throughout the book the activities encourage readers/students to apply concepts and explore the ideas and themes in each chapter. Seven case studies and an overview of three nursing models are included in this segment to allow students/readers to test out unfamiliar ideas in a safe way. They are also very necessary to the discussion and activities in Chapter 14. In addition ideas, concepts and themes can be transferred from one chapter to another. For example, in Chapter 1 you are asked what your own ideas are about health. Why do you feel healthy? As you explore later chapters you can build upon your ideas regarding health promotion. Do you perceive health promotion differently in your role as a health worker compared with other roles you may have (e.g. friend, daughter, spouse, etc.)?

Using the case studies

Wherever possible, the case studies (see Box 15.1) should be used for discussion in groups (preferably multidisciplinary). In some instances you may prefer to use patient/client situations of your own. Within the seven case studies you should use the full range of information given and note the diversity in:

- patient/client situations and backgrounds
- levels of family support
- acute and chronic care
- hospital and community settings
- all nursing branch specialities

Box 15.1 Case studies

Case study 1

Mrs Rani Patel is 31 years old and came to England 7 years ago from Pakistan when her husband Mo sent for her. Mo came to England to study and set up his own business, which he did with help from his uncle. He now owns a newsagent's shop in a run-down area of the inner city and works very long hours. The Patels do not live in this area and are very worried about being robbed; they have a large Rottweiler dog to protect them while in the shop.

When Mrs Patel came to England it was winter and she missed her family and home a great deal. She was very shy and did not have a good grasp of English. After a short while she became depressed and was diagnosed as having pulmonary tuberculosis. After extensive treatment at the local hospital outpatients' department she recovered and put on a considerable amount of weight and then conceived her daughter, Tula. Tula is now 5 years old, but was born prematurely and has moderate cerebral palsy. She attends a local authority school for children with special needs. She appears very bright but her speech is very badly affected; she is very thin and small but loves sweets!

A year ago, Tula's father's health began to deteriorate and he visited his own GP who wanted to admit him to hospital for tests, but Mo felt he could not leave his wife alone to manage the shop so he saw an Asian GP (who practised close to the shop) as a private patient. Mo was diagnosed as suffering with diabetes and was advised to test his urine daily for change.

Case study 2

Michael is a 61-year-old Irishman, born in County Cork and retaining a very strong accent which many people find difficult to understand. He came to work temporarily on the buildings in London 40 years ago. One day he intends to return to Cork for good.

He came from a large and loving family, but many years ago his parents died from cancer, and his two older brothers whom he joined in London are dead. One died in an industrial accident and the other from heart disease; both drank and smoked heavily. His only living relatives are his sisters and cousins in Australia and the USA. He has never been much of a letter writer and lost touch with them when he moved. In fact he has always been something of a loner. He lived in the same room with an Irish family for many years, but they sold up and went back to Ireland and he had to find new lodgings. Michael had great difficulty in doing this but eventually found a place in a hostel, which he hates. He feels out of place and that 'they' are only after his money.

Last week he started hearing voices and was very frightened, so much so that he saw his GP, Dr Smythe, whom he had never visited before. The doctor could not understand what he was saying. He thought Michael was rather aggressive when he began shouting and swearing when the doctor repeated the same questions. Dr Smythe referred him to the local psychiatric unit the same day. Dr Smythe was concerned about the safety of other people at the hostel and decided to contact the supervisor.

Case study 3

Mrs Vera Smith is a 62-year-old Jamaican. She met her husband Sam, also Jamaican and a civil servant, in London when they first emigrated here in the 1960s. Vera trained as an SEN at the local hospital, they both worked full time and soon bought their own home. They had two boys, Sam Junior or just Junior to the family, and Louie. The boys were 'sport mad' and were encouraged by their father to play competitively from a young age in everything from cricket to athletics. This was a source of friction in the house as Vera felt the boys should concentrate on their education.

One summer's evening, Sam Jr (15 years) and Louie (13 years) were out playing football and there was an accident. Vera received a call to go straight to the casualty department in the hospital where she now worked as a clinical manager, because her younger son had had an accident. Whilst playing, Louie had been tackled by his brother and had fallen awkwardly; he had broken his neck.

After several months in hospital including a spinal rehabilitation unit, Louie was sent home; he remained paralysed from the neck down. His mother gave up her job to care for him full time. Louie became extremely emotionally as well as physically dependent on his mother and rather manipulative; he knew if he referred to himself as 'a cripple' it would have the desired effect. Sam Sr found it very hard to cope with the situation and blamed both himself and Sam Jr. Louie is now 29 years old and Vera is still caring for him. Sam Sr died 4 years ago from a stroke. Sam Jr left home when he was 18 and moved up north; he rarely goes home.

Case study 4

Mr Peters is an 80-year-old retired businessman who lives with his youngest son and daughter-in-law and their three children in a semi-detached house in a suburban area of a large city. Mr Peters has been widowed for 12 years and his other children are scattered across the globe.

Mr Peters has glaucoma and Parkinson's disease, severely restricting his sight and ability to walk. He is totally dependent on his family for care and cannot even safely make himself a cup of tea. He is very embarrassed about being 'such a nuisance'. He never goes out alone and socialises almost exclusively through his family and old business acquaintances. His speech is also rather slurred and is not always easy to understand.

Most of the day he is alone as the children are at school or college. Both his son and daughter-in-law run a law practice in another area of the city. He used to love reading and playing chess but can no longer do these activities. Recently Mr Peters has suffered a number of falls and was taken to casualty on the last occasion. He fractured his right leg and is now awaiting surgery following admission to an orthopaedic ward.

Case study 5

Maria Williams is 59 years old and is suffering from early Alzheimer's disease; she is mildly confused and

---

Box 15.1 Continued

forgetful. She is an extremely independent person and until 1 year ago had been working full time as a telephonist. Maria lives alone in a two-bedroom first-floor council flat where she has lived for many years following separation from her husband. She has one daughter, Sheila, who is married with two school-age children and lives locally. Sheila returned to work full time when her younger child started school 2 years ago.

Neighbours have reported Maria to the local housing office as she has flooded the flat below on several occasions when she left the taps on and forgot to put the waste hose for the washing machine into the sink. Maria has been very upset and embarrassed by the neighbours' complaints and is beginning to realise that she is 'ill'.

Sheila visits regularly but is finding it difficult as her husband, Frank, resents the time she is spending with her mother and does not want to be involved. Sheila would like to take her mother to live with them but Frank will not agree and, in any case, Maria would not agree to leave her flat.

Case study 6
Bill Thompson is 79 years old and has advanced Alzheimer's disease. He lives in a fourth-floor one-bedroom council flat with his second wife Florence who is 70 years old. Florence has a daughter, Louise, by her first marriage which ended because of her first husband's violence. Bill has one son living in Australia whom he hasn't seen for many years and has always regarded Louise as his own flesh and blood.

Bill's general health is good. He eats well and is mobile; his sleep patterns vary. Florence often has disturbed nights as she is terrified that he will soil the bed while she is in it. Bill is doubly incontinent. He spends most of the day sitting in a chair talking animatedly to himself. Normally he is cheerful but at times he gets extremely distressed and sobs for hours when he realises his mother is dead. Florence finds this very upsetting and cannot console him.

She finds it very difficult to cope with Bill's deterioration, as he was always extremely fastidious about hygiene and took care with his appearance. If it

were not for the help Louise gives her, she does not know what she would do. Recently Bill has become very aggressive, particularly toward Louise as he confuses her with his first wife. He refers to her as 'that bloody bitch' and accuses them of trying to kill him. Both Louise and Florence feel that they should continue to care for Bill at home to repay him for his care to them in the past and know he would do the same for them. They have been known to the health and social services in the past and a new assessment is to be made.

Case study 7
Agnes Collins is 39 years old. She lives with her parents Bertha and Thomas Collins aged 71 and 76 years respectively. Agnes never married and has always lived at home. She has moderate learning disabilities and spends her time helping at home, shopping, cooking and cleaning. Agnes has suffered for the past 10 years with anxiety attacks and has been prescribed a low dose of a mild tranquilliser twice a day, which her GP gives her reluctantly 'when things get too much'. Recently, Agnes has been having more frequent attacks and is anxious, tearful and complaining of insomnia.

The Collins' have lived all their married life in a large four-storey house which is privately rented. Agnes was born in the house. Currently they occupy only the ground and first floors. A group of property developers have been buying houses in the area for conversion into one- and two-bedroom flats. The family normally has little contact with the landlord, but he has visited several times recently bringing a surveyor with him on the last occasion. Agnes is worried that they will have to move.

Bertha suffers from severe rheumatoid arthritis and is wheelchair-bound. She has continual pain mainly in her hands, neck and shoulders. She does not complain unless she has a particularly bad day. Over the years she has been prescribed various non-steroidal anti-inflammatory drugs with poor effect. She is reluctant to take tablets unless the pain is severe. Thomas is partially sighted and has a below-knee amputation of his right leg. This was the result of an industrial accident when he was 60 years old and he wears a prosthesis.

- multidisciplinary work
- environment.

Overview of nursing models

A brief overview is given here of three models of nursing and the stages of the nursing process (see Ch. 14) are identified within them (Aggleton & Chalmers 1986, Skinner 1994). Models provide learners with a safe 'practice domain' within which to test out new concepts and become familiar with those used in practice.

Roper, Logan & Tierney's model of nursing (1990)

View of health. Roper et al's approach to health focuses on the individual. In order to function the individual needs to be able to carry out what they call the 'Activities of Living'. The 12 Activities of Living are central to this model of nursing, which is probably the best-known in Britain and is home-grown.

The activities, which are listed in Box 15.2, relate to various forms of human behaviour. All of

> **Box 15.2 Activities of Living (Roper et al 1990)**
>
> 1. Maintaining a safe environment
> 2. Communicating
> 3. Breathing
> 4. Eating and drinking
> 5. Eliminating
> 6. Personal cleansing and dressing
> 7. Controlling body temperature
> 8. Mobilising
> 9. Working and playing
> 10. Expressing sexuality
> 11. Sleeping
> 12. Dying

them are influenced by five types of factor: physical, environmental, politico-economic, social and psychological. Roper et al also recognise that these five types of factor coexist within dependency and life-span continua (see Fig. 15.1). It is therefore possible to plot where an individual is on each continuum. Dependency recognises that at particular points in people's lives they may become dependent on others, for example young children are dependent on their parents for protection, a person who has a broken leg may need assistance to get into bed, or an elderly or disabled person may need help to socialise. This continuum is comparatively flexible in that states of dependency can alter at any point.

The life-span continuum (see Fig. 15.1) shows the normal pattern of the human life span and can be determined in a number of ways, e.g. age, developmental processes, social roles, etc. This continuum is relatively fixed. One might predict a relationship between the two continua in that,

at key points in an individual's life, dependency and life span may be matched. For instance, new babies will be extremely dependent on their mothers and also not very far along the life-span continuum. Where would you plot yourself on these continua?

What happens when health breaks down? Roper et al state that health has broken down when individuals can no longer perform the Activities of Living in their usual way. They identify five causes of problems likely to need nursing: disability/disturbed pathology; pathological/degenerative tissue change; accident; infection; and effects from the physical, psychological or social environment. Roper et al's model actively uses the nursing process approach and the stages are included here with the key elements of the model for each stage. Assessment focuses on the individual's ability to carry out the Activities of Living. Emphasis is given to the patient's usual pattern of behaviour or means of coping. The focus of care is on what the patient is not able to do. Nursing care planning is directed towards dealing with actual and potential problems and should be expressed as behavioural goals, i.e. what the patient is expected to achieve as a result of nursing intervention. These goals should be realistic and achievable. Resource implications required for nursing are also considered.

What is the role of the nurse? Nursing consists of three components: preventing, comforting, and responding (seeking). The last aspect of nursing intervention includes technical help in relation to dependence, e.g. medication, dressing, etc. All these types of intervention (implementa-

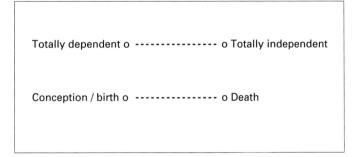

Figure 15.1 Roper, Logan & Tierney's dependency and life-span continua.

tion) may be present to varying degrees in the care of a single patient. Roper et al also include the use of other resources, e.g. other members of the primary health care team.

How is the effectiveness of nursing measured? Measurement (evaluation) is a continuous process of comparing the patient's current behaviour with the goals set at the planning stage in regard to Activities of Living. Reassessment occurs when the goals are not achieved or the model is no longer appropriate for the particular situation.

Orem's model of nursing (1980)

View of health. Health is related to an individual's right to be self-caring. This model is often referred to as the 'self-care model', and the self-care concept is central to it. Orem's view emphasises three important aspects, physiological, social and psychological, contributing to total health. This places the individual 'in the driving seat' in that people are responsible for their own health, and therefore need to fulfil their own self-care needs. This approach is therefore patient-centred, holistic and promotes health.

What happens when health breaks down? Orem defines ill health as the inability of individuals to meet their self-care needs because of demands being made on them. She states that nursing consists of helping the individual to achieve self-care again. The nurses or carers may act in a compensatory way to restore or maintain health, i.e. meet the self-care need. Orem has identified six (or eight depending on how they are listed) self-care needs which are fundamental to health (see Box 15.3)

What is the role of the nurse? The nurse's role is twofold: to promote self-care; and to act when

---

specialised care is required. The nurse needs to determine whether nursing is required, i.e. to determine whether or not the self-care needs are being met (assessment). The nurse needs to identify the reason for this deficit, i.e. is it due to a lack of skill or knowledge, or the stage of development in the patient or client? The nurse also has to assess the patient's potential ability for self-care. If nursing is required, the nurse decides with the patient or client what role the nurse will play in restoring self-care. This will be wholly compensatory, partially compensatory or educative/supportive. These decisions will be negotiated between the nurse and patient and realistic goals set (the long-term goal being self-care and particularly safe self-care): this is the planning stage.

The role the patient or client will play in achieving self-care is clearly defined in the plan; the action of the nurse and/or carers is also explained. Nursing intervention may therefore take one of the following forms (implementation):

- doing or acting for the patient or client
- guiding or directing the patient or client
- providing physical support
- providing psychological support
- providing an environment that supports development
- teaching others.

How is the effectiveness of nursing measured? Measuring the effectiveness of nursing intervention (evaluation) consists of two approaches:

- a summative approach, which is at a fixed point in time and is usually predetermined
- a formative approach, which is ongoing in nature.

By examining the goals set (which were patient-centred) and measuring what the patient has achieved in terms of safe self-care, appropriate adjustment can be made in order to set further joint goals.

Neuman's model of nursing

View of health. Betty Neuman (1982) developed her model on the basis that human beings are continually trying to make sense of their

---

> **Box 15.3   Fundamental self-care needs (Orem 1980)**
>
> - Sufficient air, water and nutrition
> - Satisfactory eliminative function
> - Activity balanced with rest
> - Time spent alone balanced with time spent with others
> - Prevention of danger to self
> - Being 'normal'

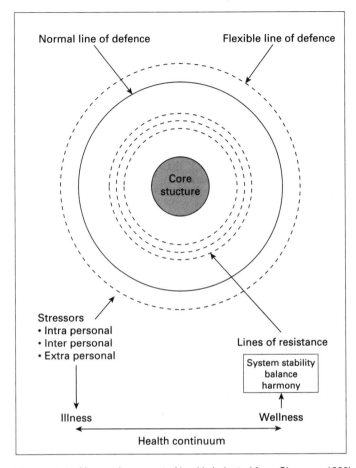

Figure 15.2   Neuman's concept of health (adapted from Chapman 1980).

environment and interpreting what is going on around them. She develops the idea that human beings are subject to stress which may be either from external sources or within the individual. She adopts a holistic approach where people react and interact with others and the environment.

The individual is a unique holistic system yet shares a common range of normal characteristics and responses. These include physiological, psychological, sociocultural, developmental and spiritual variables that form a dynamic composite whole. Neuman sees the individual as an open system interacting with, adjusting to and being adjusted by the environment. In order to survive, the individual has various unique lines of defence which protect against stressors, e.g. a core structure of survival factors, protected by

lines of resistance, by normal lines of defence and, finally, by a flexible line of defence (see Fig. 15.2).

Health is achieved when a state of inertness free of disrupting needs is achieved; this occurs through movement and adjustment. Neuman's concept of health implies a homeostatic balance. This depends on the free flow of energy between the individual and the environment. When healthy, the normal line of defence is maintained, lines of resistance are intact and basic structural elements of the system are preserved. Wellness means that there is stability of the systems and harmony with the environment.

What happens when health breaks down?   Ill health occurs when the systems are destabilised for whatever reason and there is disharmony with the environment. Society and the environment are an external source of stressors which may penetrate the normal line of defence. If this occurs it leads to ill health.

The client's systems must be assessed to identify the stressors with the client (assessment). The systems are physiological, psychological, sociocultural, spiritual and developmental, which are variables. Assessment focuses on the variables and how they affect the individual's response to stressors, how the individual responds to them and the state of the individual. Are the stressors intrapersonal (within the individual), interpersonal (between individuals) or extrapersonal (outside the individual)?

What is the role of the nurse? Nursing is required if the stress is too great (i.e. the flexible line of defence no longer provides protection against a stressor). The goal of nursing is adaptation to stress or to prevent maladaptation (i.e. restore, adapt or maintain) (planning). The goals should be negotiated with the client and be observable, measurable and ranked in order of importance. Goals may be short-term or long-term.

Nursing intervention assists the individual in reconstructing the lines of resistance or defence so that the central core of needs is protected (implementation). Pre-emptive action can be taken if a stressor is anticipated. Nurses must resolve differences in perception between them and the client before formulating a plan; nurses should not impose their judgements.

How is the effectiveness of nursing measured? Neuman's model involves identification of nursing outcomes which will be primary, secondary or tertiary or a combination of any of them (evaluation). Primary outcomes require the identification and allaying of the possible risk factors associated with the stressors. Secondary outcomes are the early identification of symptoms and interventions related to the symptoms, and tertiary outcomes focus on readaptation and re-education to prevent future occurrences and maintain stability.

Neuman's model is useful in its application to families and groups as well as individuals. It can also be used by other disciplines, due to its broad-based systems approach. Health is emphasised, and nursing seeks to achieve a maximal health approach and reconstitution. This takes place when a higher level is achieved than had previously been the case.

For further study

1. How do the named nursing models you have studied relate to:
   a. working with groups?
   b. use of the integrated approach discussed in Chapter 14?
   c. the UKCC Code of professional conduct?
   d. a philosophy of care?
2. Concerning one named nursing model, identify a specific area you would like to improve, e.g. understanding the key concepts, practising assessment.
   a. How will you rectify this?
   b. Set yourself a goal for this and record it in your portfolio.

LOCALITY PROFILING

Locality profiling is an important part of assessment and planning for the health needs of local populations. It is essential to health promotion work and to identify the resources necessary to meet health needs. Profiling can be undertaken in many ways. Here, profiling is the construction of a comprehensive picture within a defined locality usually related to health or local authority boundaries. This may be where you live or work.

What to include in a locality profile

- Details of geographical area—physical environment, main roads, etc.
- Use of boundaries—differences between health and local authority
- Demographic profile—gender, ethnic, socioeconomic issues, etc.
- Caseload profiles
- Health needs and priorities
- Availability of services for specific groups, statutory and voluntary
- Health workers

- Use of team approaches to care
- Local health initiatives

Nurses gather useful data on individuals, families and the wider community. This information provides valuable reference points for analysis of practice at the individual practitioner level and across the local population. For instance, an analysis can be made of the health facilities within a locality relative to the population needs. Or a comparison between localities can be made focusing on certain factors, e.g. physical environment, access to services for specific groups like the homeless or ethnic minorities, use of boundaries and so on. A nurse might consider the ethnic profile of the patients/clients with whom she is in contact to identify barriers to accessing the service she provides. Gaps in provision can be identified, e.g. learning disabilities.

Data sources for profile

Health workers need to locate effective and accurate sources of information to construct profiles. A useful starting point is the annual public health reports produced by health authorities usually in health promotion units. They identify health needs and priorities that have been agreed. The information can then be cross-referenced with other locality information held elsewhere. Table 15.1 shows commonly available information which can be used in profiling. Some information is more accessible than other information. Main

Table 15.1 Information sources for locality profiling

Type of information	Sources of information
Age/sex registers	GPs & FHSAs
Community profiles	Community trusts
Caseload profiles	Community trusts
Hospital inpatient and outpatient statistics	NHS trusts & RHAs
Annual public health reports	HA health promotion units
Community care plans	Local authorities
Population statistics	Local authorities & OPCS
Health authority plans	Community health councils
Voluntary sector plans	Community health councils & voluntary organisations
Housing	Local authorities
Accidents	Local authorities
Environmental issues	Local authorities

public libraries frequently provide invaluable information for profiling, particularly data produced for local authorities. However, there are limitations in using and interpreting existing data; these have been summarised in Box 15.4.

Box 15.4 Problems with data

- Inaccuracies
- Out of date
- Weak information systems,
- Not systematically collected
- Inadequate databases
- Incompatibility
- Uncollated
- Insensitive to particular groups
- Not detailed enough for thorough analysis

Activity 15.1

During the course of your study you should have collected a considerable amount of information about your locality from, for example, community care plans, public health reports, etc. Use them as a basis for this activity.

a. Identify a health need in your own locality or sphere of work. How does it relate to national and local health promotion policies?
b. Arrange an observational visit to an area connected with the problem you have identified above. For example an occupational health department in a local industry, environmental health department, sewerage disposal unit, etc.

Activity 15.2

1. Using a locality profile you have constructed, identify three groups likely to be in contact with both hospital and community services. Identify one group that may *not* be and you think should be.
2. Plan selected health promotion activities for groups using an integrated model (see Ch. 14). Consider the following dimensions in your plan: policy, legislation, environment, teamwork, gaps in provision.
3. Identify clearly the resources that would be required to carry out one of your health promotion activities, including staff involved, time required, accommodation, equipment, etc.

REFERENCES

Aggleton P, Chalmers H 1986 Nursing models and the nursing process. Macmillan, Basingstoke

Chapman C 1985 Theory of nursing: practical application. Harper & Row, London

Neuman B 1982 The Neuman systems model: application to nursing education and practice. Appleton-Century-Crofts, New York

Orem D 1980 Nursing: concepts of practice, 2nd edn. McGraw-Hill, New York

Pearson A, Vaughan B 1992 Nursing models for nursing practice. Churchill Livingstone, Edinburgh

Roper N, Logan W, Tierney A J 1990 The elements of nursing: a model for nursing based on a model of living, 3rd edn. Churchill Livingstone, Edinburgh

Skinner J 1994 Theories of nursing. Lecture notes and study materials (unpublished). University of North London

Index

Page numbers in italics refer to figures and tables, those in **bold** *refer to main entries of topics.*

A

Abortion numbers, 76
Accidents
  adulthood, 135–136
  deaths, 160
  environment, 175–176
  ethnic minorities, 45
  home, 175–176
  incidence, 22
  prevention, 21
    in childhood, 128–129
    children, 195
    elderly, 195
    exhibitions, 128
    Healthy Islington 2000, 194–195
    joint initiatives, 195
    resource pack, 195
    workplace, 195
  primary prevention, 43
  psychological distress, 179
  road traffic, 128, 175, 179, 181
Acid rain, 18
Activities
  applied, 200–206
  of living, 203
Addiction self-help groups, 106
Adolescence, **129–133**
  alcohol abuse, 131
  cognitive development, 130
  counselling, 131, 132
  drug abuse, 131
  education programmes, 131
  empowerment, 131
  homelessness, 132
  identity, 130–131
  nutritional demands, 132–133
  parental support, 130, 131
  risky behaviour, 131
  social changes, 130–131
  understanding, 130
Adulthood
  accidents, 135–136
  cancer, 134–135
  health promotion, **133–136**
  mental health promotion, 134
  outcome evaluation, 135
  positive messages, 134
  quality of life, 134
  sexual health, 136
  smoking, 135
Advocacy
  multi-ethnic project, 37
  nurses, 57
Affection needs, 100
Affective learning, 111–113
Afro-Caribbean mental health project, 107
Age profile of population, 164

Ageing, 136
Ageism, 139
AIDS
  adulthood, 136
  education in schools, 146
  later life, 139
  mass media campaign, 151, 152, 153
  prison surveys, 154
  programmes, 114
Alcohol
  adolescence, 131
  cardiovascular disease, 134
  consumption
    data, 77
    social class, 167
  costs of illness to industry, 149
  drinking patterns, 131
  health effects, 161
  misuse, 61
  pregnancy, 126
  workplace policies, 148
  see also Drinking and driving
Alma Ata Declaration (1978), 29, 96
Alzheimer's disease, 173
Ammonia, 173
Anorexia nervosa, 133
Antenatal care, access, 23
Antenatal screening, 126–127
Anxiety, 115
Architects, 182
Arthritis, 160
Asbestos, 176
Assessment
  listening, 85
  nursing, 189
Asthma
  air pollution, 172
  causal spectrum, 59
  control, 36
Attitudes
  change, 112
  communication, 88
  evaluation, 49
Audit
  care standards, 48, 49
  education, 114
  performance evaluation, 114
Authenticity, 84

B

Behaviour, 7
  adolescence, 131
  attitude link, 47
  change
    benefits, 46
    costs, 46
    evaluation, 49
    Health of the Nation strategy, 42
    HIV avoidance, 46–47
    motivation, 46
  definitions, 72
  expressed attitudes, 47

group norm effects, 99–100
  health-related, 112, 117, 161
  motives, 110
  social class, 167–168
  unhealthy, 61
Belongingness needs, 115
Bengali women's group linkworker, 84
Benzene, 173, *174*
Best interest, 56
  health promotion, 57
  moral considerations, 57
  professional nursing, **56–58**
  reactive care, 56–57
  responsibilities, 57
  UKCC code, 62
Best practice, 56
Birth rate trends, 79
Blood pressure
  cardiovascular disease, 134
  racial differences, 137
Body
  movements, 91
  orientation, 88, 90
Brainstorming, 122
Breast cancer, 135
  cost-benefit calculations, 58
  screening, 28, 43, 161
Breast self-examination, 113
Breastcare nurses, 135
Building regulations, 181
Built environment, 17, 19
  accident prevention, 21
  health status, 163
Bulimia, 133
Business interests, 55
Buzz groups, 122

C

Cancer, 134–135, 159, 160
  deaths, 161
  registration, 76
Carbon dioxide, 178, 179
Carbon monoxide, 173, *174*
Cardiovascular disease
  blood pressure, 134
  diet, 133
  exercise promotion, 129
  see also Coronary heart disease;
    Heart disease
Care, 5
  accessibility, 127
  continuity, 127
  elderly people, 21
  environment, 62, 63
  quality, 60
  women's roles, 24
  see also Community, care; Health,
    care
Carers
  health promotion, 12
  unhealthy lifestyle trap, 56
Case studies, 200–202

Catalytic converters, 180
Causal spectrum, **59**
  asthma, 59
  economy, 59
  intervention, 54
  standards, 59
Census (1991), 77
Census data, 77–78
  availability, 78
  collected, 78
  see also General Household Survey
Cerebrovascular disease, 159
Cervical cancer, 135
  screening, 28, 161
Cervical smears, 57, 59
Change
  management, 101
  resistance, 102
Change of Heart project (Northern
    Ireland), 28
Children, **126–129**
  abuse, 147
  accident prevention, 128–129, 195
  accidents in the home, 175–176
  air pollution effects, 172
  communication, 87
  developmental screening, 43
  eating habits, 128
  eating intervention, 54
  exercise promotion, 129
  health impact, 127
  nutrition, 128
  parent involvement in hospital care,
    101
  pupil-held health records, 145
  special educational needs, 145
  surveillance programmes, 127
Chlorofluorocarbons, 178–179
Chronic disease, 21–22
  primary health care, 29
Cleanliness, 19, 20
Clinical competence, 57
Clinical prevention screening
    programmes, 28
Coal mining, 176
Cognitive development in
    adolescence, 130
Cognitive learning, 111, 113
  objectives, 119
Collaboration
  inter-agency, 193
  multisectorial, 192–195
Collaborative Support Programs of
    New Jersey (CSPNJ), 116–117
Communication, **81–82**
  attitudes, 88
  children, 87
  competency, 82
  counselling, **83–84**
  education, 110
  elements, 81–82
  groups, 97
  for health promotion, **81–92**
  hearing impairment, 86–87

interpreters, 84
involvement, 99
jargon, 87
language, **84–87**
learning difficulties, 87
linguistic minorities, 84
listening, **84–87**
nonverbal, **88–92**
nurse-client, 83
skills, 82
  for helping people, *82*
  in sexual health, 136
teaching, 120–121
therapeutic, 83–84
verbal, 84
written, **87–88**
Community
  alliances, 144
  approach to health promotion, 9, **10**
  care
    chronic illness, 21–22
    collaboration, 125–126
    degenerative conditions, 21–22
    demographic change, 21
    disability, 21–22
    health promotion, **21–23**
    self-determination, 44
    self-reliance, 44
    women, 24
  caring, 9
  data gathering, 207
  development, 37
    education approach, 116
    for health approach, 45
    health promotion, 62
  empowered, 46
  general practitioner approaches, 36
  health
    groups, 105
    promotion, 9, 21, 28, **35–36**
    promotion programme
      evaluation, 49
  Health Councils (CHCs), 37
  health services
    collaboration, 126
    funding, 25
    National Health Service, 31–32
    staff, 11
  mental health teams, 103–104
  multidisciplinary teams, 103
  needs assessment, 70
  nursing and health promotion, 28,
    35–36
  personhood, 61–62
  safety, **177–178**
  social networks, 8
  teams for people with learning
    difficulties, 104
  values, 52–53
Complementary therapy, 187
Concensus, 101
Condoms, 136, 152
Confidentiality, 57
  breach, 62

Construction site noise, 175
Consumer programmes, 116–117
Consumerism, 36–37
Contagious disease controls, 58
Control needs, 100
Conversation synchronising, 88
Coronary heart disease, 133–134
  international health promotion, 28
  prevention programmes, 150
  see also Heart disease
Counselling
  adolescents, 131, 132
  antenatal, 126–127
  communication, **83–84**
  sexual health, 136
  skills, 84–85
Crisis, individual, 5–6
Cultural differences
  eye contact, 91–92
  personal space, 89
Cultural values, 52–53
Cultural/behavioural theory, 169
Cultural/materialist perspective, 169
Curing, **4–5**
Cycle routes, 175

D

Data sources, 80
Deafness, 86–87
  see also Hearing
Death
  causes, 159–160
  rate
    age-specific, 73–74
    cause-specific, 74
    morbidity proxy, 75
  talking about, 85
  unexpected, 54
  see also Mortality
Decision-making
  empowered, 46
  ethically based, 63
  health-related, 52, 110
  information, 70
  informed, 110
  participation, 64
  responsible, 60–61
Degenerative disease, 21–22
  primary health care, 29
Delegation, 101
Dementia prevalence, *79*
Demographic change
  community care, 21
  see also Population
Demonstration, 120–121
Dependency, 203
Depression in ethnic minorities, 44
Deprivation
  environmental, 178
  ill health, 42, 162
Diabetes, 127
  Asian population, 192

Diabetes (*contd*)
  self-help groups, 107
Diagnosis, listening, 85
Diet
  cardiovascular disease, 133
  change, 46
  health effects, 161
  intervention, 54
  United Kingdom, 161
Dieticians, 145
Disability, 21–22
  client-based information, 71
  prevalence, 76
  racial differences, 137
  socially constructed disadvantage,
    160
  standardised index, 74–75
  survey, 76, 77
Disabled people
  health needs, 23
  quality of life, 23
  workplace, 150
Disadvantage, 10
  habit changing, 112
  positive discrimination, 43
Disease
  complication prevention, 44
  describing, 71–72
District nurses, 25, 35
  preventive role, 41
District surveyors, 181
Doctor, clinical autonomy, 56
Domestic health, 19
Drinking and driving, 135
  mass media campaign, 151
Drop-in centres, 136
Drugs
  adolescent abuse, 131
  misuse, 127
  pregnancy, 126
  therapy, 17

E

Earth Summit on Environment and
    Development (Rio de Janeiro
    1992), 178
Eating
  disorders, 133
  habits, 128
  see also Diet
Economic factors, 8
Economic policy, 32
Education, **109–122**
  active participation, 116–117
  adult, 110
  alcohol programmes, 135
  children, 127
  Collaborative Support Programs of
    New Jersey (CSPNJ), 116–117
  communication, 110
  community development approach,
    116–117

demonstration, 120–121
empowerment, 47, 114
evaluation, 122
freeing, 109–110
goal, 110
goal-setting, 118
health curriculum, 145
health oriented programmes, 117
health-promoting, 144–146
holistic approach, 113
implementation, 119–122
initiatives, 146–147
later life, 137
lectures, 120
lifestyle, 110
manipulation, 114
mass media, **151–154**
mobilisation of activities, 23
need, 110
needs assessment, 118
new nurse, 192
nursing, 186
outreach basis, 143
parenting skills, 47
particular needs, 110
personal goals, 113
presentations, 120
principles, 117
programmes
  for adolescents, 131
  design, 113
  health promotion, 21
  health service staff, 12
Reform Act (1988), 146
road safety, 147
socio-sexual, 121
strategic aims, 119
talks, 120
see also Health, education
Educator qualities, 112
Elderly
  accident prevention, 195
  accidents in the home, 176
  health promotion, 168
  increasing numbers, 21
  inequalities in health, 168
  population, 16
  see also Later life
Emotion communication, 88
Emotional health, 109
Emotional needs, later life, 137
Empathy, 83
  touch, 90
Employees
  health promotion activities, 148
  health and safety, 149
Employment
  later life, 138–139
  support services, 139
Empowerment
  adolescence, 131
  approach to policy, 36, 37
  children, 144–145
  education, 47, 114

health promotion, 46
  notions, 61
Energy sector, 179
Engineers, public health, 181
English National Board, 130
Environment, **171–182**
  accidents, 175–176
  adjustment of individual, 205
  built, 17, 19, 21, 163
  of care, 62, 63
  community safety, 177–178
  current issues, 18–19
  deprivation, 178
  evaluation of change, 49
  green agenda, 178–179
  group learning, 121–122
  health effects, **171–177**
  healthy, 159
  home, 177
  hospital, 17
  inequality, 178
  nursing care delivery, 17
  smoking effects, 177
  workplace, 176–177
Environmental factors, 6–7
Environmental health officers, 181
Environmental level of health
    promotion, 40
Environmental professions, **180–182**
Epidemiology, 16
Epilepsy, 127
Equity, 46
  health promotion, 191–195
Esteem needs, 115
Ethics, 187
  decision-making, 63
  UKCC code, 52, 62–63, 187, 193
Ethnic minorities
  depression, 44
  health, 164–165
  infant mortality, 164
  living conditions, 45
  migrant, 164
  morbidity, 164–165
  mortality, 164
  native born, 164, 165
  nursing approach, 192
  stroke mortality, 165
Ethnicity, **164–165**
  blood pressure, 137
Evaluation, **48–49**
  community health promotion
    programme, 49
  education, 122
  nursing, 189–190
Exercise
  data, 77
  endurance, 129
  health effects, 161
  promotion, 129
  social class, 167
Experience, learning from, 115–116
Expressions, 88
Eye contact, 91

F

Facial expression, 91
Families, data gathering, 207
Family health service collaboration, 125–126
Family planning
  adolescence, 132
  nurses, 145
Feedback, 88
  principles, 82
Fire
  casualties, 176
  risk, 128
Food
  labelling, 46
  manufacturers, 45
  poisoning notification, 76
  provision of healthy, 46
Freedom of individual, 53
Fuels, alternative, 180

G

Gastric cancer, 173–174
Gender, health status, **163**
General Household Survey, 76–77
  morbidity data, 160
  National Health Service services, 162
  social class data, 167
  see also Census data
General practitioner
  community approaches, 36
  health promotion, 28, **34–35**
  multidisciplinary team, 103
  services, 31
Genetic counselling, 42, 100
Genuineness, 84
Geographical variations in health, **168–169**
Gestures, 88, 91
Global warming, 178
  motor vehicles, 179
Goal-setting, 118
Good Hearted Glasgow Campaign, 150
Good practice standards, 49
Greatest good for greatest number, 56
  population-based health promotion, 58
Green agenda, 178–179
Greenhouse gases, 178, 179
Group member
  interpretation of reality, 99
  involvement, 98–99
  perceptions, 99
Group norms
  conformation, 101
  effects on behaviour, 99–100
  power, 100
  violation, 99

Groups, **95–100**
  balanced teams, 100
  buzz, 122
  characteristics, **97–100**
  definition, **96**
  environment, 121–122
  goal establishment/achievement, 98–99
  insulation from outside influence, 101
  learning, 121–122
  needs, 100
  primary, 98
  processes, 98–100
  role effects on behaviour, 100
  secondary, 98
  self-awareness, 97
  skills, 95
  stress, 102
  teams, 102
  verbal interventions, 97
Groupthink, 101–102
Groupwork
  learning disabilities, 121
  skills, **96–97**

H

Handicap reduction, 160
Harm avoidance, 57
Health
  awareness evaluation, 49
  basic requirements, 8, 29
  belief model, 46–47
  breakdown, 203, 204, 205–206
  care
    access, 157, **161–162**, 168
    cost cutting, **55–56**
    costs, 25, 32
    ethics, 187
    expenditure escalation, 55
    hospital-dominated, 55
    nurse accountability, 192
    preventive orientation, 32
    resources, 69–70
    services, 8
    social class, 168
    values, 54
    see also Care; Health care workers
  choices, 7
  concept of homeostatic balance, 205
  curing, **4–5**
  definitions, **3–4**, 6, 55
  education, **7–8**
    primary, 42, 43
    sphere, 40–41
    types, 7–8
    see also Education
  factors outside individual control, 6–7
  hazard identification, 47
  individual choices, 6–7
  individual responsibility, 19–20

inequalities, 22–23
interests of whole population, 56
needs
  disabled people, 23
  identification, 47
nursing goal, 186
outcome determination, 23
people's views, 5
persuasion model, 45
policy
  ethically based decision making, 63
  nurses, 192
  scientific knowledge, 54
population differences, 157
positive behaviour, 96
professionals, 9, 10
protection sphere, 40
responsibility for, 7
and safety at work, 176–177
and Safety at Work Act (1974), 176
and Safety commission, 149
sector, 28
self-care in maintenance, 60
service
  access, 23
  community-based staff, 11
  hospital-based staff, 11
  staff relationships with other workers, 11–12
  users, 12
status
  evaluation, 49
  factors determining, 23
  gender differences, **163**
  inequalities, 52, 157
  surveys, 76–77
surveillance, 41
understanding of condition, 60
values, 61
see also Health of the Nation; Health promotion; Health visitors
Health care workers
  feelings for individual, 57
  health promotion, 21
  policy making, 28
  safe practice, 59
  safety at work, 150
  self-empowerment, 151
Health of the Nation strategy, 28, 33–34
  adult health promotion, 133
  behaviour change, 42
  cancers, 134–135
  childhood accident prevention, 128
  education initiatives, 146–147
  key policy objectives, 42
  medical focus, 34
  mental health targets, 134
  nurse targets, 58
  promotion of good health, 42
  responsibilities, 42
  settings, 153–154
  targets, 48

Health promotion, **3**, 6, **9**, **15–25**
  active seeking, 168
  activity levels, **70–72**
  approaches, 8
  business interests, 55
  carers, 12
  community, 9
    approach, 9, **10**
    care, **21–23**
    nursing, 28, **35–36**
  conceptualisation, 12
  economic policy, 32
  educational programmes, 12
  empowerment, 46
  equity, 9, **10**, 46
  finance-led shift, 56
  gender issues, 23–25
  general practice, 28, **34–35**
  health care costs, 25, **55–56**
  Health of the Nation strategy, 28
  health visitors, **17–18**
  hospitals, 25
  individual care, 19
  individual involvement, 30
  individual responsibility, 32, 33
  individual/personal focus, **9–10**
  inequalities, 22–23
  integrated approach, **39–41**
  integrated process, 9, **10–11**
  international programmes/policies,
    28–30
  levels, 40
  medical approach, 41
  models, 40
  multidisciplinary approach, 9, **11–12**
  National Health Service, 20–21
  nursing education/training, 15
  nursing facilitators, 12
  officers, 145
  optimum strategies, 47
  outreach basis, 143
  Peckham experiment, 20
  personal health, **19–21**
  personal involvement, 30
  planning integration, **41–42**
  policy, **36–37**
    development, **27–37**, **30–31**
    in UK, **31–33**
  portfolio development, 200
  proactive, 54–55
  psychological theory, **46–47**
  public health, 9, **10**, **16–19**, 30
  quality, 9, **10**
  radical model, **45–46**
  setting, 159, 162
  strategies, **30–31**
  time of turbulence, 9, 12
  UK policy, 28
  UK strategy, 32–33
  users of service, 12
  women in formal health sector,
    24–25
  women in informal health sector,
    23–24

Health visitors, **17–18**, 24
  empowerment of people, 41
  health promotion, 35
  information returns, 71
  need identification, 118
  partnership with parents, 127
  preventive role, 41
  safety equipment loan scheme, 128
  work principles, 18
Health/illness continuum, *6*
Healthy alliances, 34
Healthy Islington 2000, 193–195
Hearing
  impairment, 86–87
  noise pollution, 174
Heart disease, 159
  deaths, 161
  mass media campaign, 151
  see also Cardiovascular disease;
    Coronary heart disease
Heartbeat Wales, 28
Heroin, mass media campaign, 151,
    152
Highway engineers, 181
HIV
  adulthood, 136
  behaviour change, 46–47
  behavioural changes, 112
  education in schools, 146
  later life, 139
  learning materials, 111
  mass media campaign, 151, 152
  prison surveys, 154
  team community care, 103
  transmission, 131
HIV/AIDS, client-based information,
    71
Holistic approach, 45
Holistic care, 186
Holistic health promotion, 136
Homelessness, adolescence, 132
Hospital
  built environment, 17
  health care role, 10
  health promotion, 25
  health service staff, 11
  reforms, 17
Hospital-at-home schemes, 60
House
  drainage, 16
  in multiple occupation, 176
Housing, 17
  adolescents, 130–131
  contribution to health, 159
  current problems, 18
  environment, 177
  health effects, 161
  inequalities in health, 167, 169–170
  policies, 96
  provision of adequate, 45
  status data, 78
Human potential, 3
Hypothermia, 138
Hypothyroidism, 43

I

Identity, adolescence, 130–131
Ill health
  deprivation, 42
  poverty, 42
  see also Morbidity
Illness prevention, 6
Immigration Mortality Study, 164
Immunisation, 17, 42
  contribution to health, 159
Implementation
  evaluation of programmes, 49
  nursing, 189
Incentives, 58
Incidence of disease, 71–72
Inclusion needs, 100
Income, inequalities in health, 169–170
Independence, adolescence, 130
Individual responsibility
  for health, 19–20
  health promotion, 32, 33
Individuals
  constraints, 58
  crisis, 5–6
  data gathering, 207
  health promotion, 21
  holistic system, 205
  level of health promotion, 40
Industrialised countries, 29
Industry, environmental controls, 19
Inequality, environmental, 178
Inequalities in health, **157–170**
  cultural/behavioural theory, 169
  cultural/materialist perspective, 169
  factors influencing class-based, 167
  geographical variation, **168–169**
  health promotion, 167
  later life, 168
  lifestyle, 169
  social class, 165–168, 169
  trends in class-based, 166–167
Infancy, **126–129**, 127
  surveillance programmes, 127
Infant mortality, 16, 18
  ethnic minorities, 164
  rate, 74
  social class, 166
Infection notification, 58
Infectious disease rate, 16
Information
  accessing, 80
  client-based, 71
  commissioned surveys/studies, 71
  decision-making, 70
  dissemination, 48
  health promotion, **69–80**
  mortality, 73
  related of interest to health
    promotion, **77–79**
  returns from health promoters, 71
  sources, **72–77**
  sources for locality profiling, 207

Information (*contd*)
  types for health promotion, 71
Information-led intervention, 58
Informed consent, 59
  options discussion, 60
Institutions
  care, 21
  screening, 161
Integrated approach to health
    promotion, **39–41**
  health education sphere, 40–41
  health protection sphere, 40
  preventive sphere, 41
Integrated model
  of health promotion, **185–196**
  for nursing practice, 187–188
Intention to act, 47
Inter-censal estimates, 79
International programmes/policies for
    health promotion, **28–30**
Interpersonal distance, 89
Interpretation services, 57
Interpreters, 84
Intervention, causality, 54, 55
Intimate disclosure, 91
Inverse care law, 168
Inverse prevention law, 131
Inviolability feelings, 130
Involvement in health promotion, 144
Ireland, education, 146
Islington Voluntary Action Council, 194

J

Jargon, 87
Job
  satisfaction, 99
  stress, 150–151
Johari window, 97, *98*

K

Knowledge
  evaluation, 49
  imperfect, 60–61

L

Lalonde Report (1974), 29
Language, **84–87**
  difficulties, 87
  questions, 86
Later life, 136–139
  AIDS, 139
  education, 137
  emotional needs, 137
  employment, 138–139
  HIV, 139
  inequalities in health, 168
  mortality, 137–138
  poverty, 138

risk factors, 137–138
  sexual needs, 137
  sexuality, 137
  smoking, 138
  see also Elderly
Laying on of hands, 90
Lead, 173, *174*
Leadership, **100–102**
  style, 101
Learners, emotional needs, 112
Learning, **111–114**
  affective, 111–113
  cognitive, 111, 113
  diary, 116
  difficulties
    communication, 87
    community teams, 104
    involvement in meetings, 99
  disabilities, 41, 127
    community care, 44
    community housing, 133
    groupwork, 121
  evaluation, 122
  facilitation, 119
  from experience, 115–116
  group, 121–122
  levels, 111
  media, 111
  motivation, **114–117**
  objectives, 118–119
  practice, 121
  principles, 117
  psychomotor skills, 113
  reflection, 116
  styles, 113
  supervision, 121
  support, 121
Lectures, 120
Life context, **96**
Life expectancy, 136, 159
  Health of the Nation strategy, 34
Life-cycle approach to health
    promotion, **125–139**
Life-span continuum, 203
Lifestyle, 8, 9
  adolescent choice, 131
  commitment of general public, 63
  education, 110
  factors, 6, 7
  health approaches, 20
  health status, 163
  inequalities in health, 169
  intervention integration, 126
  political concensus on change, 55–56
  UK, 161
  unhealthy, 56
Linguistic minorities, 84
Listening, **84–87**
  active, 84–86
  clarifying, 85
  encouraging talking, 85
  nonverbal skills, 84–85
  paraphrasing, 85–86
  reflecting, 85

silence, 85
  summarising, 86
Living standards, 159
Local authority planners, 36
Locality profiling, 192–193, 206–207
  data sources, 207
Look after your heart (LAYH), 150
Lung cancer, 134–135
Lungs, disease resistance, 172

M

Macmillan nurses, 135
Mains sewerage, 16
Manipulation, 114
Markets, public safety, 178
Maslow's hierarchy of needs, 114–115
Mature entry programme for
    employment, 138–139
Media, 48
  advertising, 128
  changing behaviour, 152–153
  education, **151–154**
  health promotion, 144
  influence on alcohol consumption,
    135–136
  mental health, 153
Medical intervention, hi-tech, 70
Medication objectives, 119
Melanoma, 43–44, 135
Mental health, 109
  adult promotion, 134
  Afro-Caribbean group, 107
  Collaborative Support Programs of
    New Jersey (CSPNJ), 116–117
  community nurses, 145
  inequalities in health, 169
  media, 153
  personhood, 60
  primary prevention, 42–43
  prisoners, 154
  problems, 22
  secondary promotion, 44
  support group, 99
  teams
    assertive outreach approach, 104
    community, 103–104
Mental illness
  social support factors, 161
  stigma, 153
  violence, 153
  wellness goals, 113
Mental state, 4
Methane, 178
Midwife
  care, 127
  health and safety at work, 149
  outcome evaluation, 135
  partnership with parents, 127
Migration trends, 79
Montreal Protocol on Substances that
    Deplete the Ozone Layer (1987),
    179

Moral values, 52
  differing, 54
Morbidity
  causes, 160
  ethnic minorities, 164–165
  gender differences, 163
  geographical variation, 168–169
  housing, 177
  inequalities in health, 169
  measures, 75–76
  proxy, 75
  social class, 166
  United Kingdom, 160–162
  see also Ill health
Mortality
  changes, 159
  data analysis, 73–74
  ethnic minorities, 164
  gender differences, 163
  geographical variation, 168–169
  inequalities in health, 169
  information, 73
  later life, 137–138
  overall rates, 138
  patterns, 158
  proxy for morbidity, 75
  rates, 73–74
  social class, 166
  standard ratios, 74, 158–159
  trends, 79
  tuberculosis, 17
  United Kingdom, 158–160
  see also Death; Infant mortality
Motivation, anxiety, 115
Motives, 114
Motor vehicles
  pollution, 172, 179
  seat belt legislation, 19
  use reduction, 180
  see also Drinking and driving; Road
    accidents
Movement, 88, 90–91
Musculoskeletal disorders, 160

N

National Curriculum, 127, 128
  health education, 146
National Health Service
  aims, 157, 186
  business management principles,
    31
  changes, 31–32
  contracting processes, 31
  cost containment, 32
  expenditure, 162
  funding, 162
  general practitioners, 31
  health promotion, 20–21
  medical aspects, 4
  principles, 161–162
  secondary care, 162
Needle exchange schemes, 41

Needs
  assessment, **70**
  hierarchy, 115
Neoplasms, 159
Networking, professional, 182
New nurse education, 186, 192
Nightingale, Florence, 17, 186
Nitrates, 173
Nitrites, 173–174
Nitrogen oxides, 173, *174*
Noise levels, 174–175
North Karelia project (Finland), 28
Notification of disease, 76
Nottingham Patient Council Support
    Group, 99
Nurses
  accountability, 192
  advocacy, 57
  contribution to public health, 10
  data gathering, 207
  distancing from patient, 89
  education focus, 114
  empowered, 114
  environmental concerns, 19
  facilitators, 51
  health policies, 192
  health promotion, 10, 11, 21, 52, 56
  inter-agency collaboration, 193
  liaison, 96
  locality profiling, 192–193
  partnership with user, 60
  personhood, 62
  prescribing, 55
  public health role, 35–36
  relationship with other health
    workers, *194*
  reporting responsibilities, 193
  responsibility, 59
  role, 10, 11, 56, 58, 203–204
  social forces, 54
  staffing levels, 59
  supporters, 52
  target-based role, 58
  task-oriented work, 59
  teachers, 52
  time, 56
  women, 24
  working environment, 151
Nursing
  academic discipline, 186
  assessment, 189
  autonomy, 186
  care delivery environment, 17
  care planning, 203
  components, 203–204
  education, 186
  effectiveness measurement, 204, 206
  evaluation, 189–190
  facilitators, 12
  goals, 186
  health-promoting, **51–64**
  education/training, 15
  values, **52–54**
  implementation, 189

individual level of health
    promotion, 188
integrated model for practice,
    187–188
locality profiling, 206–207
models, **188–191**, 202–206
  activities of living, 203
  health breakdown, 203, 204,
    205–206
  integrated approach, 190–191
  limitations, 190
  Neuman's, 191, 204–206
  nurse role, 203–204, 206
  Orem's, 191, 204
  Roper, Logan and Tierney's, 191,
    202–204
  selection criteria, 190
  use within integrated approach,
    190–191
  view of health, 202–203, 204–205
  new, 186, 192
  outcome identification, 206
  personhood, **59–62**
  philosophy, *188*
    health promotion, **186–188**
    influences, 186–187
  planning, 189
  practice
    health promotion, **186–188**
    integrated model of health
      promotion, **185–196**
  process and integrated approach,
    189–190
  professional, 56–58, 186
  theory, 186, 187
Nutrition
  cardiovascular disease, 133
  children, 128
  demands in adolescence, 132–133
  people with learning disabilities, 133
  pregnancy, 126
  radical education, 45–46
  women's role, 24

O

Obesity, 133
  cardiovascular disease, 134
Occupational hazards, 22
Occupations
  mortality differential, 167
  social class, 165–166
Office blocks, 176–177
Organisational level of health
    promotion, 40
Osteoporosis, 129
Ostomy surgery, 106
Ottawa Charter, 9, 30, 32
Outcome evaluation, 49, 122
  in adulthood, 135
Outreach workers, 136
Ozone, 172
  layer damage, 18, 178

P

Pain, 54
Palliative care, 41, 44
Paramedic professions, women, 24
Parenthood preparation, 126
Parenting skills, 47
Parents
children's care in hospital, 101
input into children's education, 127
partnership with midwife/health
visitor, 127
support for adolescents, 131
Partner tracing, 136
Patients
advisory groups, 104
care plans, 103
compliance, 60–61
consumers, 187
Peckham Pioneer Health Centre
experiment, 20
Peer
education practices, 61
groups, 60
teaching programmes, 147
Performance feedback, 49
Perinatal mortality
rate, 74
regional inequality, 43
Personal health, **19–21**
Peckham experiment, 20
Personal skills, education, 110
Personal space, 90
Personhood, 56
commitment, 63
community, 61–62
mental health, 60
moral primacy of individual, 60
nurse, 62
partnership, 60
professional nursing, **59–62**
UKCC code, 62
Pesticides, 174
Petrol, 173
Phenylketonuria, 43
Physical health, 109
Physiological needs, 115
Planning
evaluation, 49
integrated approach, **41–42**
nursing, 189
Play areas, 45
Poisoning, accidental, 128
Policy
change evaluation, 49
development, **30–31**
making in health promotion, **27–37**
Pollution
air, 172–173, 178
industrial waste, 58
levels, 36
motor vehicles, 179
noise, 174–175

reduction, 171
water, 173–174
Population
age profile, 164
available health data, 80
census data, 76
change, 21, 78
estimates between censuses, 78–79
health in UK, **158–161**
national data application to local
populations, 79
needs assessment, 70
projections, 79
revised estimates, 79
social characteristics, 78
Population-based health promotion,
58
Portfolio
development, 199
formulation, 200
Positive health enhancement, 40–41
Positive regard, unconditional, 83
Posture, 90, 90–91
Poverty, 10, 17
health status, 33
ill health, 35, 42
later life, 138
nutrition education, 45
old age, 138
poor health, 161
strategies, 23
United Kingdom, 161
Practice nurse, 58
Pregnancy
care, 126
outcome, 23
Prenatal care, 126
Presentations, 120
Pressures, colleagues/subordinates, 63
Prevalence of disease, 72
Prevention, **5–6**, 41
Preventive health model, **42–45**
diagnosis, 43
effective treatment, 43
primary prevention, 42–43
secondary prevention, 43–44
tertiary prevention, 44–45
Preventive measures, personal
behaviour, 59
Preventive orientation of health care,
32
Preventive sphere, 41
Primary health care
access, 159
approach, **96**
community oriented, 105
importance, 29
needs assessment, 70
practice managers, 101
resources, 32
teams, 102, 103–104
adolescents, 131
patient advisory groups, 104
UK focus, 33

Primary prevention, 42–43
Priorities for health, 192
Prisons, 154
Health Service, 154
screening programmes, 161
Privacy, 89
Process evaluation, 122
Project 2000, 22, 192
Promoting Better Health (1986), 34–35
Protective clothing, 176
Psychiatric nurses, community, 35, 41
Psychological services, 145–146
Psychological theory in health
promotion, **46–47**
health belief model, 46–47
reasoned action theory, 47
Psychomotor learning objectives, 119
Psychomotor skill learning, 113
Public health
approach to health promotion, 9, **10**
collective view, 33
engineers, 181
health promotion, **16–19**
health visitors, **17–18**
nurse contribution, 10
nurse role, 35–36
nursing approach, 192
policy, 8–9, 18
health promotion, 30, 63
Public transport, 180

Q

Quality of care, 60
Quality of life, **5**
adults, 134
disabled people, 23
health education, 109
Health of the Nation strategy, 34
patient involvement in care plan,
103
transport, 179
Quarantine, 58
Questions, 86
closed, 86
open-ended, 86

R

Radical model for health promotion,
45–46
empowerment, 46
Reasoned action theory, 47
Record-keeping, 87–88
Records, 87–88
accuracy, 71
client access, 88
maintenance, 71
patient-held, 88
Reflection, learning, 116
Rehabilitation, 41, 44
service for mentally ill, 48

Relationships, children's education, 147
Report writing, 88
Resource allocation, 28, **69–70**
Respiratory disease, 159
  air pollution, 172
  deaths, 161
Risk factor intervention international programmes, **28–29**
Risk factors, later life, 137–138
Road accidents, 128, 175, 179
  cost to society, 175
  prevention, 181
Road safety
  education, 147
  improvements, 175
  officers, 181
Role play, 122

S

Sacred texts, 53
Safe sex promotion, 152, 153
Safe standards of practice, 63
Safety
  equipment, 128
  initiatives, 129
  needs, 115
    assessment, 118
  see also Road safety
Satisfaction surveys, 48
School nurse, 41, 145
  role, 147–148
Schools
  health fax, 145
  health profiles, 145
  health-promoting, **144–146**
  HIV/AIDS education, 146
  Irish, 146
  professionals for health education, 145
Science, 53–54
Scotland, education, 146
Screening
  antenatal, 126–127
  cardiovascular disease, 134
  clinical prevention programmes, 28
  contribution to health, 159
  institutions, 161
  programmes, 43
  school nurses, 148
  task-oriented, 58
Seat belt legislation, 19
Secondary care
  access, 159
  National Health Service, 162
  services, 32, 33
Secondary prevention, 43–44
  research, 43–44
  screening programmes, 43
  service provision, 43
Self-actualisation needs, 115
Self-awareness, 97

Self-care, 60
  fundamental needs, 204
  promotion, 204
Self-determination, 44
Self-development, 97, 126
Self-esteem, 60, 61
  education, 110
  generation in community, 61
  social context, 61
Self-evaluation, 82
Self-help groups, **105–107**
  Afro-Caribbean mental health project, 107
  barriers, 106
  negative impact, 106
  research, 107
  sexual health, 136
  support, 106
Self-inflicted injury, 131
Self-knowledge, 82
Self-regard, 110
Self-reliance, 44
Self-treatment teaching, 113, 114
Sensory impairment, 127
Service utilisation data, 76
Settings for health promotion, **143–154**
Sex education, Irish schools, 146
Sexual harassment, 150
Sexual health
  adulthood, 136
  promotion amongst adolescents, 130, 131
Sexual needs in later life, 137
Sexuality
  adolescents, 130
  ageing, 137
  children's education, 147
  children's knowledge, 127
Sexually transmitted diseases, 114
Sick building syndrome, 176–177
Sickle cell disease, 100, 126
  Afro-Caribbean population, 165
Sickness, reactive response, 54
Skin cancer, 43–44, 135
Smog, 172
Smoking
  adulthood, 135
  behaviour change, 117
  cardiovascular disease, 133
  client-based information, 71
  costs of illness to industry, 149
  data, 77
  disadvantaged people, 112
  environmental effects, 177
  expense to society, 58
  gender difference in health status, 163
  health promotion activity, 161
  intervention, 55
  later life, 138
  mass media campaign, 152–153
  mortality, 159–160
  passive, 58, 177
  policies, 19
  poor health, 161

pregnancy, 126
  workplace policies, 148
Social change
  adolescence, 130–131
  health impact, 159
  health promotion, 170
Social class
  classification data, 78
  health behaviour, 167–168
  health care access, 168
  inequalities in health, **165–168**, 169
  infant mortality, 166
  morbidity, 166
  mortality, 166
Social difference, ethnicity, 164
Social environment
  health status, 163
  supportive, 112
Social factors, 6–7, 8
Social health, 109
Social level of health promotion, 40
Social marketing, **47–48**
Social networks, 8, 9
  health promotion, 10
Social state, 4
Social stratification in United Kingdom, **162**
Social support, education, 110
Social workers, 36
Society's value on health, 54
Socio-sexual education, 121
SOLER, 84–85
Space
  personal, 89
  use in communication, 89
Special educational needs, 145
Speech, supplementing, 88–89
Spiritual health, 109
Standardised disability index, 74–75
Standardised mortality ratio, 74, 158–159
Staring, 92
Stoma support groups, 106
Street
  drainage, 16
  environment, 18
Stress
  noise pollution, 174
  nursing, 206
Stressors, 206
Stroke, 133–134
  deaths, 161
  ethnic minority mortality, 165
Student activities, 199, 200–206
Suicide, 131, 160
  social support factors, 161
Sulphur dioxide, 172, *174*
Support
  adolescents, 131
  antenatal, 126–127
  self-help groups, 106
  systems, 7
Surveillance programmes for infants/ children, 127

Sustainable development strategies, 178
Swimming, 128
Sympathy, 83

T

Talk, 120
  clarifying recent, 97
  developing current, 97
  encouraging, 85
  initiating further, 97
Task-sharing, 102
Tasks, group norm functions, 99
Teachers in health education, 145
Teaching
  activities, 199
  evaluation, 122
  methods, 112–113, 119–121
  objectives, 118–119
  peer programmes, 147
  plans, 111, 118–119, 121
  principles, 117
  process, 118
Teams
  building, 104–105
  collective approaches to health, 105
  community
    mental health, 103–104
    multidisciplinary, 103
    for people with learning
      difficulties, 104
  goals, 104–105
  policy development, 104–105
  working relationships, 104
Teamwork, **102–105**
  director of activity, 102
  primary health care, 102, 103–104
  special interest group, 102–103
  task-sharing, 102
Tertiary prevention, 41, 44–45
Testicular cancer screening, 43
Text telephone, 67
Thalassaemia, 126
Third World communities, 37
Total parenteral nutrition special
  interest group, 102–103
Touch, 88, 90
  caring, 90
  procedural, 90
Town planning, 180, 182
Toxic waste, 18
Traditional communities, 52–53
Traffic
  engineers, 181
  pollution, 18
Traffic-calming measures, 175

Transcultural differences, 44
Transport
  alternative methods, 180
  health, 179–180
  policies, 180
  quality of life, 179
  sector, 179
Tuberculosis, 17

U

Unemployment
  health status, 33
  inequalities in health, 167
  school leavers, 130–131
Unhealthy behaviour, interactive
  approaches, 61
United Kingdom
  age profile of population, 164
  changing, 53
  confusion, 54
  cultural diversity, 53
  diet, 161
  diversity, 54
  ethnicity, 164
  health of population, **158–161**
  health promotion policy, **31–32**
  health status, 33
  lifestyle, 161
  morbidity, 160–162
  mortality, 158–160
  poverty, 161
  questioning of values, 53
  science, 53–54
  social stratification, **162**
  sustainable development strategies,
    178
United Kingdom Central Council
  (UKCC) Code (1992), 52, **62–63**,
    187, 193
  patient-held records, 88
  treatment focus, 62
United Nations
  Convention on the Rights of the
    Child (1992), 147
  Universal Declaration of Human
    Rights, 63
Urban decay, 17
User-centred approach to policy, 36, 37

V

Vaccination, 17
Values
  clarifying, 110
  consensus, 55

health, 61
issues in health promotion, 56
society's of health, 54
Verbal interventions, 97
Victim-blaming approach, 45, 169
Violence perception of mental illness,
  153
Vocal expression, 88, 89
Voluntary sector, 36, 194

W

Ward design, 186
Warmth, 83
Water
  clean, 29
  drinking, 173
  supply, 16
Wealth, 167
Well-being, 4, 5
  nursing goal, 186
Wellness, 205
Women
  nurses, 24
  nutrition, 24
  paramedic professions, 24
  responsibilities, 24
  roles, 23, 24
  specific needs, 23
Workload of colleagues/subordinates,
  63
Workplace, **148–151**
  accident prevention, 195
  costs of ill health, 148–149
  disabled people, 150
  evaluation of health promotional
    activities, 148, 149
  health and safety, 176–177
  inequality of health, 169–170
  job stress, 150–151
  look after your heart (LAYH), 150
  nurses, 151
  office blocks, 176–177
  sexual harassment, 150
World Health Organization (WHO)
  Alma Ata Declaration, 29, 96
  European strategy ethics tragets, 52,
    63–64
  Health for All, 9, 22, 29–30, 32
  health definition, **4**, 6
  health promotion approach, 28,
    32–33
  health promotion definition, 40
  Healthy Cities, 18, 22, 30, 171
  international policy development,
    29–30
  Ottawa Charter, 9, 30, 32